The Cerebellum and Adaptive Control

The cerebellum – the region of the vertebrate brain that makes smoothly coordinated movements possible – is a remarkable machine. How it accomplishes its highly complex feats of coordination has been the subject of much inquiry; one of the preeminent theories places adaptive control at the forefront.

The Cerebellum and Adaptive Control reinforces the view that the cerebellum functions as an adaptive control system. That is, it automatically adjusts its output for such eventualities as temporary or lasting weakness of muscle. This text is the first to synthesize the substantial body of literature on the subject, combining the neuroscience of the cerebellum with the science of control theory common to electrical and computer engineers. Organized into four parts, the book examines cerebellar anatomy and physiology, cerebellar function, and models and theories, and ends with a summary and conclusions. The author's clinical perspective offers a broader view of cerebellar function beyond the basic neuroscience. An appendix demonstrates evidence supporting the adaptive control model from a detailed comparison of the cerebellum with an adaptive signal processor of the author's design and construction.

John Barlow's book is the only up-to-date work on this crucial aspect of cerebellar function. Researchers and graduate students of neurophysiology, as well as electrical and computer engineers, will find this integrated model an insightful and relevant look at the functioning cerebellum.

John S. Barlow is a neurophysiologist at the Massachusetts General Hospital and Senior Research Associate in Neurology at Harvard Medical School. He is also a former research affiliate at the Research Laboratory of Electronics at the Massachusetts Institute of Technology.

T0224522

The Cerebellum and Adaptive Control

JOHN S. BARLOW

Massachusetts General Hospital
Harvard Medical School

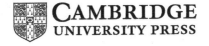

CAMBRIDGE
UNIVERSITY PRESS

CAMBRIDGE UNIVERSITY PRESS
Cambridge, New York, Melbourne, Madrid, Cape Town, Singapore, São Paulo

Cambridge University Press
The Edinburgh Building, Cambridge CB2 2RU, UK

Published in the United States of America by Cambridge University Press, New York

www.cambridge.org
Information on this title: www.cambridge.org/9780521808422

First published 2002
This digitally printed first paperback version 2005

A catalogue record for this publication is available from the British Library

Library of Congress Cataloguing in Publication data
Barlow, John S., 1925–
The cerebellum and adaptive control / John S. Barlow.
p.   cm.
Includes bibliographical references and index.
ISBN 0-521-80842-1
1. Cerebellum.   2. Adaptive control systems.   I. Title.
QP379 .B37   2002
573.8´6 – dc21   2002023394

ISBN-13 978-0-521-80842-2 hardback
ISBN-10 0-521-80842-1 hardback

ISBN-13 978-0-521-01807-4 paperback
ISBN-10 0-521-01807-2 paperback

For Sibylle Jahrreiss Barlow, my patient wife,

without whose assistance this work could not have been completed.

It seems likely that the cerebellum has some function of *proportioning* the muscular response to the proprioceptive input, and if this proportioning is disturbed, a [cerebellar] tremor may be one of the results. [emphasis added]

Norbert Wiener, *Cybernetics or Control and Communication in the Animal and The Machine*, 1948, p. 114

It is a lamentable fact that much of the available information regarding the cerebellum is still uncorrelated and difficult to understand. Not until neurophysiological and neuroanatomical data are brought in harmony and correlated with the clinical and neuropathological findings can we expect to be able to form an all-embracing concept of cerebellar function. It is hoped that the present publication will contribute toward this end.

From the Preface by Jan Jansen and Alf Brodal to the Festschrift, *Aspects of Cerebellar Anatomy*, for Prof. K. E. Schreiner in celebration of his 80th birthday, Oslo, Norway, 1954, p. 3–4

No one had any idea of how the cerebellar cortex should work or what operations it should perform with the impulses coming into it from diverse sources.

S. L. Palay, speaking of the era after Ramón y Cajal, in his Introduction to *Cerebellar Cortex*, 1974, by S. L. Palay and Victoria Chan-Palay, p. 1

In engineering control, an adaptive system is capable of adjusting its characteristics in response to changes of environmental conditions.

Matsuo Ito, *The Cerebellum and Neural Control*, 1984, p. 338

Contents

Preface

Let us consider first the exquisite design of the cerebellar cortex as a laminated rectangular lattice, a structure built with a precision only exceeded in biology by the insect eye and its connectivities. A theory of the cerebellar cortex has to incorporate this design as a key feature, and moreover has to account for the convergence onto each Purkinje cell of two quite distinctive inputs, that from the mossy-fiber input with the immense divergence (8,000) and convergence (100,000) and that from the climbing fibers where the divergence number is about 10 and the convergence number is 1. This extraordinary double innervation has been maintained through all the exigencies of evolution from primitive cerebella to the great efflorescence in mammals and birds. It is particularly remarkable that, when the cerebellar hemispheres were developed in step with the cerebral hemispheres, the inferior olive hypertrophied also. The cerebral efferents had to travel down to the medulla oblongata to excite the newly developed inferior olivary neurons for the essential climbing fiber input to the cerebellar hemispheres. (Eccles 1982, p. 607)

This book assembles evidence that the requirements of a model to meet the unique anatomical and functional features that characterize the cerebellum are currently best met by adaptive control models (or their neural net equivalents), the signal feature of which is their ability to adjust (i.e., to optimize) their own parameters automatically.

Adaptive control models – "adaptive" being the operative word – in various forms and under various names have been discussed since the 1970s, and have reached increasing levels of sophistication more recently. Adaptive controllers embody principles that result in powerful capabilities, for example, prediction of the immediate future of a signal on the basis of samples of its immediate past and generating a signal for controlling an object (e.g., a robotic arm) from the desired trajectory of the arm. These and other features of adaptive signal processors (i.e., adaptive controllers that do not have a specifically controlled object) are illustrated by means of a specific adaptive signal processor and are discussed in relation to cerebellar mechanisms. To this end, moderate amounts of background material concerning both the cerebellum (or, in the larger sense, the cerebellar system, a term intended to include such closely related structures as the inferior olive) and its mechanisms, as well as material on adaptive controllers, are surveyed but not critically reviewed (an undertaking that is beyond the scope of this book). To some extent, the book traces a twofold evolution of ideas about the cerebellum itself and about the development of models of the cerebellum. Further details regarding the content of the book are provided in Chapter 1.

Readers interested in the manner in which the theme of this book evolved over a 50-year incubation period can find more details in the Author's Note at the end of the book.

Acknowledgments

It has been a special pleasure to have worked on this book with Ellen Carlin, Assistant Editor, Life Sciences, of Cambridge University Press, New York, and with Michie Shaw, Books Project Manager, Techbooks, Fairfax, Virginia.

The author is grateful to the following publishers for permission to reproduce copyrighted figures, and in several instances, also the author's permission when specified by the publisher, as noted in the figure captions: Academic Press/Morgan Kaufmann, Orlando; Almqvist and Wiksell, Stockholm; American Medical Association, Chicago; American Physiological Society, Bethesda; Annual Reviews, Palo Alto; Blackwell Science, Ltd., Oxford; Cambridge University Press, New York and Cambridge; Cold Spring Harbor Laboratory Press, Cold Spring Harbor, NY; Elsevier Science, Oxford; Freund Publishing House, Ltd., Tel Aviv; Harcourt, Inc., Orlando; IEEE (Institute of Electrical and Electronic Engineers, Inc.), Piscataway, NJ; John Wiley & Sons, Inc., New York and Chichester; Kluwer Academic/Plenum Publishers, New York; Lippincott Williams & Wilkins, Philadelphia; Masson Editeur, Paris; McGraw-Hill Companies, New York; MIT Press, Cambridge, MA; Oxford University Press, Oxford; Prentice-Hall, Inc., Upper Saddle River, NJ; Springer-Verlag, New York and Heidelberg; and Swets & Zeitlinger Publishers, Lisse, Holland.

In addition, the author is grateful to the following authors for permission to reproduce figures for which they hold the copyright: Prof. József Hámori, Budapest, Hungary; Prof. John J. Hopfield, Princeton, NJ; and Prof. Rudolph Nieuwenhuys, Abcoude, The Netherlands.

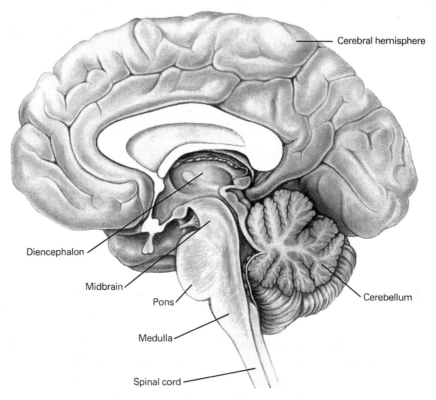

Midsagittal section of a human brain, showing the cerebellum at the lower right. (From R. Nieuwenhuys, J. Voogd, and C. van Huijzen (1988). *The Human Central Nervous System: A Synopsis and Atlas* (3rd ed.), copyright 1988, Springer-Verlag, Heidelberg, reprinted by permission of the publisher and author.)

PART ONE

ANATOMY AND PHYSIOLOGY OF THE CEREBELLAR SYSTEM

ONE

Introduction

1.1. History

In the introductory chapter of his magnificent three-volume monograph, *The Comparative Anatomy and Histology of the Cerebellum*, Olof Larsell (1967; Larsell and Jansen, 1972) provides a history of the cerebellum in its gross aspects, which reads in part as follows (additional historical details can be found in Clarke and O'Malley 1968):

Herophilus (335–280 B.C.) is usually credited with recognition of the human cerebellum as a distinct division of the brain. Aristotle (384–322 B.C.), however, calls it parencephalis, indicating that he did not regard it as part of the principal mass of the brain. The great Galen (A.D. 131–200) designated the vermis cerebelli "the worm-like outgrowth" (epiphysis scolexoides). The arbor vitae [the treelike set of outlines of white substance seen on a median section of the cerebellum] was described by Thomas Willis (1664) in his *Cerebri Anatome* as "ramificatio cerebelli ad foramen arboris." The latter author also suggested that the cerebellum presides over the involuntary movement of the body, whereas the cerebrum controls those movements brought about by volition. The first good drawing of the vermis was publishes by Heister (1717), but Vesalius (1543) had already included in his *Fabrica* rather crude illustrations of the entire cerebellum which are in striking contrast to his beautiful figures of muscles, bones, and other structures. Haller (1777) described the cerebellar hemispheres under the name lobi, and Malacarne (1780) gave a detailed description of the entire organ. Many of the terms which Malacarne introduced are still in use. He also described the surface folia or "laminette," giving their total number as 500 to 780. In the cerebellum of an idiot, he found only 340 folia, leading him to conclude that intelligence depends on the number of cerebellar folds. . . .

The earlier studies of the cerebellum in animals were largely experimental in execution. Rolando (1809) removed the cerebellum in fishes, reptiles, and mammals, described the disturbances of voluntary movements that resulted, and

3

pointed out that cerebellar ablation does not affect sensation. Flourens (1844) confirmed and extended Rolando's observations, emphasizing the exaggeration of tendon and antigravity reflexes and the curious stiff-legged locomotion, with retraction of the head that followed ablation of the cerebellum in birds. [Purkinje's original description of the pear-shaped cell somata was made in Prague in 1837; see also Brazier 1988]. Ferrier (1876) reported his observations on the responses of the eyes, head, and neck to electrical stimulation of the cerebellum in dogs. Luciani (1891) described the results in the dog of complete removal of the organ, and Sherrington (1900) defined the cerebellum as the "head ganglion of the proprioceptive system," holding that it functions as a whole because it deals with the musculature of the body as a whole rather than with individual muscles. This concept was the dominating influence in cerebellar physiology for more than forty years.

During the last decade of the nineteenth century a new approach toward an understanding of the organ was begun by studies on its comparative anatomy and its embryonic development. The first article to appear in the *Journal of Comparative Neurology* was a comparative paper on the cerebellum by C. L. Herrick (1891).

There have been many attempts in the past to characterize the essential function of the cerebellum, of which the one by C. J. Herrick (1924b; the two Herricks were brothers) can serve as an example:

The cerebellum is primarily the balancing brain, controlling posture, regulating and coordinating all movements of precision of the skeletal musculature, and maintaining muscular tone. Its stabilizing influence may be compared with the action of a gyroscope on a large steamship, ensuring the steady progress of the vessel in its course by compensating the buffeting of wind and waves. The role of the cerebellum is that of proprioceptive adjustor.

According to Dow and Moruzzi (1958 p. 4), it was Flourens (1824, 1842) who introduced the concept of the function of the cerebellum as coordinating movements. Thus, after cerebellar ablation, the possibility of executing movements remained, but the coordination of these movements was lost.

1.2. The Cerebellum at Present

Ito (1984) published a magnificent, comprehensive, treatment of the cerebellum, which was preceded by that of Eccles, Ito, and Szentágothai (1967), and before that, by the book of Dow and Moruzzi (1958). Subsequently, a vast additional literature on the cerebellum has emerged and continues to appear, seemingly at an ever-increasing rate. For example, eight full papers, 43 open peer commentaries, and the responses to the latter by the authors of the full papers, under the general topic, "Controversies in neuroscience IV: Motor learning and synaptic plasticity in the cerebellum" (Bell, Cordo, and Harnad 1996), are included in the September 1966 issue of *Behavioral and Brain Sciences* (Vol. 19, No. 3). Two issues of *Learning and Memory* (Vol. 3, No. 6, and Vol. 4, No. 1) were devoted to the cerebellum as were paired issues of

Trends in Neurosciences (Vol. 21, No. 9, Sept. 1998), and *Trends in Cognitive Sciences* (Vol. 2, No. 9, Sept. 1998). In an interesting short autobiographical note, Ito (1999) briefly traced the history of the discovery of the inhibitory action of the cerebellum, the evolution of the concept of synaptic plasticity, and its demonstration experimentally.

1.3. The Perspective of This Book

The present work, the focus of which is the question of the cerebellum as an adaptive controller, has a relatively narrow perspective. Correspondingly, in the background to this main theme, only the most directly relevant aspects are considered, for the most part. In no way is a comprehensive treatment of the cerebellum intended or attempted. Some repetition can be found; this is partly intentional, to emphasize important points, and partly unintentional.

In Part I (Anatomy and Physiology of the Cerebellar System – a term used here to include the cerebellum itself, its nuclei, and the inferior olive), a brief treatment of the evolutionary or comparative anatomical aspects (Chapter 2) of the cerebellum is given. In the chapter on anatomy and physiology of the cerebellar cortex itself (Chapter 3), somewhat greater emphasis is placed on the former than on the latter. In subsequent chapters, emphasis is placed on those connections and components of the cerebellar system that appear to be of particular importance in relation to the question of cerebellar mechanisms (e.g., the mossy fibers; Chapter 4), the inferior olive and associated climbing fibers (e.g., the mossy fiber and climbing fibers constituting the major input systems to the cerebellar cortex; Chapter 5), the cerebellar nuclei (Chapter 6), which together with the vestibular nuclei constitute the output system of the cerebellar cortex, and the nucleocortical and nucleo-olivary pathways (Chapter 6).

In Part II (Cerebellar Functions), limited aspects of cerebellar mechanisms are discussed, including synaptic plasticity (Chapter 7) as a specific mechanism of cerebellar adaptability (adaptive control), the vestibulocerebellum (Chapter 8) as the simplest form of cerebellar function, cognition and imaging studies (Chapter 9), and conditioning and timing (Chapter 10). To include human disease in the survey of actual or presumed cerebellar function, aspects of cerebellar pathology and pathophysiology and their clinical manifestation are included (Chapter 11). Specialized cerebellar-like structures in certain fish (i.e., the valvula and the electroreceptive lateral lobe and the mammalian dorsal cochlear nucleus), which are found in these animal groups in addition to a true cerebellum, are included (Chapter 12) because of their resemblance in certain respects to the cerebellum itself, even if the functions of these organs and their relationship to the cerebellum remains unclear in part.

In Part III (Models and Theories), as background to the consideration of adaptive control models of the cerebellum, a relatively limited survey of a number of nonadaptive theories and models (the two terms are used more or less interchangeably) of cerebellar function are discussed (Chapter 13). A review of the closely related topics of adaptive control and neural nets (Chapter 14) follows. Several specific features of adaptive controllers are next illustrated in an adaptive controller (adaptive signal processor) of the author's own design and construction (Chapter 15). A survey of several adaptive control models of the cerebellum then follows (Chapter 16).

In Part IV (Summary and Conclusions), a selective recapitulation of material in earlier chapters is presented, together with a detailed comparison between an adaptive signal processor and the vestibulo-ocular reflex as an example of the operation of the cerebellar system (Chapter 17). Some remaining questions are also discussed. In sum, the marshalled evidence that the cerebellum can be considered at least in part as an adaptive controller appears to be very strong. At the same time, however, the cerebellar system itself appears to lack the capability of true prediction, for which a specific time mechanism would be required. The site of the latter capability, perhaps distributed in location, remains unclear.

TWO

Comparative Anatomy of the Cerebellum

If we can discover what functional factors were primitively concerned in the initial differentiation of the cerebellum from preexisting bulbar structures and some of the steps by which additional functional systems of diverse kinds were drawn into the cerebellar complex, some light may be shed on the great problems of the analysis of higher cerebellar functions.   (C. J. Herrick 1924b)

It is from the standpoint that a brief survey of the circumstances under which the cerebellum and its Purkinje cells developed in phylogeny could shed some light on the evolution of its organization and functions in higher forms that this review, mostly from classical sources, is presented. This survey is based primarily on the following sources: Ariëns Kappers, Huber, and Crosby (1960), Crosby (1969), Herrick (1924a, 1924b), Larsell (1967), Larsell and Jansen (1972), Llinás (1969), Llinás and Hillman (1969), Nieuwenhuys (1967), Schnitzlein and Faucette (1969), Butler and Hodos (1996), and Nieuwenhuys, ten Donkelaar, and Nicholson (1998). Some additional aspects of comparative anatomy of the cerebellum are included in Chapter 12, which discusses cerebellar-like structures in certain fish, including the valvula of mormyrid fish, the electrosensory lobe, and the mammalian dorsal cochlear nucleus.

2.1. Origins of the Cerebellum

Larsell (1967; pp. 6–7) summarized the early phylogeny of the cerebellum as follows:

The primitive predominantly vestibular and lateral-line organ cerebellum of the lampreys [eel-like fish with a round mouth] is continued in the sluggish urodeles [tailed amphibians] and higher forms as a laterally situated vestibular and lateral-line subdivision, medial to which develops a corpus cerebelli whose fiber tract connections are quite different. The corpus cerebelli receives proprioceptive and other sensory impulses and becomes the predominant feature of the cerebellum in the vertebrates above the sluggish urodeles, as well as in the active types of fishes such as selachians [sharks, skates, and rays] and teleosts [bony fish].

Microscopically, it is evident that precursors of Purkinje cells arose amid granule cells, first irregularly in location and then in a progressively layered fashion: the layer of Purkinje cells. The Purkinje cells themselves progressively developed extensive dendritic trees that increasingly become confined to a single plane, through which the parallel fibers (the axons of granule cells) thread, initially in a somewhat random fashion but increasingly at right angles, not unlike the wires strung on the cross-arms of telephone poles of former times.

In a departure from the main trend of cerebellar evolution, the valvula (Chapter 12) develops in association with the lateral line organs and electrosensory system of certain fish, becoming large enough to cover the rest of the brain. In the detailed anatomy of this unusual structure, the molecular layer (constituted of the parallel fibers and apical dendritic tree of the Purkinje cells), as well as the layer of Purkinje cells themselves, becomes greatly folded or foliated. The granular layer of granule cells, however, does not participate in this folding, nor do its axons bifurcate; the parallel fibers arise directly from the granule cells. This arrangement must be of special significance in relation to the processing of data from lateral line organs and electroreceptors, perhaps in the capacity of phased arrays for beam forming (Chapter 12).

The origin of the cerebellum in close association with nuclei of the eighth (vestibular) nerve and the lateral line nerves perhaps suggests that this part of the cerebellum originated as a means of carrying out some type of transformation of the coordinate system of input data from the vestibular organ and the lateral line organs. Bullock (1969) suggested that the function of the cerebellum might be along the lines of an organ primarily computing and representing, in some analogue fashion, an image of the relations of the body in space. In this connection, it is relevant to note that, in the counterpart of the vestibular system among manmade navigation systems (i.e., the so-called strap-down or vehicle-oriented inertial navigation systems), such a transformation of coordinates must be carried out by a central computer on the basis of the input data from the motion sensors (angular, rectilinear; Barlow 1964, 1966; Siouris 1993; see also Chapter 12). It should be noted that this part of the cerebellum in lower forms, and its counterpart in higher forms (as the flocculonodular lobe), is slightly different in its histology from the main body of the cerebellum (corpus cerebelli). Thus, Brodal (1967) pointed out that the mossy fibers in the flocculus and nodulus (and also the caudal part of the uvula and the dorsal paraflocculus) of the cat, vestibular fibers terminate with more profuse branching and a greater number and density of terminal globules than is the case with the "classical" (nonvestibular) type of mossy fibers. A relatively greater number of Golgi cells appeared to be associated with these "vestibular" mossy fibers.

2.2. Fish

In vertebrates, the cerebellum develops from two bilaterally symmetrical formations located dorsally at the upper end of the medulla oblongata (the rhombencephalon),

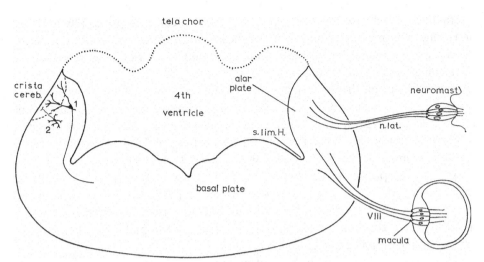

Figure 2.1. Diagrammatic transverse section through the upper medulla oblongata of a lamprey, showing (on the right) the similarities between receptor cells of the lateral line nerve and the vestibular nerve, and (on the left) the crista cerebellum or prototype cerebellum with a precursor Purkinje cell (1) and granule cell (2). crista cereb., crista cerebellaris; n. lat., nervus lateralis; tela chor., tela choroidea; s. lim. H., sulcus limitans of His. (From Nieuwenhuys 1967; reprinted by permission of the author.)

in the region of termination (in their respective nuclear complexes) of the fibers from the eighth or vestibular nerve and the lateral line nerves. This area is sometimes termed the area octavolateralis. Thus, the oldest afferent paths to the cerebellum are those of the vestibular and, in fish (and also in amphibia), of the lateral line systems. This area is also the area of termination of the trigeminal nerve. This arrangement is illustrated in Figure 2.1 for the lamprey (a member of the cyclostomes, that is, eel-like fish having a round suctorial mouth and having a brain length of 1 centimeter). The lamprey is the lowest form in which there is a clearly distinguishable cerebellum. Whether still lower forms of vertebrates possess a cerebellum (e.g., the myxinoids, the most primitive living vertebrates) has been an issue of much debate (Nieuwenhuys 1967).

In bony fish (teleosts), it has been proposed that the cerebellar auricles, which receive a large input from the vestibulolateral line system, constitute the vestibulo-cerebellum and are the homologues of the flocculonodular lobe of higher vertebrates, whereas the corpus cerebelli, receiving spinocerebellar and tectocerebellar fibers, is the homologue of the vermis of higher vertebrates (Ariëns et al. 1960).

It is relevant to note that the labyrinth (the three semicircular canals together with the saccule and utricle) and the lateral line organs of lampreys (*Petromyzontidae*) have a remarkable structural, as well as functional similarity, which is evident from the right side of Figure 2.1. An important difference between the two structures is that the arrangement of the lateral line organs is such that they are sensitive to relative motion of the fluid surrounding the animal, whereas the labyrinths, having basically the same sensing mechanism, are sensitive to fluid, the endolymph, which is trapped in the labyrinths. Thus, by means of detection of the motion of fluid, the lateral line organs detect the occurrence of external currents, principally to detect and locate other moving animals, whereas the labyrinth serves to provide information concerning the animals' own equilibrium of the body and orientation in space (i.e., concerning gravity and inertia).

It is evident that these two types of information, which can be considered proprioceptive and exteroceptive, respectively, are complimentary, a point that will be relevant to a consideration (following) of the question of function of the primitive cerebellum. It should be noted that another part of this primitive cerebellum receives additional inputs (e.g., tectocerebellar and spinocerebellar; Nieuwenhuys 1967).

In adult lampreys, the vestibulolateral lobe receives input from the vestibular apparatus and the lateral line organs, whereas the corpus cerebelli (cerebellar body) receives spinal, bulbar, and trigeminal fibers. This major division of the cerebellum into two parts is continued in higher forms. In fishes and amphibia, precursors of the cerebellar nuclei can be recognized.

Histologically, the area of the brain of lampreys in which the two nerves (vestibular and lateral line) terminate consists principally of small granular cells that have a few short dendrites and a laterally directed axon that bifurcates longitudinally (Fig. 2.1, left side, 2). These bifurcated axons are the forerunners of the parallel fibers. Scattered among the granular cells are larger neurons having long dendrites extending in the same direction as the axons of the granule cells (Fig. 2.1, left side, 1), with axons that may curve downward and medially. These are the precursors of the Purkinje cells. The neuropil zone of intermixing of the axons of the granular cells and the dendrites of the larger cells is termed the crista cerebellaris or cerebellar crest, also known as the molecular layer. The two intermingled cell types form a cell layer. The small granule cells are equivalent to those in higher forms, and change little in phylogeny. The larger cells have been considered, as just mentioned, to be the precursors of Purkinje cells. It should be noted, however, that true Purkinje cells are characterized, among other features, by the fact that their dendrites branch in a single plane, whereas the dendritic tree of the larger cerebellar cellular elements is not confined to one plane (Nieuwenhuys 1967).

The cerebellum of cartilaginous fish (sharks and rays) is considerably larger than, and much further differentiated than, that of the round-mouth fish (cyclostomes), and the larger ones display grooves in the cerebellum, the number of which increases with the size of the body. It is also in this group of fishes that the Purkinje cells spread their dendrites, which are covered with numerous spines, in a single plane. Of particular note is the fact that the cartilagenous fishes have an olivocerebellar system, which accompanies the caudal portion of the spinocerebellar tract toward the body of the cerebellum (corpus cerebelli). The olivocerebellar fibers originate from the contralateral inferior olive and terminate in all parts of the body of the cerebellum.

2.3. Amphibia and Birds

In comparison with the salamander (Urodela, or tailed species), frogs (Anura, or tailless species) show a much more massive and more highly differentiated development of the cerebellum. This applies particularly to the Purkinje cells, which now

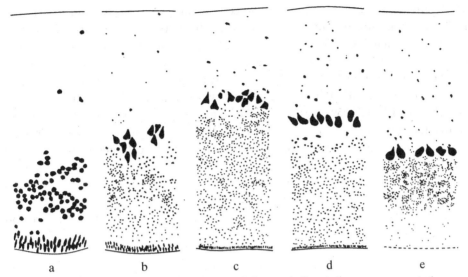

Figure 2.2. Sections showing the cell picture of the cerebellum of some representative vertebrates: (a) lamprey, (b) lungfish, (c) turtle, (d) lizard, and (e) pigeon. Note the progressive
trend toward strict layering of the Purkinje cells from (b) to (e), and the diminution of size of
granule cells after (a). (From Nieuwenhuys 1967; reprinted by permission of the author.)

constitute a distinct zone between the granular and the molecular layers (see Fig. 2.2
for the general trend toward layering). Further, the dendrites of the Purkinje cells are
clearly oriented in a sagittal plane and show a more complex ramification (see Fig. 2.3
for the general trend). In crocodiles, the cerebellar cortical afferent and efferent

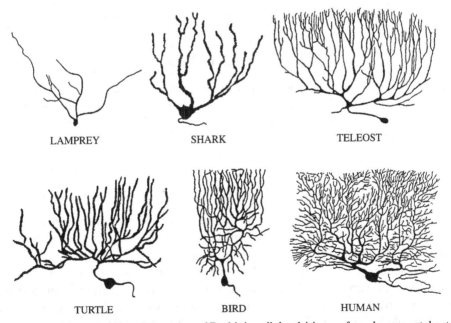

Figure 2.3. The progressive elaboration of Purkinje cell dendritic tree from lower vertebrates
to humans. (From Nieuwenhuys 1967; reprinted by permission of the author.)

axons are not scattered among granule cells, as in turtles, snakes and lizards, but rather are concentrated into a deep white matter between the ventricular surface and the granular layer. Accordingly, it can be said that crocodiles possess a true cerebellar cortex, as do birds and mammals.

It is of interest that, in the frog, primary vestibular nerve fibers project as climbing fibers directly onto the Purkinje cells in the vestibulolateral line or auricular lobe (Precht and Llinás 1969); vestibular fibers thus appear to be the first nonolivary source for climbing fibers for this type of cerebellar afferent in phylogeny. Primary vestibular fibers also terminate as mossy fibers on granule cells in the auricular lobe and activate Purkinje cells through the parallel fiber system in the frog. In contrast, in the cat cerebellum, for example, primary and secondary vestibular inputs end as mossy fibers exclusively.

The cerebellum of birds differs from that of reptiles by being more massive and more complexly fissured.

2.4. Afferent Fiber Systems to the Cerebellar Cortex

Llinás and Hillman (1969) suggested that, whereas the climbing fiber system appears to represent a very primitive input to the cerebellar cortex, which has not changed very much in phylogeny, the mossy fiber granule cell system has undergone large changes. Among these changes is the large development of the molecular layer in higher vertebrates and the enormous increase in the number of synapses between parallel fibers and Purkinje cells as well as the development of inhibitory cells in the molecular layer (i.e., the stellate and basket cells, as well as the Golgi cells of the granule layer).

2.5. The Flocculonodular Lobe

The vestibular apparatus is closely related to the phylogenetically ancient flocculonodular lobe of the cerebellum. The latter is therefore sometimes referred to (somewhat inaccurately) as the "vestibulocerebellum"; it is also sometimes referred to as the archicerebellum.

2.6. Phylogeny of the Vestibulo-Ocular System

In their overview of the evolution of hindbrain visual and vestibular mechanisms in relation to oculomotor function, Baker and Gilland (1996) suggested that retinal and inertial signals (concerned respectively with movement of the world and the organism itself, including gravity) would have been selected (some 450 million years ago) by primitive brain stem–cerebellar circuitry because of their invariant relationship with the environment. Hence, the early octavolateral organization, including vestibular nuclei, would lead to an integrated inertial and visual coordinate system.

2.7. Phylogeny of the Cerebellar Nuclei

Cerebellar nuclei have not been recognized with certainty in any species of fish (Fig. 12.7, right); a single deep nucleus has been identified on each side in the frog (compare Fig. 12.7, left), possibly a forerunner of the fastigial and interpositus nuclei (Altman and Bayer 1997, pp. 20–22). The emergence of a precursor in frogs of the later deep nuclei may suggest an association with the emergence of amphibians as land species.

THREE

Anatomy and Physiology of the Cerebellar Cortex

> There has been a successful analysis of the neuronal interactions in the cerebellar cortex (Eccles 1973), but this does not help to any appreciable extent in the attempt to develop an understanding of the mode of operation of the cerebellum in the control of movement. At the best it can form the basis for building models. (Eccles 1977b)

In view of the limited scope of this book and the correspondingly limited treatments of cerebellar anatomy and physiology, the following books and papers may be cited as supplementary sources: Brodal (1981); Brodal (1998); Eccles (1973, 1977b); Gilman, Bloedel, and Lechtenberg (1981); Ito (1984); Kandel, Schwartz, and Jessell (1991); Lechtenberg (1981); and Rothwell (1994).

The anatomical aspects of this chapter are based primarily on Brodal (1981); Eccles, Ito, and Szentágothai (1967); Ghez (1991); Ito (1984); Paley and Chan-Palay (1974); Palkovits, Magyar, and Szentágothai (1972); Parent (1996); and Ramón y Cajal (1995), supplemented in many instances from more recent publications. A synopsis of cerebellar anatomy appears in Voogd and Glickstein (1998). Further aspects of cerebellar system anatomy that are particularly relevant to the topic of adaptive control are considered in subsequent chapters: the mossy fibers (Chapter 4), the climbing fibers and their source, the inferior olive (Chapter 5), and the cerebellar nuclei and their efferent pathways (Chapter 6).

3.1. Anatomical Aspects of the Cerebellar Cortex

As depicted in Figure 3.1 the cerebellum can be divided into three functional parts, each having its distinctive connections with the brain and spinal cord: the vestibulocerebellum, the spinocerebellum, and the cerebrocerebellum (Ghez 1991), which correspond roughly to the successive stages of evolution of the cerebellum that were

A Outputs

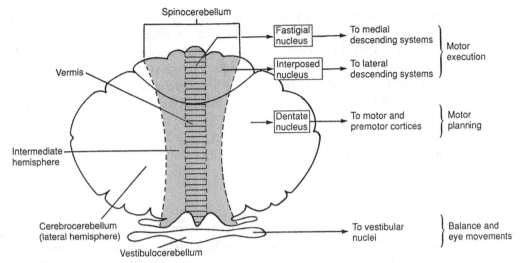

B Inputs

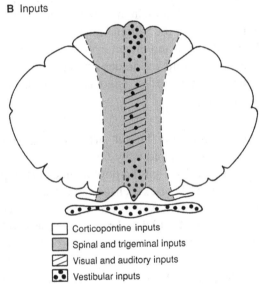

Figure 3.1. Schema of the three functional divisions of the cerebellum (the vestibulocerebellum, the spinocerebellum, and the cerebrocerebellum) with their outputs (A) and inputs (B). (From Ghez 1991, in: Kandel, Schwartz, and Jessells (eds.), *Principles of Neural Science, 3rd edition*, copyright 1991, The McGraw-Hill Companies, reprinted by permission of the publisher; see also Ghez and Thach [2000].)

outlined in Chapter 2. (In the following paragraphs concerning the major divisions of the cerebellum, "input" refers to the mossy fiber input, one of the two principal afferent pathways to the cerebellar cortex, the other being the "climbing fibers," which are discussed later.)

3.1.1. Major Divisions of the Cerebellum

The Vestibulocerebellum. The vestibulocerebellum, or flocculonodular lobe, has no corresponding (deep) cerebellar nucleus; it receives directly from the vestibular nuclei, and its output, from Purkinje cells of the cerebellar cortex, projects back directly to the vestibular nuclei in the medulla (bottom part of Fig. 3.1A). In conjunction with the vestibular nuclei, the vestibulocerebellum controls eye movements in relation to body position and movements (vestibular reflexes), and axial musculature.

Thus, Purkinje cells located in discrete zones of the flocculus are part of different pathways concerned with the regulation of specific components of compensatory eye movements (De Zeeuw et al. 1994).

The Spinocerebellum. The spinocerebellum, so named because much of its input originates in the spinal cord, comprises the medial (vermis) and intermediate parts of the cerebellar hemispheres (center part of Fig. 3.1A). It receives sensory information from the periphery (proximal and distal parts) and from the primary motor and somatosensory cortex, in register with that from the periphery. The Purkinje cells of the vermis project to the fastigial nucleus, and those in the intermediate zone project to the interposed nuclei (Chapter 6). In turn, the fastigial nucleus controls the medial (mainly axial and proximal musculature), and the interposed nuclei control the lateral (mainly distal musculature) components of the descending motor pathways in the execution of limb movements, including their ongoing aspects. Both nuclei include projections to the motor cortex.

The Cerebrocerebellum. The cerebrocerebellum (lateral parts of Fig. 3.1) comprises the lateral part of the cerebellar hemispheres and is by far the largest part of the cerebellar cortex. Its input is derived entirely from the pontine nuclei (Chapter 4), which receives projections from the cerebral cortex (sensory and motor cortex and from premotor and posterior parietal cortex, as well as other parts of the cerebral cortex, which are detailed in Chapter 9). The Purkinje cells of the cerebrocerebellum project to the dentate nucleus and thence via the thalamus (ventrolateral nucleus) to the premotor cerebral cortex and to additional regions of the cerebral cortex (Chapter 9). The dentate nucleus also projects to the parvocellular (small-cell) part of the red nucleus and thence to the inferior olive. In relation to motor control, the cerebrocerebellum is considered to be concerned with planning, initiation, and timing of movements, but in recent years, a role in cognitive function has also been implicated (Chapter 9).

The cerebellum can be divided in other ways. Thus, the adult mammalian cerebellum consists of a series of lobules oriented primarily in the mediolateral plane, and the lobules can be grouped into three lobes: anterior, posterior, and flocculonodular (Hawkes and Eisenman 1997). The three lobes are sometimes designated as the spinocerebellum, pontocerebellum, and vestibulocerebellum, respectively, referring to the major afferent system that projects to each lobe. At higher resolution, the adult mammalian cerebellum is subdivided into an elaborate, reproducible array of parasagittal stripes and transverse zones. Because the stripes and zone boundaries are orthogonal, they subdivide the cerebellum into a patchwork grid.

3.1.2. Surface Dimensions and Uniformity

If completely unfolded in its anteroposterior dimension, the human cerebellum would extend about 1 meter; its width would be only about one seventh of a meter, a much smaller extent, because most folia (leaves) run transversely (Braitenberg and Atwood 1958, Braitenberg, Heck, and Sultan 1997; Brodal 1981). Although there are some regional differences, particularly as concern the older flocculonodular lobe (as mentioned below), the detailed structure of the cerebellar cortex is remarkably uniform, according to the results of most anatomical and biochemical procedures. However, newer techniques such as use of monoclonal antibodies can unmask an underlying biochemical heterogeneity (e.g., multiple overlapping classes of Purkinje cells) beneath a uniform cytology (Gravel et al. 1987).

3.1.3. Layers and Cell Types

Embryology. Neurons of the cerebellar cortex are known to arise from two well-separated germinative layers (Schilling 2000). The inhibitory Purkinje neurons, the sole output (projection) neurons, arise from the neuroepithelium lining the roof of the fourth ventricle, from whence they migrate outward to reach their final position. In contrast, the excitatory cerebellar granule cells, which project onto Purkinje cells, arise from the external granular layer, a secondary germinal layer located on the surface of the cerebellar anlage, from which they migrate inwardly past the Purkinje cells to their final position, within the (internal) granule cell layer. The precursors for inhibitory cerebellar cortical interneurons (i.e., basket and stellate cells, in particular) arise from the neuroepithelium of the fourth ventricle and migrate outward to reach their final positions, much like the Purkinje cells. In contrast to Purkinje cells, however, the interneuronal precursors continue to proliferate during their migration.

Between the surface of the cerebellar cortex and the underlying white matter, there are three layers (Fig. 3.2) as follows (the dimensions are for the adult cat): the outermost, *molecular layer* (of about 300 mu [300–450 mu in man]), the *Purkinje cell layer* or, more exactly, the layer of Purkinje cell bodies (each of dimensions 50–70 mu by 30–35 mu), and the innermost *granular layer* of varying thickness, from 100 mu or less in the depths of the folia to 400–500 mu at the top of the folia (Fig. 13.1), the latter lying next to the white matter.

Among these three layers (Fig. 3.2), the principal neurons of the cerebellar cortex are distributed: (1) the output *Purkinje cell* (Purkinje layer; Herndon 1963; Viets and Garrison 1940); (2) the input *granule cell* (granular layer), and three types of interneurons, including (a) the *Golgi cell* (granular layer), (b) *basket cell* (molecular layer), and (c) *stellate cell* (molecular layer); and (3) the *unipolar brush cell.* An

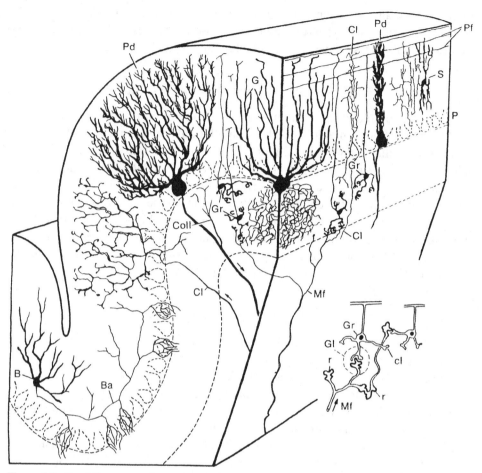

Figure 3.2. Semidiagrammatic representation of part of a cerebellar folium to show the main elements of the cerebellar cortex and their topographical relationships and orientation. Note especially the arrangement of the Purkinje cell dendrites (Pd) and basket cell axons (Ba) in the transverse plane of the folium and the longitudinal arrangement of the parallel fibers (Pf). Other abbreviations: B, basket cell; Cl, climbing fiber; Coll, recurrent collateral of Purkinje cell; G, Golgi cell; Gr, granule cell; Mf, mossy fiber; P, Purkinje cell; Pd, Purkinje cell dendrites; Pf, parallel fibers; S, stellate cell. Inset, lower right: diagrammatic illustration of the relation between the rosettes (r) of the mossy fibers (Mf) with the dendritic "claws" (cl) of the granule cells (Gr) in a glomerulus (Gl). The bifurcation of the granule cell axons to form parallel fibers are shown at the top. Other elements of the glomerulus are not shown. (From Brodal 1981, adapted from Hámori and Szentágothai 1966; reprinted with permission from A. Brodal, *Neurological Anatomy in Relation to Clinical Medicine (3rd ed.)*, copyright 1981 by Oxford University Press; and Springer-Verlag and Prof. J. Hámori.)

additional type of cell, the *Lugaro cell*, is less well established. It lies in the granular layer close to the Purkinje cell layer, and contacts by recurrent Purkinje collaterals and by axons of granule cells or parallel fibers have been reported. Its targets have not been established and its function is unknown (Ito 1984; Palay and Chan-Palay 1974).

Purkinje Cells. The Purkinje cells number approximately 1,500,000 in cats and 15,000,000 in humans. The cell bodies of these inhibitory cells are flask shaped, and their axons penetrate through the granular layer (in which recurrent collaterals may be given off that may branch repeatedly and extend transversely with respect to the axis of the folia, often for a considerable distance) and continue into the white matter to terminate in the cerebellar nuclei (where a single Purkinje cell may contact approximately 35 nuclear cells) or in the vestibular nuclei. The recurrent collaterals are generally presumed to terminate on the proximal dendrites of the Purkinje cells and, in cats at least, on basket and Golgi cells. (It may be noted that the recurrent inhibition derived from Purkinje cells is monosynaptic because Purkinje cells are themselves inhibitory, whereas recurrent inhibition derived from the neocortical pyramidal cells is necessarily disynaptic because pyramidal cells are excitatory.)

The extensively branched apical dendritic tree, which extends outward into the molecular layer, is quite flattened, being confined almost to a single plane perpendicular to the longitudinal axis of the folium. Its thickness approximates about one twentieth its other dimensions (15–20 mu vs. 300–400 mu). The distal dendritic branches are covered with spines (thorns), with which, generally speaking, afferent excitatory fibers make contact. In contrast, inhibitory inputs (from stellate cells and other Purkinje cells) usually end on the proximal smooth shafts of dendrites.

To study the formation of cerebellar lamination and differentiation of Purkinje cells in the absence of their extracerebellar afferents, Tauer, Volk, and Heimrich (1996) used combined immunocytochemical and Golgi electron microscopic techniques and organotypic cultures of immature cerebellar tissue. It was found that the lamination (layering) was retained in the majority of cultures, and most Purkinje cells were aligned. The authors concluded that the Purkinje cells in organotypic cultures send their axons to the correct target region independently of their local position, but the orientation of the dendritic tree and differentiation is influenced by the cellular environment and by specific synaptic interaction.

Basket and Stellate Cells. Of the interneurons in the molecular layer (i.e., basket and stellate cells), 40% were found by Mann-Metzer and Yarom (2000) to be electrically (electrotonically) coupled, from which it was suggested that these interneurons form local networks that give rise to synchronized activity. Such electrical synapses and intrinsic currents were demonstrated to form a highly modifiable communication pathway.

Climbing Fiber Synapses onto Purkinje Cells. Climbing fiber synapses have several features that make for an extremely powerful excitatory effect (Fig. 3.2); activation of a Purkinje cell by its climbing fiber (Fig. 3.3) invariably results in a (complex) spike (Fig. 3.8). The disposition, on the Purkinje cell dendritic tree, of the inhibitory synapses of the stellate cells also has a strong effect, not to mention that of the basket cells, which synapse primarily around the initial segment of the Purkinje cell axon.

The primary and secondary dendritic branches of Purkinje cells receive climbing fibers, whereas the tertiary "spiny branchlets" are the site of parallel fiber synapses

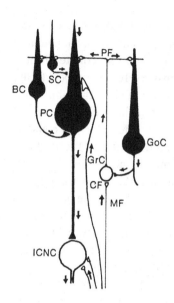

Figure 3.3. Simplified diagram of the most significant neuronal connections in the cerebellar cortex. Cells and terminals shown in black are inhibitory. Abbreviations: BC, basket cell; CF, climbing fiber; GoC, Golgi cell; GrC, granule cell; ICNC, intracerebellar nuclei; MF, mossy fiber; PC, Purkinje cell; SC, stellate cell. See also text. (From Eccles 1966; in: Granit (ed.) *Muscular Afferents and Motor Control*, copyright 1966, Almqvist and Wiksell, Stockholm; reprinted by arrangement with the publisher.)

(Ito 1984). The parallel fiber input (see below) induces "conventional" Na^+ spikes ("simple spikes"), whereas climbing fiber activity results in large CA^{++} spikes with a long duration ("complex spikes").

Granular Layer. The granular layer contains the cell bodies of Golgi cells (see below) together with a large number of the small (cell body: 5–8 mu), densely packed, *granule cells*. The total number has been estimated to be of the order of 10^{10}–10^{11}, more than any other type of neuron. The granule cells are the only neurons in the cerebellar cortex having an excitatory output (with the exception of the unipolar brush cells; see below), and they excite all the other cells in the cerebellar cortex. Structurally, they have 4 or 5 (range 2–7) short dendrites that end with clawlike expansions, the glomeruli (rosette) or cerebellar isles (Fig. 3.2, inset), which are contacted ("grasped") by endings of mossy fibers (see below). Dendrites from more than one granule cell may contribute to a given glomerulus. However, it is evidently quite unusual for dendrites to be shared between two mossy fibers. It has been estimated that there are as many 20 granule cells in synapse with a mossy fiber rosette.

Unipolar Brush Cells. Recently, the existence of another type of cell in the granular layer has become identified: the unipolar brush cell (UBC; Fig. 3.4; Mugnaini, Diño, and Jaarsma 1997), which is characterized by a single dendrite that terminates with a brushlike tip of dendrioles to receive mossy fiber terminals, thus constituting a giant glutaminergic (excitatory) synapse (Nunzi and Mugnaini 2000). The latter, which represent the main synaptic apparatus of the UBC, articulate tightly with a single mossy fiber rosette to form a glomerular array having extensive synaptic contact, one of the largest in the vertebrate central nervous system.

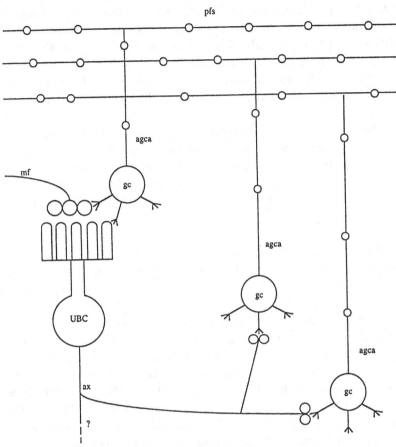

Figure 3.4. Schematic diagram of the mossy fiber–unipolar brush cell–granule cell pathways using dendrodendritic synapses (left) and axodendritic synapses (right). mf, mossy fiber; UBC, unipolar brush cell; ax, UBC axon; agca, ascending granule cell axons; pfs, parallel fibers. Question mark denotes the unresolved question of whether the UBC axon, in addition to providing local terminal branches, projects outside the granule cell domain. (From Mugnaini, Diño, and Jaarsma 1997; reprinted from *Progress in Brain Research*, copyright 1997 by Elsevier Science; reprinted with permission from the publisher.)

A single mossy fiber stimulus evokes a prolonged train of action potentials in the UBC, which is presumably distributed to postsynaptic targets (Nunzi and Mugnaini 2000). Such a potentiation is attributed to a combination of a fast excitatory postsynaptic current (EPSC) and a slow EPSC (Slater, Rossi, and Kinney 1997). The UBCs, which are densely concentrated in folia of the vestibulocerebellum, receive mossy fiber inputs from at least two sources: primary vestibular fibers from otolith and canal organs, and secondary vestibular fibers from the vestibular nuclei/prepositus hypoglossi complex (Diño et al. 2000). Inhibitory input to the UBCs originates from inhibitory (GABAergic) Golgi cell axons. UBCs are provided with axons that bear synaptic endings situated at the center of glomeruli, similar to cerebellar mossy fiber afferents. UBC axons thus form a cortex–intrinsic fiber system that provides a substantial number of (unorthodox) mossy rosettes in the vestibulocerebellum, and provides excitatory innervation to granule cells, other UBCs, and presumably also Golgi cells. The UBCs were considered to be putative interneurons of the cerebellar granular layer and to represent perhaps an extraordinary device for feedforward, excitatory links along the mossy fiber pathways, thus prolonging and enhancing the effect of the mossy fiber input on Purkinje cells.

UBCs were also found to be present in the spinocerebellum, but rare or absent in the lateral cerebellum (which receives a prominent input from the pontine nuclei). Accordingly, it was suggested that UBCs may be important for the modulation of reflex mechanisms and sensorimotor transformations, but perhaps unsuited for neuronal circuits involved with cognitive functions (Mugnaini, Diño, and Jaarsma 1997).

Parallel Fibers. The unmyelinated (or thinly myelinated) axons of granule cells ascend into the molecular layer (Fig. 3.2), where they may synapse with Purkinje cells before bifurcating in a T-shaped manner, the two branches extending as parallel fibers for a short distance in either direction along the long axis of the folium (thus the name), across the dendritic trees of the Purkinje and other cells.

The length of parallel fibers (expressed as the sum of the lengths of the two branches), a parameter that is important for some theories of cerebellar function (Chapter 13), has long been of interest (e.g., Braitenberg and Atwood 1958; Braitenberg, Heck, and Sultan 1997; Brand, Dahl, and Mugnaini 1976; Dow 1949; Mugnaini 1983; Pichitpornchai, Rawson, and Rees 1994; Schild 1980; Smolyaninov 1971; Thach, Goodkin, and Keating 1992). Some of the earlier determinations ranged appreciably in value (about 2–10 mm), as did the depth in the molecular layer of the parallel fibers, but greater agreement has occurred in recent years. Taking into account that the parallel fibers closer to the outer surface of the molecular layer (which would then make contact with the more distal parts of the Purkinje cell dendritic tree) are somewhat longer than those near its base (i.e., near the layer of Purkinje cell bodies), Brand, Dahl, and Mugnaini (1976) found an average value of 6 millimeters in the cat, with a range of 5 to 7 millimeters.

From measurements in chickens and monkeys, Mugnaini (1983) found that the length of parallel fibers can reach a length of approximately 6 millimeters, which is consistently longer than the width of single efferent cortical strips (0.5–1 millimeters). It was also found that in these two species, the longer parallel fibers are situated in the outer molecular layer, becoming progressively shorter toward the Purkinje cell layer, a finding opposite those of some earlier authors.

From a survey of determinations, Braitenberg, Heck, and Sultan (1997) provided a range of 4.7 to 6 millimeters for the combined length of the two parallel fiber branches of one granule cell axon.

It should be noted, however, that there are variations, not only in length of the parallel fibers, but also in their diameter and in the density of varicosities (which correspond to the presence of synapses with Purkinje cells) along the length of a

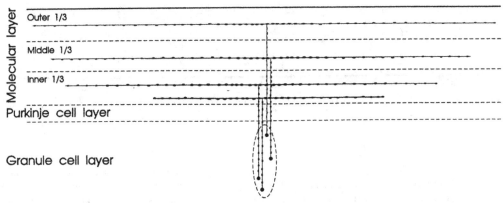

Figure 3.5. Summary diagram indicating the relative lengths and diameters of the parallel fibers in the different thirds of the molecular layer, and the relative size and spacing of the varicosities along both the parallel fibers and the ascending axons. (From Pichitpornchai, Rawson, and Rees 1994; in *J. Comparative Neurol.* Vol. 342, copyright 1994 Wiley-Liss, Inc., a subsidiary of John Wiley & Sons, Inc.; reprinted by permission of the publisher.)

given parallel fiber, as shown in Figure 3.5. There are also variations in the ascending segment of the granule cell axons prior to their bifurcation to form parallel fibers. These variations would of necessity introduce some differences and nonlinearities in conduction velocities, and perhaps in the local variations of densities of parallel fiber–Purkinje cell synapses.

The essentially perpendicular arrangement of the transverse input mossy parallel fibers and the longitudinal Purkinje (as output), basket, and stellate cells (longitudinal) in the cerebellar cortex has been reemphasized by Voogd and Ruigrok (1997).

Cohen and Yarom (2000) pointed out that the parasagittal organization of the cerebellar cortex that is imposed by the climbing fiber input overlaps that of the corticonuclear projections, thus suggesting a functional organization.

The parallel fibers make synaptic contact with the dendritic spines of the Purkinje cells, as well as with stellate, basket, and Golgi cells. According to one estimate, some 200,000 parallel fibers make contact with a single Purkinje cell in the cat and 250,000 cells in the human. According to another estimate, of the 400,000 parallel fibers passing through the dendritic tree of a Purkinje cell, only 80,000 make synaptic contact. In any event, a given Purkinje cell is under the influence of a large number of granule cells. Conversely, a given parallel fiber has been estimated to pass through from 450 to 1,100 Purkinje cells along a folium, but if synapses are made with only one in three to five Purkinje cells, the number could decrease to about 100 or even less.

Golgi Cells. Already mentioned, the Golgi cells resemble Purkinje cells in some respects (Fig. 3.2) in that they are large and have branching dendritic trees that extend outward into the molecular layer; their number approximates that of the Purkinje cells. The dendritic tree of the Golgi cell, however, extends in all directions (about three times as far as the Purkinje dendritic tree) rather than being confined to

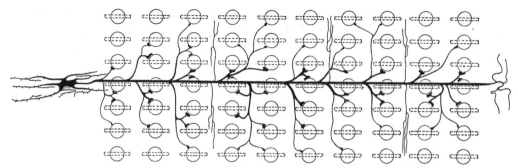

Figure 3.6. Matrix of Purkinje neurons (cell body indicated by circle, dendritic tree by bar) potentially reached by descending axon branches of a basket neuron. The whole matrix and arborization is seen from the surface. The thin side branches of the basket axon and the terminal branching, running in the longitudinal direction of the folium, have an ascending course and probably terminate in the molecular layer. (From Szentágothai 1965; reprinted by permission of Prof. Szentágothai's heirs [by courtesy of Prof. Hámori].)

the transverse plane of the folium, as is the case for the Purkinje, stellate, and basket cells. Parallel fibers form excitatory synapses with the Golgi cell dendrites, which are also contacted by other afferents (e.g., Golgi cell dendrites that remain in the granular layer may be contacted by mossy fibers directly). The axons of Golgi cells, which are extensively branched, make synaptic contact with dendrites of granule cells at the glomeruli, as already mentioned. Recurrent Purkinje axons synapse onto Golgi somata. The granule cell to Golgi cell ratio is of the order of 5,000 to 1.

Molecular Layer. The molecular layer, the most superficial layer, is dominated by fibers; the relatively few neurons in this layer, which are located just above the level of the Purkinje cell bodies, are the *stellate cells* and *basket cells*. The dendrites of both cell types, like the dendrites of the Purkinje cells, which are in the same layer, are oriented in the transverse plane of the folium and receive collaterals of climbing fibers.

Basket Cells. The dendritic tree of the basket cells (Fig. 3.2, B), like that of the Purkinje cells, is transverse to the folium, but as already mentioned, is not as flattened as that of the Purkinje cell. At times, the dendrites of the two cell types appear in regular alternation. The axon of the basket cells (Fig. 3.2, Ba) passes for some distance across the folium just above the Purkinje cell bodies, giving off descending collaterals at right angles, which surround Purkinje cell bodies like a basket, making synaptic contact with an average (in the cat) of about 10 Purkinje cells (Fig. 3.6), and contacting about 3 Purkinje cells in both directions along the longitudinal axis of the folium (in the cat), for an average total of some 30 Purkinje cells. Horizontal axonal segments of the basket cells also contact dendrites of Purkinje, basket, and stellate cells.

The descending axons of the basket cell axons and their arborizations form a unique plexus, termed pinceau, or (artist's) paintbrush, around the initial segment of Purkinje axons, thus forming an axoaxonic (inhibitory) synapse, an uncommon structure elsewhere in the vertebrate brain. Although the pinceau would initially seem to constitute a powerful inhibitory structure, its actual effect has yet to be clarified completely.

As a result of this arrangement, the basket cells, which are only slightly more numerous than Purkinje cells (by 15–20%), can act on a series of Purkinje cells across the folium and to a lesser extent, along it. This arrangement is in contrast to the parallel fibers, which activate a series of Purkinje cells along, rather than across, the folium. It is to be emphasized that the inhibitory effects of basket cells are on Purkinje cells that are arrayed laterally (with respect to the long axis of the folium) from the locus of the basket cell's dendritic tree, thus providing inhibition to off-axis Purkinje cells. In contrast, stellate cells (see the following) provide primarily on-axis inhibition to Purkinje cells and to the more distal parts of the Purkinje cell dendritic tree. The parallel fibers that synapse with basket and stellate cells may not necessarily be the same ones that synapse with Purkinje cells.

Stellate Cells. The stellate cells, which lie in the outer two thirds of the molecular layer, have a cell body and a dendritic arborization that is smaller than those of the basket cells. Like the basket cells, the dendritic tree of stellate cells is oriented transversely to the long axis of folia. Also like basket cells, the stellate cells receive synapses principally from parallel fibers, and their axons – coursing transversely to the axis of folia (although not as far as the basket cell axons) – synapse principally with Purkinje cells in its immediate vicinity, the more so the more superficial the stellate cell in the molecular layer. The stellate cell axons form synapses only on dendritic shafts of Purkinje cells, whereas basket cells form baskets around the Purkinje cell somata and pinceau around their initial segment, as already mentioned. (The more highly structured basket cell is a more recent development in phylogeny than is the stellate cell.) The ratio of stellate to Purkinje cells is estimated to be about 1:17.

Inhibitory Mechanisms: Golgi Cells vs. Basket Cells. From the preceding account, it is evident that Golgi cells are inhibitory to granule cells and that basket cells are inhibitory to Purkinje cells, but the manner of the inhibition in the two instances is different. These two types of cells are diagrammed in Figure 3.7, originally from Ramón y Cajal (1995). The inhibition by the Golgi cells occurs at the level of the glomeruli; the inhibitory effect of the Golgi synapses counteracts the excitatory effect of the mossy fiber synapses. The inhibitory synapses of the basket cells on the Purkinje, in contrast, are on the initial segment of the Purkinje cell axon; the excitatory synapses of (primarily) the parallel fibers are on the Purkinje cell dendritic tree. It seems likely that there is a significant functional difference between these two arrangements for delivering inhibition, perhaps related to the extremely small size and great number of the granule cells. (It should be noted that the Golgi cells are also inhibitory to stellate and basket cells.)

Starting from the point that Golgi cells, being inhibitory, exert both a feedback and a feedforward inhibition of granule cell activity, De Schutter, Vos, and Maex (2000) and Vos et al. (2000) concluded that Golgi cells (in relation to the mossy

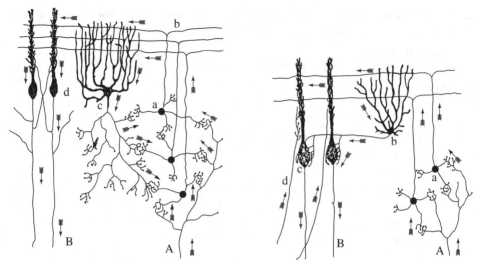

Figure 3.7. Two diagrams from Ramón y Cajal showing, on the left at top, a Golgi cell with its synapses onto the glomeruli of three granule cells, and on the right at top, a basket cell with its synapses onto two Purkinje cells. Both cell types receive their input from the parallel fibers. Arrows indicate direction of impulses. Legends for left side: A, mossy fiber; a, granule cell; b, parallel fiber; c, Golgi cell; d, Purkinje cells; B, Purkinje axons (note recurrent collaterals). Legends for right side: A, mossy fiber; a, granule cell; b, basket cell; B, Purkinje axon; c, Purkinje cells; d, climbing fibers. See text. (From Eccles, Ito, and Szentágothai 1967; in: Eccles, Ito, and Szentágothai, *The Cerebellum as a Neuronal Machine*, copyright 1967, Springer-Verlag New York, originally from Ramón y Cajal 1911 [Figs. 103 and 104]; [English translation, 1995 by N. Swanson and L. W. Swanson, Oxford University Press.]; reprinted by permission.)

fiber–granule cell–parallel fiber network) perform poorly as gain controllers at time scales of interest for cerebellar motor control. However, these authors suggested that beams of Golgi cells were being synchronized by common parallel fiber inputs (in contrast to the earlier suggestion of parallel fiber beams at the level of Purkinje cell activity proposed by Eccles et al. [1967]), which may result in lateral inhibition by Golgi cells, and also in a tight control over the timing of granule cell spikes, which could implement a temporal code.

3.1.4. Afferent Fiber Systems of the Cerebellar Cortex: Climbing Fibers and Mossy Fibers

There are primarily two kinds of afferent fibers to the cerebellar cortex (the intracortical terminations of which have already been considered): the mossy fibers (Chapter 4) and the climbing fibers (Chapter 5). Both give off collaterals to the cerebellar nuclei. The function of the (excitatory) collaterals of the mossy fibers and of the climbing fibers, which project to the cerebellar nuclei, and the nature of their interaction with the (inhibitory) fibers from the Purkinje cells, has long been of interest (e.g., Thach 1972).

Climbing Fibers. Moderately thin and myelinated, the climbing fibers pass undivided from the inferior olive, through the cerebellar white matter and the molecular layer, and to the level of the Purkinje cells. Electrophysiological and anatomical studies indicate that branches of a single fiber can divide and innervate different lobules of the cerebellar cortex in a parasagittal distribution (i.e., longitudinally) to synapse with 10 to 15 Purkinje cells. In maturity, only a single (branch of a) climbing fiber innervates a given Purkinje cell, in contrast to the immature state, during which there is multiple innervation (up to four climbing fibers per Purkinje cell) of which all but one normally recede in the course of maturation (Chapter 11).

The branch of a climbing fiber for a given Purkinje cell follows closely and winds ivylike along its dendritic branches, making contact with the dendritic spines of the latter, thus forming the basis of an extensive and powerful excitatory synaptic action. These synapses are confined to the inner two thirds of the molecular layer. As previously mentioned, some of the collaterals of climbing fibers may end on neighboring Purkinje cells, stellate cells, basket cells, and Golgi cells, although the presumed excitatory synaptic action on Golgi cells, and also on granule cells, has evidently not been substantiated.

In humans, there is a total of about 1 million neurons for both inferior olives, as compared with about 15 million Purkinje cells, for a ratio of 1 to 15.

In contrast to the extensive branching of the mossy fibers (described following), the climbing fibers ascend, as just mentioned, undivided from the inferior olive through the white matter of the cerebellum to the Purkinje cell layer.

Mossy Fibers and Their Terminations. These fibers, which derive their name from their moss like terminals in the granular layer, are thick and heavily myelinated, and therefore can be expected to possess a conduction velocity higher than that of the thin climbing fibers. Unlike the climbing fibers, all of which arise from a single source (the inferior olive, Chapter 5), mossy fibers arise from numerous sources (Chapter 4). In contrast to the above-noted, limited branching by climbing fibers in the vicinity of the Purkinje cell layer of the cerebellar cortex to a small group of Purkinje cells, mossy fibers give off collaterals, as many as 20 or 30, along their entire course through the white matter, not just in the folia in which they largely terminate. Having entered the cerebellar cortex, mossy fibers branch repeatedly; one fiber may supply two or even more folia. In their final course, they give off many collaterals, which, like the final branches, end in the granular layer as a cluster of small endings, forming what are often referred to as rosettes (glomeruli), as previously described. The mossy fibers remain (thinly) myelinated up to their preterminal portions. Their terminal or synaptic endings interdigitate with, and form synaptic contacts with, the clawlike dendritic terminations of the granule cells (Fig. 3.2, inset), as described above. As just mentioned, rosettes are surrounded by granule cell dendrites and Golgi cell axon terminals, forming glomeruli. Thus, mossy fiber rosettes and Golgi cell axon terminals are the presynaptic elements of glomeruli, and granule cell dendrites are the postsynaptic elements of glomeruli, the mossy fiber terminations being excitatory and the Golgi terminals inhibitory. One mossy fiber has been estimated to make contact with some 450 granule cells. Mossy fiber terminals also synapse onto the somata of Golgi cells.

Trajectories of Single Climbing (Olivocerebellar) and Mossy Fibers. In a study of trajectories of single olivocerebellar and of mossy fibers in the rat, it was found (Shinoda et al. 2000; Sugihara, Wu, and Shinoda 1999) that there were approximately 250 swellings (synapses) on single climbing fibers, a result that was basically similar to the results of previous authors. At least 91% of the olivocerebellar fibers examined had collaterals to the cerebellar nuclei, and all the mossy fibers (from the lateral reticular nucleus) projecting to the cerebellar cortex had collaterals to the cerebellar nuclei. The nuclear collaterals of climbing fibers were thinner than the climbing fibers themselves. (In contrast, it was noted that many mossy fibers originating from the pontine nuclei lacked nuclear collaterals.) The broadness of cerebellar cortical innervation by single lateral reticular nucleus axons contrasted with a single zonal projection of olivocerebellar axons. The latter, besides terminal arborization around Purkinje cell thick dendrites, had terminals that surrounded Purkinje cell soma, fine branchlets that extended transversely in the molecular layer, and thin retrograde collaterals that reentered the Purkinje cell and granular layers. The authors concluded by indicating that further information is needed for understanding the functional interactions at nuclear efferent neurons among Purkinje cell inputs from widely distributed cortical areas innervated by a single mossy fiber and nuclear inputs from a collateral of the same mossy fiber. The existence of collaterals to the cerebellar nuclei from mossy fibers and from climbing fibers en route to the cerebellar cortex has not been without controversy (Shinoda et al. 1977).

3.1.5. Divergence and Convergence in the Cerebellar Cortex

According to one calculation (Palkovits, Magyar, and Szentágothai 1972), the extent of divergence or spread in the mossy fiber input to the cerebellar cortex can be estimated in the following way. From measurements at the base of the folia, the ratio of fibers is as follows: one-sixth Purkinje axons, one-sixth climbing fibers, and four-sixths mossy fibers. Therefore, the ratio of mossy fibers to Purkinje cells is 4:1. Within a given folium, one mossy fiber breaks up into some 16–17 mossy rosettes (glomeruli). From earlier data, the granule cell–glomerulus ratio is 27–28:1, and the mossy fiber–granule cell ratio is about 1:460. Correspondingly, because the granule cells have each 4.17 dendrites on average, the average mossy rosette is contacted by some 112 granule cell dendrites (460/4.12). The number of granule cells belonging to one Purkinje cell ($1792 = 16 \times 112$) is capable of transmitting impulses from four mossy fibers (because there are four mossy fibers for each Purkinje cell) and their 68 (17×4) rosettes (glomeruli), whereas the parallel fibers, of an assumed length of 2 mm, penetrate the dendritic trees of 225 Purkinje cells (spaced at 0.008 mm). Because the parallel fibers establish synapses with only every one fifth of these Purkinje cells, the calculated number of parallel fibers–Purkinje spine synapses would be 80,640 per Purkinje cell ($1792 \times 225/5$). This estimate is in good agreement with an independent count of the Purkinje dendritic spines of 91,600. (Note that the assumed length of parallel fibers of 2 mm is now considered an underestimate, as mentioned earlier in this chapter; today's estimate of a length of 6–7 mm would bring the total estimate of parallel fibers per Purkinje cell more closely in line with other more recent estimates on the order of 200,000.)

These estimates do not, however, take into account the branching of mossy fibers in the white matter before entering the cerebellar cortex. It is also the case that granule cells activated by any given mossy fiber are likely to be widely dispersed in the granular layer within the distribution territory of that mossy fiber. Likewise, the parallel fibers of these granule cells will be at correspondingly different depths in the molecular layer, impinging on different branches of the dendritic tree of the same, or even different, Purkinje cells. Moreover the 2-mm parallel fiber length is an underestimate, as indicated above. The consequence is that the Purkinje cell would likely be presented with samples of the same mossy fiber discharge in several different parts of its dendritic tree at the same time. It is also clear that each mossy fiber entering the white matter from below distributes to a large field of cortex, which overlaps extensively with that of its neighbors (Palay and Chan-Palay 1974).

Under certain simplifying assumptions, a ratio of mossy fiber–Purkinje cell within the folia of 4:1 has been estimated for the cat, which, in view of the very much larger ratio for parallel fibers to Purkinje cells, could perhaps suggest that an interpolation or vernier process of some kind takes place in the cerebellar cortex.

There are certain differences among mossy fibers and their terminations according to their sources of origin (e.g., with respect to their degree of branching within the granular layer; Brodal 1967, 1981; Brodal and Drabløs 1963).

In addition to the extracerebellar origins of the mossy fibers and the climbing fibers, a portion of the mossy fibers originate from the cerebellar nuclei, thus constituting a feedback loop to the cerebellar cortex. These nucleocortical fibers are considered in greater detail in Chapter 6. There are also fibers originating from the cerebellar nuclei that terminate as inhibitory synapses in the inferior olive, which completes another feedback loop to the cerebellar cortex, in this instance via the inferior olive; these are also considered further in Chapter 6.

3.1.6. Layering of Granule Cells and Parallel Fibers

As previously mentioned, the disposition of granule cells in the granular layer is such that the more deeply lying cells give rise to the more deeply lying parallel fibers in the molecular layer, and the more superficial cells in the granular layer are associated with the more superficially lying parallel fibers (Fig. 3.5). Further, the thickness of the more deeply lying parallel fibers has been reported to be appreciably greater than that of the more superficially lying ones (1.0 mu vs. 0.1 to 0.2 mu), a difference that at least to some extent is reflected in the length of the parallel fibers at different levels in the molecular layer. The density of parallel fibers in the molecular layer (which in cross-section appears to be an almost crystalline-like array; see Fig. 12.5 for the extreme case of the valvula) is increased by the fact that no space is taken up by neuroglial cells. The ratio of granule cells to Purkinje cells is of the order of 5,000 to 1, but estimates vary appreciably. In addition to (excitatory) synapses onto the dendrites of Purkinje cells, parallel fibers also form (excitatory) synapses with Golgi, stellate, and basket cells.

Efficacy of Parallel Fibers vs. Vertical Segments of Granule Cell Axons. In relation to possible mechanisms of function of the cerebellar cortex, an important question, as mentioned earlier, is that of the relative importance of the distribution on Purkinje cells of the different segments of axons of granule cells (i.e., the ascending [vertical] segment vs. the parallel fiber segment). If the ascending segment is more important and the branched parallel fiber from the same granule cell has an appreciably weaker effect, then the impact of a given granule cell will be primarily on those Purkinje cells that directly overlie it (i.e., with which the vertical segment of the granule cell has synaptic contact). However, if the two parallel fibers from such a granule cell have a major impact on Purkinje cells, then the effect of the granule cell could in principle make itself felt for the full extent of the parallel fibers. From their study of this question, Garwicz and Andersson (1992) found that synaptic activity does spread along the parallel fibers, as far as 1.5 mm outside the mossy fiber termination area.

In this connection, in a study of the spatial effects of excitatory amino acids in the rat cerebellar cortex using optical imaging of a voltage-sensitive dye (Grinvald et al. 1988) in conjunction with stimulation of the cerebellar cortex, Elias, Yae, and Ebner (1993) found discrete "beams" of optical activity consistent with extracellular recordings. The authors concluded that the optical signal was not due to the evoked parallel fiber activity but was mainly generated by postsynaptic targets.

3.1.7. Other Afferent Fibers to the Cerebellar Cortex

The fibers to the cerebellar cortex from the nucleus locus coeruleus and the raphe nuclei and their effects (Brodal 1981; Brodal 1998; Ito 1984; Kandel, Schwartz, and Jessell 1991; Parent 1996) are generally not included in this overview.

3.1.8. Cerebellar Cortex vs. Cerebral Cortex: Differences and Similarities

Oscarsson (1979) emphasized that the cerebellar cortex, unlike the cerebral cortex, is remarkably uniform, and differences in its cytoarchitectonics (structure) cannot be used for its parcellation into regions with different functions. Thus, functional differentiation depends largely or exclusively on differences in the afferent and efferent connections. Similarly, Sotelo and Chédotal (1997) pointed out that the cerebellar cortex differs from the cerebral cortex by one major cytoarchitectonic feature: the former is characterized by its striking uniformity, whereas the latter varies over its extent (i.e., cytoarchitechtonic areas) and can be divided into numerous distinct layers. However, further analysis of both cortices based on input/output arrangement suggests that both, despite their individual specifications, are organized according to common principles. That is, both are parcellated into narrow sagittal zones – the

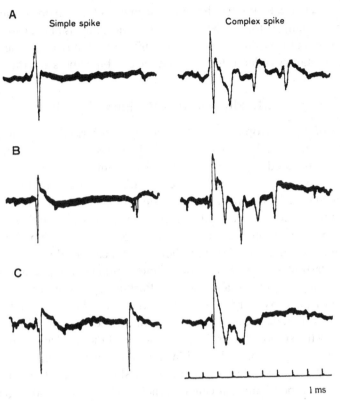

Figure 3.8. Simple and complex spikes of three sample Purkinje cells (A, B, C), recorded extracellularly from the cerebellar cortex of a rhesus monkey. (From Mano, Kanazawa, and Yamamoto 1989; In: Strata (ed.) *The Olivocerebellar System in Motor Control*, copyright 1989, Springer-Verlag, Heidelberg; reprinted by permission of the publisher.)

microzones of the cerebellum are comparable to the modular columnar organization of the neocortex.

3.2. Physiological Aspects of the Cerebellar Cortex

To reiterate, the most significant connections among the neurons of the cerebellar cortex and the afferent and efferent fibers are shown highly schematized and simplified in Figure 3.3. The climbing fibers, originating from the inferior olive (not shown) terminate as monosynaptic excitatory synapses onto the dendritic spines of the Purkinje cells, covering most of the dendritic tree and invariably evoking a complex spike consisting of one to four or five individual spikes (Fig. 3.8). The mossy fibers, however, indirectly excite the dendritic trees of Purkinje cells via the dendritic glomeruli of the granule cells and their axonal branches in the form of the parallel fibers. As previously mentioned, the latter also excite the dendrites of the Golgi cells, which in turn inhibit the granule cells, basket cells, and stellate cells, the latter two also being inhibitory. The stellate cells inhibit the dendritic tree of the Purkinje cells, whereas the basket cells inhibit the initial segment of the axon of the latter. The output of the Purkinje cells, which terminates on the neurons of the cerebellar nuclei (and on neurons in the vestibular nuclei), is inhibitory. That is, these nuclear neurons also receive excitatory collaterals from both the climbing fibers and the mossy fibers.

3.2.1. Physiology of the Purkinje Cell

From studies of the electrophysiological properties of Purkinje cell somata and dendrites in mammalian (adult guinea pig) cerebellar slices, Llinás and Sugimori (1980a, 1980b, 1992) concluded that (1) sodium and calcium conductances (channels) in Purkinje cells are largely confined to the somatic (cell body) and dendritic membranes, respectively; (2) parallel fibers activate primarily the spiny branchlets of the Purkinje dendritic tree, either directly through the vertically ascending portion of the granule cell axon or through the horizontal compartment of the parallel fibers, via synaptic contacts from up to 200,000 parallel fibers for each Purkinje cell; (3) this postsynaptic depolarization is restricted to the fine terminals of the dendritic branches and, via a cascade-like effect, activates the Purkinje cell soma to generate simple spikes (Fig. 3.8); (4) GABAergic receptors on the soma (for basket cells) and on the dendritic tree (for stellate cells) have a shunting effect; (5) climbing fibers, which cover primarily the smooth (i.e., spineless) portion of the dendritic tree, activate the latter more or less synchronously, and in turn, the soma, to generate fast (as high as 400 Hz) inhibitory postsynaptic potentials (IPSPs) at the postsynaptic target cell terminals (e.g., cerebellar nuclear cells). In their review, Llinás and Sugimori (1992) stated that they believe that the climbing and parallel fiber systems time-share the Purkinje cell but are not completely independent of one another functionally. It may be mentioned that Brodal and Kawamura (1980) believed that physiological evidence existed indicating that the input to the cerebellum from many or even all sources (i.e., cutaneous, visual, vestibular, etc., and from the cerebral cortex and other regions) reaches it both via climbing and via mossy fibers (i.e., that there is a dual input).

Normally, the Purkinje cell is activated by either parallel or climbing fiber input. Because the climbing fiber has many contacts with the Purkinje cell, a very large (e.g., 25 mV) excitatory postsynaptic potential (EPSP) results; it is the most powerful synapse in the central nervous system (Rothwell 1994). A brief burst of spikes follows (Fig. 3.8), and then a long repolarization phase with possibly additional spikes superimposed. The dendritic Ca^{2+} conductance, and the Na^+ and K^+ conductances of the soma and axon, participate in this activity. A single action potential arriving via a climbing fiber invariably produces a complex spike in a Purkinje cell. In contrast, the parallel fiber input to a Purkinje cell is much weaker and produces a graded EPSP. The resulting action potentials (if any) are termed simple spikes, and probably do not entail activation of the dendritic Ca^{2+} conductance (Rothwell 1994).

De Schutter and Bower (1994a, 1994b) reiterated several interesting points of contrast between the parallel fiber and climbing fiber systems: (1) each contacts a different and non overlapping region of the Purkinje cell dendrite: climbing fiber synapses are made on the thick, smooth, proximal dendrites of the cell, whereas the granule cell synapses (i.e., parallel fiber synapses) are restricted to the small spine-covered tertiary dendrites (the spiny branchlets); (2) each of these systems generates different postsynaptic effects in the Purkinje cell: climbing fiber activation evokes a large all-or-none Ca^{2+}-dependent dendritic action potential, whereas parallel fiber (granule cell) inputs are considered to generate more classical dendritic EPSPs and to produce fast Na^+ spikes as the Purkinje cell output.

De Schutter and Bower (1994a, 1994b), by adding simulated climbing fiber and parallel fiber excitatory synaptic inputs to a basic computer model of the Purkinje cell, were able to replicate both complex spikes and simple spikes, provided there were inhibitory synaptic inputs to the Purkinje cell from basket and stellate cells.

Using a fluorescent indicator to image voltage in combination with synaptically activated sodium transients in Purkinje cells, Lasser-Ross and Ross (1992) found that fast sodium action potentials resulted in large increases in internal sodium concentration in the soma and axon, but not in the dendrites, consistent with the results of the above-mentioned physiological experiments of Llinás and Sugimori (1980a, 1980b).

Resolution of Purkinje Cells (Minimum Activation of Dendritic Spines). In relation to the "resolution" of single Purkinje cells, Denk, Sugimori, and Llinás (1995) determined that the smallest unit of active electrical response is a single spine, rather than a spiny branchlet; hence, the spine has to be considered the fundamental unit in Purkinje cell integration. These researchers pointed out that, considering that each of the 10^7 Purkinje cells in a human brain contains as many as 100,000 spines, the cerebellum would be provided with 10^{12} computational elements.

Reciprocal Trophic Interaction Between Purkinje Cells and Climbing Fibers. A reciprocal trophic interaction between climbing fiber terminal arborizations and Purkinje cells was reported by Strata et al. (1997), such that when the climbing fiber is missing, the Purkinje cell undergoes a hyperspiny transformation and becomes hyperinnervated by parallel fibers. However, this change was found to be reversible; the climbing fiber-deprived Purkinje cell is able to elicit sprouting of nearby intact climbing fibers and the new arbor is able to restore synaptic connections fully.

Bistability in Purkinje Dendrites. Using ion channels, Yuen, Hockberger, and Houk (1995) modeled the possibility of bistability in Purkinje cell dendrites, pointing out, among other aspects, that the hysteresis inherent in bistability is equivalent to short-term memory without changes in synaptic weight (as in long-term depression [LTD]). Independent bistability in several dendritic branches would, in turn, result in multi-stability of the Purkinje cell.

Basis of Fluctuation of Purkinje Inhibitory Postsynaptic Currents in Stellate and Basket Cells. In exploring the possible origins of the appreciable fluctuation in inhibitory postsynaptic currents in Purkinje cells arising from stellate and basket cells, Vincent and Marty (1996) concluded that the major source of the fluctuation is localized within the axonal arborization of presynaptic neurons. The concerted release of several presynaptic vesicles appeared necessary. That is, such multiquantal events were considered to result from fluctuations in presynaptic depolarization, or from fluctuations in a regenerative calcium-ion amplification mechanism.

3.3. Organization of the Cerebellar Cortex in Relation to Other Structures

3.3.1. Connections Among Cerebellar Cortex, Cerebellar Nuclei, and Cerebral Cortex

The lateral cerebellum (cerebrocerebellum, Fig. 3.1) receives inputs mainly from the cerebral association cortex and projects primarily via the dentate nucleus to areas 4 and 6 of the cerebral cortex (via the ventrolateral thalamic nucleus), whereas the intermediate cerebellum receives inputs mainly from the sensorimotor cortex and also from the periphery and projects primarily via the interpositus nucleus to the same cortical areas. This finding suggests that the pyramidal tract neurons in area 4 constitute the common paths from the cerebral cortex (Shinoda et al. 1993). The cerebellar cortex also receives the same inputs from the cerebral cortex as do the cerebellar nuclei, the resulting temporal and spatial modulation by the Purkinje cells of the excitatory inputs to the cerebellar nuclei, thus providing the organized output signal that results in finely controlled movement, according to Shinoda et al. (1997).

3.3.2. Microzones and Microcomplexes of the Cerebellar Cortex: Functional Units

The cerebellar cortex itself can be divided into a number of independent sagittal zones, termed microzones (of, e.g., 1 mm in width in the cat) which, with its group of nuclear neurons, forms the operational unit of the cerebellum, perhaps comparable with the cell column of the cerebral cortex, but with less distinct borders (Andersson and Oscarsson 1978; Oscarsson 1979, 1980). As specified by Ito (1984), a microcomplex is composed of a cerebellar microzone (i.e., a set of Purkinje cells), projecting to a distinct group of target (i.e., nuclear) neurons, and receiving two kinds of inputs from mossy fibers and climbing fibers, the output being carried by the deep nuclear cells. Both mossy fibers and climbing fibers supply collaterals to the nuclear cell group and pass on to the corresponding microzone of cerebellar cortex.

On the basis of newer methods of molecular biology applied to the cerebellum, an estimate of the size of basic cerebellar modules of as small as about 100×150 microns has been made, corresponding in the mouse cerebellar cortex to some 4,000 modules total, or 40 Purkinje cells and their associated interneurons for each module (Hawkes 1997). It was suggested by this author that in higher species, the size (but not the number) of modules would be expected to increase with increasing cerebellar surface area, at least for the parasagittal boundaries.

3.4. Molecular Biology of the Cerebellum: Its Compartmentation and Cell Types

In addition to the better known compartmentation of the Purkinje cells and the molecular layer, Ozol and Hawkes (1997) drew attention to the substantial evidence indicating that the granular layer is subdivided into a large number of highly reproducible modules. Based on this evidence, the authors argued that the cerebellum consists of many hundreds of reproducible structural/functional modules, and that a modular organization is a prerequisite for the efficient parallel processing of information during motor control.

Reviews of some aspects of the genetic basis for normal and abnormal development of the cerebellum and its cell types (e.g., global and subcellular levels of compartmentalization, sagittal vs. rostrocaudal compartmentalization) have appeared (Goldowitz and Hamre 1998; Oberdick, Baader, and Schilling (1998). (Genetic aspects of the cerebellum are discussed more extensively in Chapter 11.)

3.5. Cerebellar Modulation of Sensory Responses

Generalized effects of stimulation of the cerebellar cortex have been reported. Thus, as a result of stimulating the cerebellum (especially Lobulus V, VI, and VII of the vermis), Crispino and Bullock (1984) found systematic modulation (enhancement or depression, with a characteristic time course) of sensory-evoked potentials (visual, auditory, somatosensory) in midbrain, thalamus, and cerebral cortex of the rat. The authors concluded that these effects were clearly associated with the cerebellum itself rather than with adventitious spread of the cerebellar stimulation.

3.6. Special Techniques: Voltage-Sensitive Dyes and Optical Imaging

In their review of the use of voltage-sensitive dyes and optical recordings, Ebner and Chen (1995) included a summary of studies using this technique for investigating the cerebellum. The authors indicated that the technique has several distinct advantages for investigating the cerebellum: its uniformity and simplicity (e.g., only five basic types of neurons, only two major input channels [mossy and climbing fibers]), the thinness of the cerebellar cortex (1 mm) so all three cortical layers (molecular, Purkinje cell, and granular layer) can be optically evaluated temporospatially.

Using a special array recording system for optical imaging of voltage-sensitive fluorescent dyes in an isolated cerebellar preparation to reveal the temporal and spatial flow of cell somata and dendritic (but not axonal) inhibitory and excitatory activity within a 50×50 or 100×100 mu surface of cerebellar cortex down to as deep as the granule cell layer, Cohen and Yarom (2000) reported that white matter (i.e., mossy fiber) stimulation elicited a patch of activity throughout which activation is simultaneous, whereas surface (i.e., parallel fiber) stimulation resulted in a beam of activity that propagates along the parallel fiber system. These results were considered to be in accord with the hypothesis of Llinás (1982), showing that the ascending part of the granule cell axons, rather than the parallel fiber system, provides the main drive to Purkinje cells.

Cohen and Yarom (2000) concluded that the basic, independent modules of the cerebellar cortex consist of a localized group of granule cells and Purkinje cells above them, with the feedback inhibition of the Golgi cells and the feedforward inhibition of the stellate cells regulating the activity of each module. In this view, mutual interactions among the different modules occur in the sagittal axis via the long-range axons of the molecular layer interneurons, and in the mediolateral axis via the parallel fibers, the latter interactions, arising from disinhibition, being far more significant and efficient over a much broader time window in comparison with the mediolateral interaction via the parallel fibers, which are rather weak and are efficient only within a narrow time window. Cohen and Yarom (2000) also pointed out that the parasagittal organization of the cerebellar cortex imposed by the climbing fiber input overlaps that of the corticonuclear projections and suggested a functional organization.

FOUR

The Mossy Fiber Afferent System

In this chapter and in Chapter 5, a brief overview is presented of the principal origins of, respectively, the mossy fibers and the afferent fibers to the inferior olive. The information below is distilled mainly from Brodal (1981); Bloedel and Courville (1981); Ekerot, Larson, and Oscarsson (1979); and Brodal (1998).

The termination sites of the climbing fibers from the inferior olive and the mossy fibers in the cerebellar cortex are, with few exceptions, quite different. Although both types of excitatory fibers are ultimately derived from a variety of sources, the climbing fibers, so far as is known, take their immediate origin entirely from the inferior olivary nucleus (the inferior olive), whereas the mossy fibers do not similarly pass through a single nuclear structure.

The mossy fibers conduct impulses relatively rapidly, branch extensively, and influence many Purkinje cells via the granule cells. However, the excitatory effect on each Purkinje cell is weak so the conjunctive action of many mossy fibers is required to fire the Purkinje cells at rates of 50–500 per second.

4.1. Vestibulocerebellar Afferents

The vestibulocerebellar afferents terminate in the flocculus and nodulus, the ventral part of the uvula, and the paraflocculus, and provide inputs to the cerebellum that are undoubtedly important for automatic regulation of posture and movement of the head, trunk, and limbs (Fig. 3.1).

Primary Vestibular Fibers. The primary vestibular fibers are fibers from the vestibular end-organs (semicircular canals and otolith organs), which have been traced to the vestibulocerebellum and the fastigial nucleus. The terminals of the primary vestibular fibers are appreciably more concentrated than mossy fiber terminals elsewhere in the cerebellar cortex. In addition, they give off fine short collaterals that also terminate within the granular layer.

Secondary Vestibulocerebellar Fibers. The secondary vestibulocerebellar fibers arise from portions of the medial and descending vestibular nuclei and, in general, project to the same areas of the cerebellar cortex as the primary vestibular fibers. (There may also be some indirect projections of primary and secondary vestibular fibers to the cerebellar cortex by way of certain brain stem sites, e.g., the lateral reticular nucleus.)

4.2. Spinocerebellar Pathways

The mossy fiber afferent systems to the cerebellar cortex and their collaterals to the cerebellar nuclei can be divided into two groups: the one consisting of direct pathways projecting from the spinal cord and pontine nuclei, and the other consisting of projections from the spinal cord and cerebral cortex via the precerebellar reticular nuclei. Generally speaking, the *direct spinocerebellar and pontocerebellar* projections convey information to the cerebellum from the spinal cord and the cerebral cortex, respectively. In contrast, the *reticulocerebellar* systems convey information to the cerebellum that reflects the integration of inputs from ascending and descending pathways onto neurons within the precerebellar reticular nuclei. In fact, most stimuli activate both the direct and the indirect pathways to the cerebellum.

Of the *direct spinocerebellar systems*, the *dorsal spinocerebellar tract* (DSCT), arising from Clark's column in the spinal cord (see also Chapter 14), conveys impulses from proprioceptors: muscle spindles, tendon organs, pressure receptors in the hairless pads, and from touch and pressure receptors in the hairy skin and joint receptors. Clearly, the dorsal spinocerebellar tract carries modality – and topographically – specific (i.e., small receptive field) information about the lower extremities and the lower trunk. The *cuneocerebellar tract* (arising from the lateral cuneate nucleus) is the counterpart of the dorsal spinocerebellar tract for the upper trunk, forelimbs, and neck. Both tracts enter the cerebellum via the inferior cerebellar peduncle.

The *ventral and rostral spinocerebellar tracts*, although they are also direct paths from spinal cord to cerebellum, differ from the tracts just considered. The fibers of the *ventral spinocerebellar tract* are on the whole much thinner. They appear to convey impulses from tendon organ or from muscle spindle afferents. Their receptive fields are evidently large, and they are subject to descending influences (e.g., facilitated by the pyramidal tract and inhibited by reticulospinal paths). They enter the cerebellum partly via the inferior and partly via the superior cerebellar peduncles. They evidently convey information that is already highly integrated at the spinal level, in contrast to the more topical information conveyed by the dorsal spinocerebellar and cuneocerebellar tracts just mentioned. Correspondingly, the information conveyed by the latter tracts is apparently distributed to much smaller cerebellar areas than those from the ventral and rostral spinocerebellar tracts, perhaps indicating that the mossy fibers of the latter tracts branch more extensively.

There remains to be mentioned the less well-established *trigeminocerebellar pathway*, for which the mesencephalic trigeminal nucleus is an intermediate station, being concerned with the mediation of proprioceptive impulses from the face.

To illustrate some of the complexity that attends the above-described systems, the following can be cited. In recordings from awake behaving monkeys, van Kan,

Gibson, and Houk (1993) found that mossy fibers provide the intermediate cerebellum with position, velocity, and direction information about movement of individual forelimb joint, perhaps derived from efference copy and the usual afference. The discharge patterns of Golgi cells were noted to be quite different from those of mossy fibers; all Golgi cells showed a phasic discharge without tonic components. The output signals from the nucleus interpositus suggested that the intermediate cerebellum incorporates position and velocity information from individual joints, together with other inputs, into phasic signals relating to coordinated movements of the entire limb. In this connection, Horne and Butler (1995) suggested that the cerebello–thalamo–cortical pathway receives a form of efference copy from the motor cortex and compares this message with that derived from peripheral afferents concerning the actual progress of the movement.

4.3. Fractured Somatotopy

From probing the vermal area of the cerebellar cortex (crus I and crus II) in rats by means of microelectrode micromapping methods, Shambes, Gibson, and Welker (1978) found that cutaneous mechanoreceptors terminate within columnar assemblies of granule cells appearing as individual patches, which in turn make up mosaics. The somatotopic organization of single patches was precise, but among the mosaics it was fractured. Thus, small regions of the body surface project in an orderly pattern to small patches (of about 1 mm diameter) of the cerebellar cortex; however, the same body patches were repeated many times across the cerebellar cortex, interspersed with patches representing different areas of the skin (Stein and Glickstein 1992).

In relation to the question of connectivity (i.e., the detailed pattern of termination of fibers on the group of neurons to which they project), Ji, Jin, and Vogel (1997), using wheat germ antiglutinin-horseradish peroxidase labeled spinocerebellar mossy fibers, reached the conclusion that the connectivity (i.e., sites in the cerebellar cortex of terminal fields) of mossy fibers is determined by the granule cells, rather than by Purkinje cells, as had been suggested earlier.

Diffuse rather than localized proprioceptive responses to passive hindlimb joint rotation were found from Purkinje cells in the cerebellar vermis of anesthetized cats by Gray, Perciavalle, and Poppele (1993), which the authors considered to be in accord with the principle of fractured somatotopy.

4.4. Interconnections Between Mossy Fiber and Climbing Fiber Systems

Evidence indicating the existence of connections between the mossy fiber and climbing fiber systems (i.e. between the cuneocerebellar and cuneo-olivary neurons, as well as a possible cerebral cortical influence on this link) has been obtained (Rubia 1992).

4.4.1. Newer Techniques in the Study of Fiber Systems

In addition to classical anatomical techniques, newer ones have been brought to bear on the study of fiber systems of the cerebellum. For example, Neutral Red, a pH-sensitive dye (an acidic shift indicating increased fluorescence) used to determine pH in neurons was reported by Chen, Hanson, and Ebner (1998). These authors electrically stimulated parallel fibers in the cerebellar cortex of rats. It was found that a significant portion of the fluorescence change was of intracellular origin and reflected activation of parallel fibers and their postsynaptic targets. It was suggested that optical imaging using this dye should prove useful for neuronal activity mapping.

4.5. The Precerebellar Nuclei

Precerebellar nuclei refers to nuclei that give off most of their efferent fibers to the cerebellum. (The inferior olivary nucleus, which gives off the climbing fibers, is considered in Chapter 5.)

4.5.1. The Pontine Nuclei

The massive pontine nuclei constitute the most important relay for pathways from the cerebral cortex to the cerebellum and also for some afferent fibers arising from elsewhere (e.g., the superior and inferior colliculi, the ventral nucleus of the lateral geniculate body, and from the cerebellar nuclei). It is said that the pontine nuclei also receive inputs from all cerebellar nuclei: the dentate (lateral), anterior interposed (interpositus), and fastigial. In the human, there are some 20 million cells in the pontine nuclei on each side.

The afferents to the pontine nuclei from the cerebral cortex include all four lobes (frontal, temporal, parietal, occipital), the largest portion being from the sensorimotor region which is somatotopically organized in the pontine nuclei, but with representation as well from the visual region. It should be emphasized that the fibers from the cerebral cortex to the pontine nuclei are not merely collaterals of the corticospinal tract, for the latter are said to be outnumbered by 20 to 1 by the former in humans. The organization (localization) of both the cerebral fibers in the pontine nuclei and of the projections from the latter to the cerebellar cortex is rather precise, although with overlap.

Multiple Inputs to the Basilar Pontine Nuclei. Usually considered to be relay in nature, the basilar pontine nuclei, representing the largest input to the cerebellum, evidently have a more complex organization, having GABA-ergic (inhibitory) inputs from multiple sources in the brain stem as well as intrinsic local-circuit GABAergic cells, in addition to the input from the cerebral cortex (Milaihoff et al. 1992).

4.5.2. The Reticular Nuclei

Other sources of mossy fibers to the cerebellum include the *reticular tegmental pontine nucleus*, the *lateral reticular nucleus*, and the *paramedian reticular nucleus*, all of which can be considered as precerebellar nuclei.

Reticular Tegmental Pontine Nucleus. The reticular tegmental pontine nucleus receives input from the cerebral cortex (the primary sensorimotor cortex) and the cerebellar nuclei. Quantitatively, the most important input to the nucleus comes from the cerebellar nuclei via the superior cerebellar peduncle. The nucleus can therefore be considered a link in a cerebello–reticulo–cerebellar feedback system, although not point to point. It is the only one of the reticular group of nuclei that does not receive an input from the spinal cord.

Lateral Reticular Nucleus. Situated just lateral to the inferior olive, the lateral reticular nucleus receives afferents principally from the spinal cord, and also from the magnocellular part of the red nucleus and the cerebral cortex. Its efferents to the cerebellum pass via the inferior cerebellar peduncle.

Paramedian Reticular Nucleus. Located in the medial medulla, the paramedian reticular nucleus receives afferents from the spinal cord, the fastigial nucleus, the cerebral cortex, and perhaps the vestibular nuclei.

With the exception of the reticular tegmental pontine nucleus, the reticular group of nuclei can be viewed as loci for conjoint action on the cerebellar cortex by spinal and cerebral cortical influences.

Perihypoglossal Nucleus. As its name suggests, the perihypoglossal nucleus is in the immediate vicinity of the hypoglossal nucleus (the nucleus for the 12th cranial nerve) and may also be mentioned as a precerebellar nucleus and source of mossy fibers.

Of the preceding sources of mossy fibers, all give off collaterals to the cerebellar nuclei. The collaterals of the *rubrocerebellar projection* are in contrast exclusively to the cerebellar nuclei.

4.5.3. The Cerebellar Nucleocortical Fibers

This important feedback path from the cerebellar nuclei to the cerebellar cortex in the form of mossy fibers is discussed in Chapter 6.

FIVE

The Inferior Olivary System and the Climbing Fibers

In view of the importance attached to the climbing fibers and the inferior olivary nucleus (also termed the inferior olivary complex, inferior olive, or simply IO) in a number of theories of cerebellar function (Chapters 13, 14, 16, and 17), its anatomy and physiology is surveyed in some detail (see also Chapter 6).

The sequence of topics in this chapter is as follows: organization of the inferior olivary nucleus itself; its afferent input from the periphery; projections to it from other structures (e.g., the cerebellar nuclei); and finally, the climbing fibers (i.e., the output system from the inferior olive to the cerebellar cortex with their collaterals to the cerebellar nuclei). The chapter closes with a consideration of theories of function of the inferior olivary nucleus and a discussion of modulation of sensory (peripheral) input to the inferior olive. For purposes of differentiation, arbitrarily, *afferent* refers to input derived from the periphery, whereas *projection* refers to input derived from or directed to another brain structure (e.g., cerebellar cortex or nucleus).

5.1. The Inferior Olivary System

5.1.1. Organization of Inferior Olivary Nucleus

The inferior olive is a folded gray mass in the medulla, lying just above and slightly lateral to the pyramidal tracts (Fig. 5.1), and consists of a principal olive and dorsal and medial accessory olives. The principal olive (Fig. 5.2, bottom, 4) is a folded narrow band of cells in which a ventral and a dorsal lamella can be distinguished. The axons from the cells cross the midline and enter the cerebellum in the contralateral restiform body (inferior cerebellar peduncle). Brodal (1981) worked out an ingenious remapping of the folded inferior olive into a single plane.

Cell Types. Microscopically, the olivary neurons according to Golgi studies in several species (Scheibel and Scheibel 1955; Scheibel et al. 1956) are of two principal

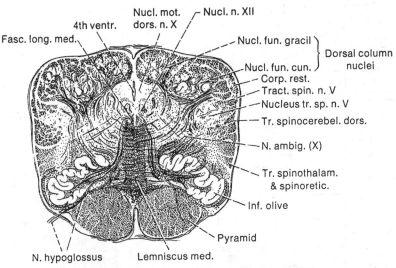

4th ventr. Nucl. mot. dors. n. X Nucl. n. XII Fasc. long. med. Nucl. fun. gracil Dorsal column nuclei Nucl. fun. cun. Corp. rest. Tract. spin. n. V Nucleus tr. sp. n. V Tr. spinocerebel. dors. N. ambig. (X) Tr. spinothalam. & spinoretic. Inf. olive Pyramid N. hypoglossus Lemniscus med.

Figure 5.1. The inferior olive (lower right and left) in a drawing of a transverse section through the caudal part of the medulla oblongata in man. (From Brodal 1981; *Neurological Anatomy in Relation to Clinical Medicine (3rd ed.)*; copyright 1981, Oxford University Press; reprinted by permission of the publisher.)

types (Fig. 5.3). The first, the more typical olivary neurons, have highly ramified and spatially more limited spherical dendritic trees (Type II), and were found in the phylogenetically newer principal olivary nucleus and rostral halves of the accessory nuclei. Their dendritic fields were about as extensive as those of Purkinje cells. Indeed, it could be said that the dendritic arborizations of inferior olivary neurons of this type are as chaotic as those of Purkinje cells are orderly. The second type of cell, with large, simple, and relatively unramified dendritic patterns (Type I), was taken to be more primitive, and tended more to be found in the accessory olives.

Types of Afferent Terminations. Among the afferent terminals (Fig. 5.4), in addition to a bushy type (the most frequent), a heavy rosette-bearing type and a thinner bouton type were seen. The overlapping, conelike distribution of terminal axons (Figs. 5.4A and 5.5a, b, and d) among the tightly packed highly ramifying dendritic arbors (Fig. 5.3) was considered, on the one hand, to lose the identity of a given input (i.e., so the dendritic receptive nets function as highly uncritical transmitters of information) and, on the other hand, enhance the probability of synchronous firing of rather large numbers of cells (Scheibel and Scheibel 1955). The bushy afferents were considered to be well suited to provide for activation of relatively large cell populations, whereas the other two types were thought to perhaps serve to fractionate activity in such ensembles. A hypothetical diagram showing possible relationships among the various types of afferent axonal terminals and neurons is reproduced in Figure 5.6.

According to Armstrong (1974), neighboring arborizations of the most common bushy type are so heavily overlapped that they preclude a high degree of

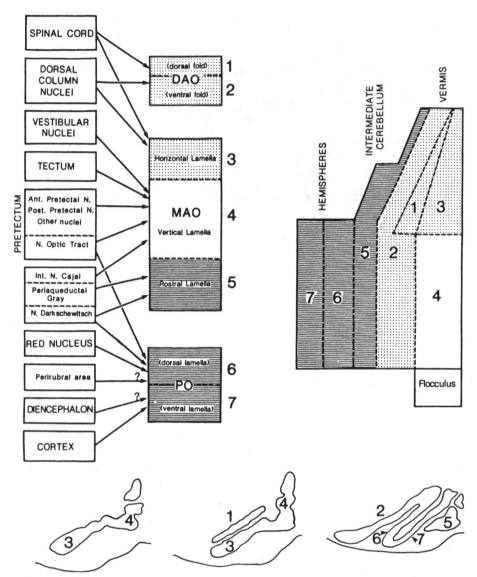

Figure 5.2. Schematic diagram of lamellar and zonal distribution of olivary afferents and efferents. The two lamellae (folds) of DAO (dorsal accessory olive; 1 and 2) and the horizontal lamella of MAO (medial accessory olive; 3) appear to receive afferents mainly from the spinal cord and dorsal column nuclei while projecting to the anterior vermis and parts of intermediate cerebellum. The medial MAO (vertical lamella; 4) receives from the vestibular and visual areas, and projects to the posterior vermis and the flocculus. The rostral lamella of MAO and both lamellae of PO (principal olive) receive projections from higher centers and send fibers to the lateral hemispheres. In the lower part of the figure, three drawings of the inferior olive demonstrate the lamellae corresponding to their sagittal zones of projection in the cerebellum. (From Azizi and Woodward 1987; *J. Comparative Neurol.* Vol. 263, copyright 1987, Wiley-Liss, Inc., a subsidiary of John Wiley & Sons, Inc.; reprinted by permission of the publisher.)

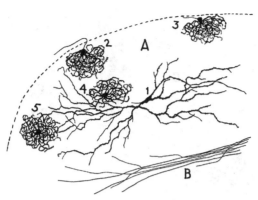

Figure 5.3. Portion of main olivary nucleus. A, grey matter; B, white matter; 1, large neuron with unramified dendrites; 2 and 3, peripherally located cells with fan-shaped arbors; 4 and 5, centrally located cells with spherical dendrite arbors. Neuron 1 is classified as Type I, neurons 2–5 as Type II. Two-week-old human infant. Golgi × 220. (From Scheibel and Scheibel 1955; in: *J. Comparative Neurol.* Vol. 102, copyright 1955, Wiley-Liss, Inc., a subsidiary of John Wiley & Sons, Inc.; reprinted by permission of the publisher; See also Ruigrok et al. 1990.)

topographical localization within the nucleus. Similarly, from their extensive study on the inferior olive (i.e., medial accessory olive [MAO]) of the cat, Ruigrok et al. (1990) reiterated the distinction between two types of cells in the inferior olive drawn earlier by Scheibel and Scheibel (1955; Fig. 5.3): Type I, with sparsely branched dendrites that radiate away from a usually small cell body, and Type II (located more rostrally) in the MAO, with dendrites that branch frequently, forming a ball-like structure that overlaps with those of perhaps 100 other olivary neurons.

Most, if not all, of the spines of both type I cells (characterized by dendrites that run away from the soma) and type II cells (characterized by dendrites that tend to turn

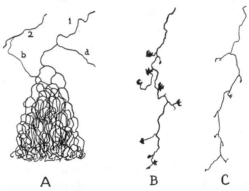

Figure 5.4. Terminal patterns of axons afferent to the inferior olive. (A) Bushy arbor formed by terminating axon 1. Collateral b, from fiber 2 also contributes to the plexus, whereas collateral a of fiber 1 probably contributes to an adjacent plexus. (B) Rosette-bearing heavy afferent fiber. (C) Bouton-bearing fiber of moderate or fine caliber. (Rapid Golgi method, 7–10-day-old kitten material, at same magnification.) (From Scheibel, Scheibel, Walberg, and Brodal 1956; *J. Comparative Neurol.* Vol. 106, copyright 1956, Wiley-Liss, Inc., a subsidiary of John Wiley & Sons, Inc.; reprinted by permission of the publisher.)

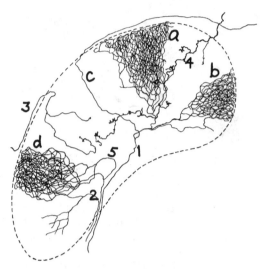

Figure 5.5. Patterns of afferent fibers in inferior olive; 1, 2, and 5, parent axons for bushy arbors a, b, and d; c, collateral that leaves inferior olive without terminating; 3, fine fiber with simple bouton endings, probably from region of medial longitudinal fasciculus; 4, heavy afferent fiber with bouton clusters and rosettes. Ten-day-old kitten. Golgi method × 440. (From Scheibel and Scheibel 1955; in *J. Comparative Neurol.* Vol. 102, copyright 1955, Wiley-Liss, Inc., a subsidiary of John Wiley & Sons, Inc.; reprinted by permission of the publisher.)

back toward the soma) were found to be located within olivary glomeruli (complex synaptic arrangements). Further, all glomerular spines received both a GABAergic (inhibitory) and non-GABAergic (probably excitatory) synaptic input (de Zeeuw, Ruigrok, Holstege, Jansen, and Voogd 1990).

It appeared that cells with more compact dendritic arborization are of a more advanced type (Fig. 5.3, cell types 2–5). Interestingly, no cells of this type were found in the phylogenetically oldest subdivision of the olivary complex (i.e., the rostral pole of the medial accessory olive; the cap of Kooy), which projects to the flocculonodular lobe of the cerebellum. According to Armstrong (1974), citing Kooy, there is an inferior olive in all vertebrates with the possible exception of cyclostomes (Chapter 2), although in fishes and reptiles the nucleus consists of a diffuse group of cells that do not have the ovoid form characteristic of the mammalian olivary cell.

Of the three fiber terminal types (Fig. 5.4), it was suggested that the heavy rosette-bearing afferents may represent recently developed rapidly transmitting systems, whereas the bushy afferents, distributed more widely within the olive, may represent a more ancient and generalized type of afferent system (Scheibel et al. 1956). In humans, there are about 1,000,000 total cells for both olives, as compared with about 15,000,000 Purkinje cells (Armstrong, 1974).

Rutherford and Gwyn (1980) reported, in the squirrel monkey, a pattern similar to the ones described above (i.e., of two types of dendritic arborization – the one having dendrites curling around the soma in a "ball-like" pattern and the other having dendrites streaming away from the soma; Fig. 5.3). By electron microscopy, these authors found axosomatic synapses to be of the symmetrical (inhibitory) type,

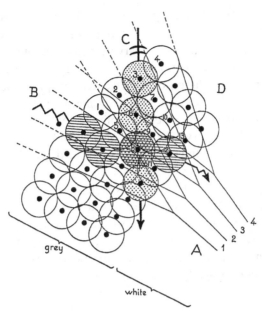

Figure 5.6. Hypothetical diagram showing possible relationships among the various types of afferent axonal terminals and neurons of the inferior olive. A, Bushy afferents arborize in overlapping patterns within the olivary cell pool, D, Rosette-bearing heavy afferent fiber, C, and bouton-bearing fiber, B, course obliquely through the pool, each establishing synaptic relations with small numbers of cells. Cells 1 through 13 are probably capable of being directly activated by an impulse train in bushy afferent 3. However, of this group, cells 3, 6, and 8 are also assumed to receive synaptic contributions from fiber C and cells 8 and 12 from fiber B. It is suggested that such fractionation of olivary cell ensemble 1 through 13 may provide an anatomical substrate for selective patterns of activations. (From Scheibel and Scheibel 1955, in: *J. Comparative Neurol.* Vol. 102, copyright 1955, Wiley-Liss, Inc., a subsidiary of John Wiley & Sons, Inc.; reprinted by permission of the publisher.)

whereas axodendritic synapses, which occurred at all levels of the dendritic tree, were of the asymmetrical (excitatory) type. Gap junctions (the morphological correlate of low-resistance pathways between neurons, see below) were encountered in all three divisions of the inferior olive. Intrinsic neurons (i.e., confined to the olive itself) were considered to be quite rare, at best. (This finding contrasts with that for the cerebellar nuclei, where intrinsic neurons [which are inhibitory] are found.) However, among the conclusions drawn by King (1980) from studies on opossum and cat were the following: (1) olivary neurons do not receive a primary input on their cell bodies or proximal dendrites (which differs from the findings just mentioned); (2) the majority of cerebellar and midbrain/thalamic axons terminate within synaptic clusters (rosettes), in contrast to spinal afferents, which contact primarily dendritic shafts; and (3) the locations of neurons that mediate olivary IPSPs were not identified.

Cellular Locations of Terminations. As for type of synapse, Sotelo, Gotow, and Wassef (1986) found in the rat that inhibitory axonal terminals established conventional synapses with dendrites (94% of samples) or with cell bodies (6%), of which 84% were type II (inhibitory) synapses and only 16% were type I (excitatory). Inhibitory terminals were found in the glomeruli characterizing the olivary neuropil, within which formations of olivary neurons were electrotonically coupled through dendrodendritic gap junctions (see below). This arrangement suggested to the authors a synaptic modulation of the electrical coupling such that the release of the inhibitory transmitter GABA, by increasing nonjunctional membrane conductance, could shunt the coupling between olivary neurons. However, only a small proportion of the GABA innervation of the olive would be involved in the synaptic control, because only 14% of the GAD (glutamaic acid decarboxylase, the GABA-synthesizing enzyme)-positive terminals analyzed were in a glomerular location, with all the fibers arising presumably from the cerebellar nuclei. Such a functional decoupling of selected gap junctions could be responsible for spatial organization of the olivary electrotonic coupling. These authors (Sotelo, Gotow, and Wassef 1986) also concluded that the inferior olive appears to be composed solely of projecting neurons, without interneurons. (Concerning the question of intrinsic rhythmic activity of inferior olivary neurons, see Chapter 13.)

5.1.2. Afferent Pathways to the Inferior Olivary Nucleus

By classical techniques, the afferent fibers to the inferior olive were found to originate mostly from the spinal cord, as well as from the cerebral cortex, the red nucleus, the mesencephalic reticular formation, the superior colliculus, the pretectum, and importantly, from the cerebellar nuclei (Fig. 5.2). For simplicity, the three parts of the inferior olive, namely, the principal olive, the medial accessory olive, and the dorsal accessory olive, are considered as a single unit. However, Kaufman et al. (1996), using the technique of retrograde transneuronal (transsynaptic) migration of virus particles or virions (e.g , alpha-herpes), in combination with immunohistochemical detection for studies of connectivity, found a large number of sources of inputs to the vestibulocerebellum (i.e., flocculus, paraflocculus, uvula, nodulus) via the inferior olive.

Fibers from the limbs are the best known and ascend to the olive via what may be termed the *ventral funiculus spino-olivary pathway* (also known as the direct spino-olivary pathway) and the *dorsal funiculus spino-olivary pathway*, which have relays in the dorsal column nuclei and receive fibers from the dorsal funiculi. Both pathways are activated by flexor reflex afferents. Other possible sources of afferents to the inferior olive from the caudal brain stem include the spinal trigeminal nucleus, the external cuneate nucleus, the lateral reticular nucleus, the reticular formation, and the vestibular nuclei (see below).

The cerebellar nuclei (Chapter 6), except for the fastigial nucleus, at least in the cat, provide the most widely distributed input to the inferior olive, although the most massive input appears to originate from a cell group in the dorsomedial part of the mesencephalon.

Other brain stem structures from which projections to the inferior olive arise include the superior colliculus, the pretectum, and certain mesencephalic nuclei (including the nucleus interstitialis, nucleus of Darkschewitsch, and the interstitial nucleus of Cajal). There are some projections from the caudate nucleus, only questionably from the globus pallidus, but evidently not from the putamen.

A final, but important, source of projections to the inferior olive derive from the *cerebral cortex*, of which all regions contribute (at least in the cat), but preponderantly the sensorimotor region (see also Chapter 9).

Berkley and Worden (1978) found several regions of overlap in the inferior olive of somatosensory and motor inputs. Cells were found that responded to activation of both the cerebral cortex and the spinal cord, a finding of possible relevance to the concept of the inferior olive as a comparator (see below).

In general, the terminations from this great diversity of sources in the different parts of the inferior olive (i.e., the principal olive and the dorsal and medial accessory olives) appears to be topographical (i.e., well localized, although with some overlap). For example, afferents from spinal cord overlap only partially with those from cerebral cortex, whereas afferents from spinal cord overlap extensively with those from mesencephalic afferents.

From their studies on the rat, Azizi and Woodward (1987) concluded that the inferior olive can be divided into three functional regions on the basis of their common afferents and efferents (Fig. 5.2): (1) the dorsal accessory olive (DAO) and caudal medial accessory olive (MAO) form a somatic sensory zone; (2) the medial area of the MAO is the visual-vestibular zone; and (3) the principal olive (PO) in conjunction with the rostral MAO is the third zone integrating inputs from higher centers.

Afferents from Vestibular Nuclei to Inferior Olive. In an anatomical study, Balaban and Beryozkin (1994) traced pathways from the vestibular nucleus to the inferior olive (the dorsal cap of Kooy), and suggested that such pathways represent a feedback link in the olivo–flocculo–vestibular loop that coordinates activity in the left and right flocculus and nodulus during horizontal head movements. The effect would be to facilitate the execution of conjugate vestibulo-ocular and optokinetic reflexes. The feedback projection from the prepositus hypoglossi nucleus to the inferior olive was proposed by Strata, Rossi, and Tempia (1995) to function conjointly with the brain stem saccadic neural integrator (Robinson 1989) formed by the medial vestibular and prepositus hypoglossi nuclei in such a way as to improve the dynamic performance of the integrator and for its adaptive capabilities.

5.1.3. Types of Afferent Signals to Inferior Olive

According to Armstrong (1974), the olive receives a large input from receptors located in the limbs, including cutaneous mechanoreceptors, joint afferents, and Golgi tendon organs (but evidently not from muscle spindles), as well as from the sensorimotor cortex, midbrain (red nucleus), periaqueductal gray, etc., and also from the visual and vestibular systems. In alert cats, Gellman, Gibson, and Houk (1985) found that IO cells responded about evenly to cutaneous stimulation and proprioceptive stimulation. The former included light touch, puffs of air, vibration, stroke, slip, or pinching a fold of skin; the latter, passive displacement of a limb, joint rotation, sharp taps near a tendon or muscles, or squeeze of a muscle. The proprioceptive cells were surprisingly unresponsive to self-produced stimuli. The latter authors viewed their results as being consistent with the hypothesis that inferior olivary neurons function as somatic event detectors responding particularly reliably to unexpected stimuli.

In the cat, Saint-Cyr (1983) concluded that there appeared to be no projection to the olive arising from neocortical areas representing the distal limb muscles, only for those areas representing axial and proximal forelimb muscles, which suggested that neocortical–olivo–cerebellar projections play a preponderant role in the cerebellar control of posture.

5.2. Projections to the Inferior Olive

5.2.1. Projections from Cerebellar and Vestibular Nuclei

Projections to the inferior olive from the cerebellar nuclei (except for the fastigial nucleus) terminate mainly in the principal olive. This finding, although controversial for a time (see Chan-Palay 1977, p. 366, for a history of this question), is now well established in a number of species. The terminations are highly ordered, and thus constituting a feedback loop such that the cerebellum could have the capacity to monitor its own activity, in particular, the excitation of the Purkinje cells (Armstrong 1974; Asanuma, Thach, and Jones 1983b; Brodal and Kawamura 1980; Courville, de Montigny, and Lamarre 1979; Graybiel et al. 1973; Kalil 1979; McCrea, Bishop, and Kitai 1978; Swenson and Castro 1983).

The cerebello-olivary connections, all of which originate from the cerebellar nuclei (except for the fastigial nucleus), are probably as specifically organized as the olivocerebellar projections (i.e., the patterns of the two are reciprocals of one another, according to Brodal and Kawamura [1980]). These authors viewed the presence of fibers from the cerebellar nuclei to the olive as indicating the existence of a feedback system to the olive from the cerebellar nuclei by which the latter may influence the action exerted by the olive on the cerebellar nuclei as well as on the cerebellar cortex.

Direct (Inhibitory) and Indirect (Excitatory) Nucleo-Olivary Projections. Legendre and Courville (1987) found that the cerebello-olivary fibers were not collaterals of the cerebellothalamic projection, and that there are thus two different populations of neurons in the cerebellar nuclei that give rise to these distinct efferent projections. Among other differences, the cells of origin of the cerebello-olivary fibers were smaller by almost a factor of two. A small fastigio-olivary projection was found, in addition to the known lateral (dentate) and interpositus projections. These authors raised the question of whether olivo-nuclear fibers (i.e., collaterals of climbing fibers) terminated on the smaller cells of origin of the nucleo-olivary projection (thus constituting a "reverberating" loop); they also raised the question of whether Purkinje cell axons may terminate on these same smaller cells in the nuclei.

In the rat, the different GABAergic projections to the inferior olive (IO), which arise largely in the cerebellar nuclei and the vestibular nuclei, conform to the olivo-cerebellar and cerebellar corticonuclear compartments; therefore, these compartments can be extended to include the GABAergic efferent systems to the IO (Nelson and Mugnaini 1989). It follows, in the view of these authors, that GABA modulation of climbing fiber activity is an important feature of cerebellar control of movement.

Dietrichs and Walberg (1989) pointed out that, if the cerebellar nucleo-olivary projection is entirely GABAergic and thus inhibitory, then the olivocerebellar neurons may be inhibited by the cerebellar nucleo-olivary fibers, whereas disinhibition could occur through the Purkinje cells acting on the cerebellar nucleo-olivary neurons.

De Zeeuw, Ruigrok, Holstege, Jansen, and Voogd (1990) concluded that the cerebellar nuclear projection to the IO is derived from rather small cells with thin axons, whereas larger cerebellar nuclear cells, besides terminating in the thalamus, also provide a projection to mesodiencephalic regions from which the excitatory olivary projections are derived. It was further concluded that the combined GABAergic and non-GABAergic input to glomerular spines are consistent with the hypothesis that they may modulate the electrotonic coupling of olivary cells (see below), and at the same time, their firing frequency in a timing-sensitive way.

In addition to a GABAergic inhibitory input to the inferior olive (medial accessory olive MAO) from the cerebellar nuclei (i.e., the interpositus), de Zeeuw et al. (1989) reported evidence of another GABAergic input of noncerebellar origin and raised the question of whether the noncerebellar input may regulate the excitability of IO cells, whereas the cerebellar nuclear input modulates synchronous firing via its effect on the gap junctions among IO cell dendrites.

Summarizing their own and the work of others, De Zeeuw, Ruigrok, Holstege, Jansen, and Voogd (1990) pointed out that in the cat there are two major afferent systems to the medial accessory olive (MAO) and also to the principal olive (PO): a GABAergic (inhibitory) input derived from cerebellar nuclei, and a non-GABAergic (excitatory) innervation from the mesodiencephalic junction.

Projections from Vestibular Nuclei. The existence of a GABAergic input to the inferior olive from the vestibular nuclei was reiterated by De Zeeuw, Wentzel, and Mugnaini (1993); these authors concluded that the ubiquitous combined GABAergic and non-GABAergic input to the olivary glomerular spines is consistent with the hypothesis that they may serve to modulate the electrotonic coupling of olivary cells and, at the same time, modulate their firing frequency in a manner sensitive to timing. In this connection, De Zeeuw, Ruigrok, Holsteg, Shalekamp, and Voogd (1990) found that the axon hillock and initial segment of cells of the IO give rise to spines that are located within glomeruli and that are mainly innervated by GABAergic (65%) as well as non-GABAergic terminals. These authors suggested that the synaptic input to the axon hillock may be involved in inactivating (resetting) the cell, in regulating the oscillatory firing frequency, and/or in a timing-sensitive operation.

Of particular interest, in relation to the later consideration of the vestibulo-ocular and optokinetic reflexes (Chapter 8), is the question of GABAergic and non-GABAergic inputs to that part of the inferior olive that exerts visual control of eye movements (i.e., the dorsal cap of Kooy), which is continuous with the median accessory olive. De Zeeuw, Wentzel, and Mugnaini (1993) found that, in rat and rabbit, the dorsal cap receives a major input from the nucleus prepositus hypoglossi. In

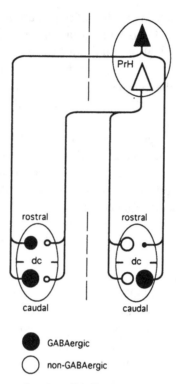

Figure 5.7. Schematic diagram showing distribution of GABAergic and non-GaBAergic projections from the nucleus prepositus hypoglossi (PrH) in the ipsilateral and contralateral, caudal and rostral dorsal cap (DC) (of Kooy) in the rat. The surface areas of the different GABAergic and non-GABAergic terminal fields (black and white circles) are meant to represent differences in the relative proportions of the two terminal populations (not the sizes of the individual boutons). (From De Zeeuw, Wentzel, and Mugnaini 1993; in *J. Comparative Neurol.* Vol. 327, copyright 1993, Wiley-Liss, Inc., a subsidiary of John Wiley & Sons, Inc.; reprinted by permission of the publisher.)

turn, the dorsal cap sends climbing fibers to Purkinje cells in the flocculonodular lobe. These authors found that the principal electron microscopic features of the dorsal cap are the same as those of other olivary subdivisions. Thus, the neuropil contains glomeruli (synaptic clusters) and extraglomerular synaptic fields. The neurons are coupled by gap junctions, and this nucleus contains numerous GABA-positive and GABA-negative axon terminals (Fig. 5.7).

In pursuing earlier indications that the cerebellar nuclei provided an (indirect) excitatory as well as a direct inhibitory (GABAergic) effect on the inferior olive, De Zeeuw and Ruigrok (1994) concluded that the indirect cerebellar projection to the inferior olive via the midbrain nucleus of Darkschewitsch is disynaptic and excitatory. It was further concluded that the direct GABAergic terminals from the cerebellar nuclei contact the same individual spines in the olivary glomeruli as the excitatory mesodiencephalic terminals, indicating that the indirect excitatory pathway could act in conjunction with the direct cerebellar GABAergic input, as shown in Figure 5.8.

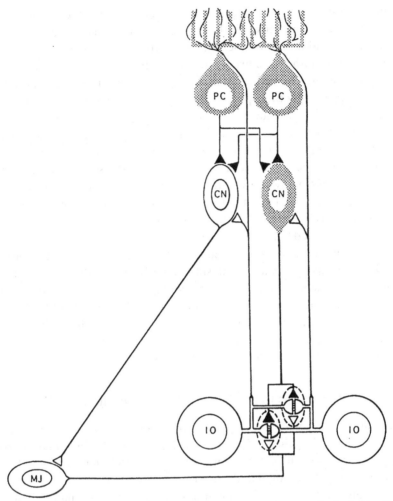

Figure 5.8. Diagram of the neuropil in the medial accessory olive and principal olive (bottom), and its relation with the cerebellum (top) and mesodiencephalic junction (MJ, left side). All olivary spines (half circles) are located within glomeruli (dotted circles), and are innervated by both an excitatory mesodiencephalic and an inhibitory cerebellar terminal (white and black triangles, respectively). The olivary axons provide climbing fibers to the Purkije cells (PC) in the cerebellar cortex and collaterals to both the GABAergic and excitatory cerebellar nuclei (CN) neurons. The GABAergic projection neurons in the cerebellar nuclei project exclusively to the inferior olive (IO), whereas a substantial part of the excitatory projection neurons in these nuclei innervate the neurons in the mesodiencephalic junction that in turn project back to the inferior olive. The excitatory and inhibitory neurons in the cerebellar nuclei can receive input from the same Purkinje cell axon. Small lines between olivary spines indicate the dendrodendritic gap junctions by which they are electronically coupled. (From De Zeeuw, Simpson, et al. 1998; reprinted from *Trends in Neurosciences* Vol. 21, copyright 1998, Elsevier Science; reprinted by permission of the publisher.)

Teune, van der Burg, and Ruigrok (1995) found in rats that cerebellar nuclear projections to the red nucleus and those to the inferior olive originate from separate populations, and that consequently, these two pathways may transmit different information. These authors confirmed the finding that the neurons projecting to the magnocellular part of the red nucleus are mainly found in the interposed nuclei, whereas those projecting to its parvocellular part are predominantly located in the lateral (dentate) cerebellar nucleus.

Ruigrok and Voogd (1995) emphasized the presence of the two pathways from cerebellar nuclei to the inferior olive: the first, excitatory, via nuclei at the mesodiencephalic junction thence to the inferior olive, and the second, a direct (nucleo-olivary), GABAergic pathway, the latter having an important role in regulating the degree of electrotonic coupling among olivary neurons (probably by a shunting mechanism), thus rendering them more difficult to activate by incoming afferent volleys. These authors suggested that such coupled olivary neurons, once activated, however, may develop membrane potential oscillations that are electrotonically conveyed to neighboring neurons (see below), and subsequently, during the depolarizing phase of the oscillation, result in a more easily triggered rebound or long-latency response.

Horn, van Kan, and Ruigrok (1996) found that the inhibitory (GABAergic) effect from nuclear cells on inferior olivary cells reduced the sensitivity of the latter rather than reduced the receptive fields, which could be expected were the inhibitory effect on the regulation of inferior olivary gap junctions.

5.2.2. Projections to the Inferior Olive from the Red Nucleus

As a preliminary, the two parts of the red nucleus should be differentiated: a caudal, magnocellular (large-cell) division, which receives afferents mainly from the interpositus nucleus of the cerebellum, and the parvocellular (small-cell) division, which receives input predominantly from the cerebral cortex. The magnocellular red nucleus gives rise to the rubrospinal tract, projecting contralaterally to several brainstem sites and to neurons in all segments of the spinal cord. In contrast, the parvocellular division projects only to the ipsilateral inferior olive, a connection that first appears in quadrupedal reptiles (Keifer and Houk 1994).

Courville and Otabe (1974) reported finding fibers from the parvocellular region of the red nucleus to the inferior olive in the macaque. A correlation of the rubro-olivary projection with the distribution of the olivo-cerebellar projection, together with the fact that the dentate nucleus is the source of efferent cerebellar fibers terminating in the parvocellular portion of the red nucleus, indicated to these authors that the rubro-olivary fibers are a link in reciprocal connections between the red nucleus and the cerebellar cortex.

5.2.3. Other Projections to the Inferior Olive

Inhibitory Inputs to Olivary Dorsal Cap of Kooy and Ventrolateral Outgrowth. The rostral dorsal cap (of Kooy) and the ventrolateral outgrowth (VLO) of the inferior olive, from which climbing fibers to the Purkinje cells of the flocculonodular lobe of the cerebellum originate, and which are involved in the visual control of eye movements, have been shown in the rabbit to receive a GABAergic (inhibitory) input from the ventral dentate nucleus of the cerebellum and also from a group of cells known as the dorsal group y. (The nucleus prepositus hypoglossi (PrH) is the major source of GABAergic input for the dorsal cap of Kooy [De Zeeuw, Gerrits, et al. 1994]).

5.3. Ultrastructure

In an ultrastructural (electronmicroscopic) study (De Zeeuw, Ruigrok, Holstege, Schalekramp, and Voogd [1990]), it was found that the GABAergic input to the olivary cell bodies was partly derived from a noncerebellar source, whereas the GABAergic terminals apposed to the axons appear to be derived from the cerebellar nuclei. Axonal spines, like dendritic spines, receive a combined inhibitory and excitatory input. Both GABAergic and non-GABAergic terminals were seen on both type I and type II olivary neurons, but terminations on the axons of type I neurons were mainly on the axonal shafts, whereas most of the terminations on axons of type II neurons were on axonal spines.

In another ultrastructural study (De Zeeuw, Holstege, et al. 1990), at least one third of labeled glomeruli (rosettes) appeared to contain both cerebellar nuclear (i.e., inhibitory) terminals and mesodiencephalic (nucleus of Darkschewitsch and reticular tegmental nucleus [of Bechterew]) (i.e., excitatory) terminals. In many cases, the terminals from both afferent systems contacted the same dendritic spines. The authors suggested that the timing between these two afferents in the rostral medial accessory olive (MAO) and principal olive (PO), which project to the cerebellar hemisphere and give off collaterals to the posterior interposed and dentate nucleus, may be important in relation to the function of the olivocerebellar system, in particular, in relation to a timing function.

5.4. Gap Junctions (Electrotonic Coupling) Among Inferior Olivary Cells and Their Modulation

In their structural study of electrotonic coupling in the inferior olive (IO), Sotelo, Llinás, and Baker (1974) found that gap junctions (the morphological correlate of low-resistance pathways between neurons) occurred mainly among dendritic profiles in the central core of the glomeruli. It was suggested that the synaptic input to the glomerulus may serve to produce a functional block of the coupling interactions among IO neurons. From the companion electrophysiological study (Llinás, Baker, and Sotelo 1974), it was concluded that the inferior olivary nucleus may act as a command center whose pattern of activity may be determined by the synchronous firing of the IO neurons.

De Zeeuw et al. (1989) found direct evidence for the cerebellar nuclear origin of the GABAergic terminals associated with gap junctions, which they considered to be involved in the regulation (i.e., shunting) of electrotonic coupling by which particular sets of parasagittally oriented Purkinje cells in the cerebellar cortex are synchronously activated. Although the vast majority of the GABAergic axodendritic terminals were found to originate in the cerebellar nuclei, the remainder were considered to suggest the existence of a noncerebellar GABAergic projection to the IO. Moreover, the authors found that one half of the terminals located strategically next to gap junctions were non-GABAergic; thus, the role of these terminals was unclear.

Modulation of the effective electrotonic coupling among olivary neurons by the cerebellar nucleo-olivary projection, resulting in ensembles of olivary neurons having synchronized activity, was reported by Lang, Sugihara, and Llinás (1996). These authors studied this question, using picrotoxin (which resulted in an increase in the average firing rate, synchrony, and rhythmicity of spontaneous complex spike activity, and a shift of the neuronal oscillation frequency to lower frequencies), and using kainic acid lesions of the cerebellar nuclei (which resulted in increased average complex-spike firing rates). It was concluded that the combination of the cerebellar and olivary nuclei may form the basis for a flexible and sophisticated motor coordination system able to help generate the many distinct movements that organisms are capable of performing.

5.5. Dendritic Lamellar Bodies in Relation to Gap Junctions

A new neuronal organelle, the dendritic lamellar body (DLB), which is associated with dendrodendritic gap junctions in the IO (and elsewhere in the brain), was recently described (De Zeeuw, Hertzberg, and Mugnaini 1995; De Zeeuw and Koekkoek 1997). Investigation of DLBs showed that lesions of the cerebellar nuclei (in rats and rabbits) reduced the density of lamellar bodies, the number of lamellae per lamellar body, and the density of gap junctions in the inferior olive, whereas the number of olivary neurons was not significantly reduced (De Zeeuw, Koekkoek, et al. 1997). Further, pairings of Purkinje cell complex spikes tended to occur more frequently in areas of cerebellar cortex having a higher density of lamellar bodies, and synchrony of Purkinje cell simple spikes tended to occur when there was synchrony of complex spikes. Thus, these results appear to point toward a close association between dendritic lamellar bodies and dendrodendritic gap junctions.

Against a background of reports of an association between dendritic lamellar bodies and dendrodendritic gap junctions, the question of an association between dendritic lamellar bodies and complex spike synchrony in the olivocerebellar system was investigated by De Zeeuw, Koekkoek, et al. (1997) by examining the effect on complex spike synchrony of lesions of the cerebellar nuclei in rats and rabbits. In the first part of the study, lesions were made in the cerebellar nuclei that resulted in a reduction of the density of lamellar bodies, number of lamellae per lamellar body, and density of gap junctions in the IO, without any significant decrease in the number of olivary neurons. In the second part of the study, the association between lamellar bodies and electrotonic coupling was evaluated by comparing degrees of synchrony of complex spikes in different Purkinje cell zones of the flocculus that receive their climbing fibers from olivary subnuclei having different densities of lamellar bodies. It was found that complex spike synchrony of Purkinje cell pairs receiving their climbing fibers from an olivary subnucleus with a high density of lamellar bodies was significantly higher than that of Purkinje cells receiving their climbing fibers from a subnucleus with a low density of lamellar bodies. Because the density of DLBs in the IO is higher than in any other part of the brain, the importance of electrotonic coupling via dendrodendritic gap junctions in the function of the olivocerebellar system seemed evident (De Zeeuw, Koekkoek, et al. 1997).

5.6. Compartmental Model of Electrophysiological Properties of the Inferior Olive

As a step in exploring the functions of the inferior olive, Schweighofer, Doya, and Kawato (1999) constructed a biophysical model of the olivary neurons to examine their unique electrophysiological properties. Studies included investigation of the role of electrical (electrotonic) coupling (via gap junctions) in two coupled spiking cells. Depending on the coupling strength, the hyperpolarization level, and other factors, the cell spikes could be in-phase, phase-shifted, or antiphase, or could exhibit a complex desynchronized spiking mode. The authors concluded that these simulation results supported the counterintuitive hypothesis that electrical coupling can desynchronize coupled IO cells.

5.7. Serotonin and the Inferior Olive

A possible role for serotonin (5-hydroxytryptamin, 5-HT) as a physiological enhancer of the timing of motor function via its effect on the IO (i.e., by increasing the average firing rate of inferior olivary neurons, while slowing their oscillation frequency and increasing the coherence of their oscillations) was suggested by Sugihara, Lang, and Llinás (1995). (Serotonin originates principally from the raphe nuclei in the pons and medulla, and axons of raphe neurons (1) terminate as mossy fiber rosettes in the granular layer, (2) terminate diffusely throughout all layers of the cerebellar cortex without specialized junctions, and (3) pass directly to the molecular layer where they bifurcate like parallel fibers and synapse with cerebellar interneurons, but not with Purkinje cells [Parent 1996].)

5.8. Efferent Projections of the Inferior Olive – Climbing Fibers

5.8.1. Climbing Fiber Collaterals to the Cerebellar Nuclei: Olivonuclear Projection

The inferior olivary complex – the principal olivary nucleus, in particular – provides a considerable output, via collaterals, to the cerebellar nuclei, which, as noted above, is reciprocated by a massive and organized nuclear olivary outflow, at least for the

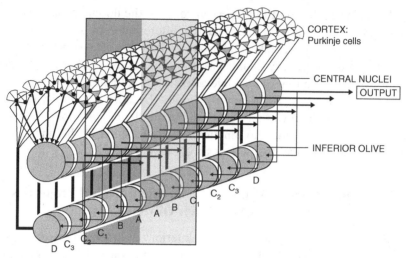

Figure 5.9. The cerebellum as a machine: cerebellar efferent modules. Each module consists of a longitudinal strip of Purkinje cells that project to a particular central cerebellar nucleus. These Purkinje cells and the corresponding nucleus receive fibers from a part of the inferior olive. Each module has its own nuclear efferents; collateral projections feed back into the inferior olive. Six symmetrically disposed, independent modules are presented on each side of the midline. (Note the nucleo-olivary feedback loop; however, the nucleocortical feedback loops are not shown.) (From Voogd and Bigaré 1980; in: Courville, de Montigny, and Lamarre (eds.), *The Inferior Olivary Nucleus: Anatomy and Physiology*, copyright 1980, Lippincott Williams & Wilkins; reprinted by permission of the publisher and Prof. Voogd, the author.)

lateral (dentate) and interpositus nuclei (Chan-Palay 1977). In this connection, Chan-Palay (1977) drew attention to a remarkable resemblance between the neurons of the nuclear border in the dentate nucleus (Figs. 6.2 and 6.3), and the neurons located at the periphery of the principal olivary nucleus (Fig. 5.3), which delineate the margins of the nucleus by turning their dendritic arborizations internally (compare also Fig. 5.9). The question was raised of whether such a similarity in the geometry and orientation of dendritic arborizations between the two structures reflects their intimate relation in connectivity, structure, and function (Chan-Palay 1977).

The electrophysiological importance of collaterals to the cerebellar nuclei from climbing fibers (as well as from mossy fibers) was stressed by Llinás and Mühlethaler (1988), who, following electrical stimulation of the cerebellar cortex or the underlying white matter, recorded excitatory and inhibitory postsynaptic potentials (EPSP–IPSP sequences) in cerebellar nuclear neurons. The EPSPs were elicited by direct activation of collaterals of climbing (or of mossy) fiber afferents; the IPSPs followed direct or orthodromic Purkinje cell activation. The integrity of the olivocerebellar system was tested with harmaline, which had powerful synaptic effects on nuclear cells.

5.8.2. Projections from the Inferior Olive to the Vestibular Nuclei

Changes in unit activity from neurons in the medial vestibular nucleus in response to reversible (i.e., cooling) and irreversible lesions in the inferior olivary nuclei were studied in rats by de'Sperati, Montarolo, and Strata (1993). The authors found that there was both a decrease in the firing rate and a modulation of amplitude in the vestibular units to natural labyrinthine stimulation (i.e., sinusoidal rotation). The results were interpreted as supporting the hypothesis that the IO, by virtue of the effect of a change in its firing rate on Purkinje cells, may regulate online the gain of reflexes under cerebellar control.

5.8.3. Feedback from Climbing Fiber Collaterals to the Inferior Olive via Nuclear Inhibitory Neurons

De Zeeuw, Van Alphen, et al. (1997) found that olivary axon collaterals (i.e., climbing fiber collaterals to the cerebellar nuclei) innervate not only non-GABAergic neurons in the cerebellar nuclei, but also GABAergic nucleo-olivary cells, thus establishing a direct feedback loop to the IO.

On the basis of tracing and electrophysiological experiments in rats and cats, Ruigrok (1997) reiterated the apparently precise topographical and reciprocal relationship between the olivary and cerebellar nuclear masses, the olivary projection to the cerebellar nuclei being strictly contralateral and originating as (excitatory) climbing fiber collaterals. The author further suggested that the inhibitory (GABAergic) nucleo-olivary feedback serves primarily to couple olivary neurons, thereby increasing the firing threshold of the coupled ensemble of olivary cells.

5.9. Parallels Between Olivocerebellar and Corticonuclear Projections

Voogd and Bigaré (1980), summarizing the work of the Leiden group (Groenewegen and Voogd 1977; Groenewegen, Voogd, and Freedman 1979), reported, in results obtained primarily from cat, that the corticonuclear and the olivocerebellar connections were essentially similar (i.e., olivocerebellar and corticonuclear fibers were found to use the same compartments in the white matter on their way to or from longitudinal strips of Purkinje cells and to terminate in the central cerebellar nucleus contained within such a particular compartment; Fig. 5.9). This arrangement is in contrast to the mossy fiber system, which terminates in more or less transversely oriented, partially overlapping areas, as mentioned previously. These authors (Voogd and Bigaré 1980) pointed out that the efferent modules are certainly not completely independent of one another because they may be interconnected at the level of the inferior olive and the cerebellar nuclei. In relation to Figure 5.9, it is relevant to note again that the ratio of Purkinje cells to nuclear cells is 30:1 in the rat and 14:1 in the monkey (Chan-Palay 1977, p. 378). It may also be recalled that feedback from nuclear cells to the inferior olive (Fig. 5.9) is evidently both excitatory and inhibitory, and the feedback to the cerebellar cortex from nuclear cells via mossy fibers (not included in Fig. 5.9), is also both excitatory and inhibitory (cf. Chan-Palay 1977, p. 379). (This question is also considered in Chapter 6.)

5.10. Parasagittal Banding on the Cerebellar Cortex

With the aid of optical imaging using the pH-sensitive dye, Neutral Red, in combination with peripheral (ipsilateral face) stimulation, Hanson, Chen, and Ebner (2000) found a parasagittal banding on the rat cerebellar cortex; the banding was shown to result from climbing fiber activation. The bands were highly frequency dependent, being most strongly elicited by stimulus frequencies in the range of 6–8 Hz, and having a large fall-off for higher and lower frequencies. Stimulation of the contralateral IO also resulted in the activation of parasagittal bands having frequency-response characteristics similar to those for the face stimulation. The authors considered that the results confirm that a parasagittal banding pattern is a dominant feature of the functional architecture of the cerebellar cortex, and that the frequency tuning observed supports the hypothesis that the climbing fiber system is involved with timing.

5.11. Cerebellar "Modules"

In a series of experiments combining electrophysiological and bidirectional tracer techniques, Apps and Garwicz (2000) studied spatially separate paravermal zones (C1, C3) that form a functionally coupled system involved in the control of voluntary limb movements, for which a series of "modules" was postulated. Each module is defined by (1) a set of olivary neurons with similar receptive fields, (2) the cortical microzones innervated by these neurons, and (3) the group of deep nuclear neurons upon which the Purkinje axons from the microzones then converge. The results indicated that corticonuclear convergence between parts of the two zones is in close proportion to the corresponding olivocerebellar divergence, which is entirely consistent with the modular hypothesis. It was further suggested that this arrangement would be well suited for combining a uniform climbing fiber input with input from sets of mossy fibers having different characteristics, thus allowing parallel processing of an array of different mossy fiber signals. This, the authors indicated, could constitute an important structural substrate for the integration of cerebellar control of skilled movements via the rubrospinal and corticospinal tracts (e.g., Thach, Kane, et al. 1992) with other aspects of its control of motor behavior, such as the coordination of posture and locomotion (cf. e.g., Thach, Goodkin, and Keating 1992, and Fig. 13.6).

5.12. Reciprocity of Olivo-Cerebellar, Olivo-Nuclear, and Nucleo-Olivary Projections

In a detailed anatomical study, Ruigrok and Voogd (2000) found that the olivary projection (as collaterals of the climbing fibers) to the cerebellar nuclei is strictly reciprocal to the nucleo-olivary projection. From this finding, it was suggested that the olivonuclear projection adheres to the organization of the climbing fiber projection to the cerebellar cortex and to the corticonuclear projection, thus establishing and extending the detailed micromodular organization of the connections between IO and cerebellum. The authors added, however, that the interaction of the various constituents of the cerebellar modules, as well as their activation by the mossy fiber system, is still a matter of conjecture.

5.13. Dual Olivocerebellar Loops

De Zeeuw, Simpson, et al. (1998) pointed out that there are two nucleo-olivary loops. In the first, a given olivary subnucleus projects (contralaterally) to Purkinje cells and gives off collaterals to the nuclei that receive its main Purkinje-cell input from the same cerebellar cortical zone (or zones). The cerebellar nuclei in turn project, with inhibitory fibers, to the same olivary subnucleus from which they received collaterals, the basic unit of such a loop being termed a cerebellar module, in their terminology. A second loop, according to these authors, is superimposed on the first, and is termed the olivocerebellar mesodiencephalic loop. Excitatory cerebellar nuclear cells project in part to the mesodiencephalic junction, where several nuclei (the parvocellular red nucleus, nucleus of Darkschewitsch, and the nucleus of Bechterew) project in turn to the IO with excitatory fibers. Because all the neurons in this loop are excitatory, there is the potentiality of a reverberating (oscillatory) loop, with possible control by inhibitory neurons (e.g., Purkinje cells).

5.14. Hypotheses of Functions of the Inferior Olive

5.14.1. Oscarsson's Comparator Hypothesis

Oscarsson (1980) concluded that experimental observations suggest that different olivary regions receive a specific input from the sensorimotor cortex to match the spinal input with respect to uni- or bilaterality and somatotopical organization. This concept became known as Oscarsson's comparator hypothesis. Further, against a background of considering each sagittal zone (at least in the anterior lobe of the cerebellum) as a functional unit that presumably controls a particular motor mechanism, Oscarsson (1980) reiterated the comparator hypothesis. In Figure 5.10, the lower motor center consists of interneurons in brain stem or cord, which could be a reflex arc, a link in descending motor paths, or a collection of neurons responsible for such motor patterns as stepping or scratching. The hypothesis assumes that the olive monitors and compares the activity at several points, and detects unexpected perturbations, on the basis of which the cerebellum sends corrective signals either directly to the lower motor center, or indirectly via thalamus and motor cortex.

At the same time, Oscarsson (1980) pointed out some difficulties with the comparator hypothesis, principally including the low rate of impulse activity in the climbing fibers (seldom greater than 1 per sec), and the variability in the latency of the climbing fiber response to stimulation of afferent fibers to the IO. Nonetheless, he

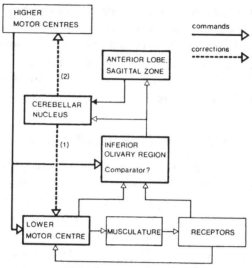

Figure 5.10. Oscarsson's comparator hypothesis for the inferior olive. The diagram is centered around the functional unit consisting of a sagittal zone with its olivary region and cerebellar nucleus and the lower motor center controlled by this unit (thick outlines). It is assumed that the olivary region monitors commands from higher motor centers, the activity these commands evoke in the lower motor center, and the resulting movement. By comparing information from these sources, the olive would detect perturbations of the commands introduced in the lower center by reflex activity and pertubations in the evolving movement due to unexpected changes in load or resistance. Information about these perturbations might be used by the sagittal zone to send signals of correction either directly to the lower motor center (path 1) or to the higher centers (path 2). (Note that the mossy fibers are not included in the figure.) Further explanation in text. (From Oscarsson 1980; in: Courville, de Montigny, and Lamarre (eds.), *The Inferior Olivary Nucleus: Anatomy and Physiology*, copyright 1980, Lippincott Williams & Wilkins; reprinted by permission of the publisher.)

considered the hypothesis consistent with concepts of the cerebellum as a seat of motor learning in which the olive plays a fundamental role of evaluating the correctness of a motor act and, through its action, modifies heterosynaptically the transmission through the granule cell–Purkinje cell synapses that are coactivated with the climbing fibers.

5.14.2. Modifications of the Comparator Hypothesis

In the review by Simpson, Wylie, and De Zeeuw (1996) concerning climbing fiber signals and their possible function(s), several points were made. In the error-detection role for the inferior olive that was a modification of Oscarsson's (1980) earlier concept of it as a comparator of command signals from higher centers with those from the periphery (interneuronal activity in the spinal cord), it was considered unlikely that the signals of intention and of achievement are conveyed only through the descending and ascending projections, respectively, to the IO because these inputs generally do not converge on the same olivary neurons. Rather, a comparison would be much more likely to occur between the ascending and descending inputs (which are all excitatory), on the one hand, and the inhibitory projection from the hindbrain, on the other hand. Each dendritic spine of an olivary neuron receives both an inhibitory input from a hindbrain center (i.e., cerebellar nuclei, vestibular nuclei, nucleus prepositus hypoglossi, solitary nucleus, dorsal column nuclei) and an excitatory input from the spinal cord, brain stem, mesodiencephalic junction, or cerebral cortex.

In their review of the microcircuitry and possible functions of the IO, including learning and timing of movements, and comparison of intended with achieved movements, De Zeeuw, Simpson, et al. (1998) concluded that the IO is capable of functioning in both motor learning and motor timing, but not with achieved movements in the sense originally proposed by Oscarsson (1980). However, the IO was considered to be capable of selecting and transmitting error signals. The authors based their conclusions on recent findings indicating that the descending and ascending projections to the IO generally do not converge on the same olivary neuron, as mentioned above. However, in view of the (unique) arrangement, whereby each dendritic spine of an olivary neuron receives an inhibitory input from one of the hindbrain regions (which include the cerebellar nuclei, vestibular nuclei, nucleus prepositus hypoglossi, and solitary nucleus) and an excitatory input (from the spinal cord, brain stem, mesodiencephalic junction, or cerebral cortex), it seemed to the authors that a comparison within the IO would be much more likely to occur between the excitatory descending and ascending excitatory inputs, on the one hand, and the inhibitory projections derived from the hindbrain, on the other hand, as summarized above.

5.14.3. Other Hypotheses Concerning Functions of the Inferior Olive

Simpson, Wylie, and De Zeeuw (1996) also considered, in some detail, several other hypotheses concerning the function of the IO and the associated climbing fibers (including gain-change, as "teachers," as a "timing device") and came to the conclusion that the function of the climbing fiber input to the cerebellum remains an enigma. Concerning climbing fibers and cerebellar learning, the authors concluded from their own studies in the flocculus that the error message is, in effect, necessary but not sufficient to ensure plasticity.

Bloedel and Bracha (1998) drew attention to several aspects of the behavior of climbing fibers, including (1) signaling the occurrence of an unexpected sensory stimulus during the course of a movement (i.e., a discrepancy or mismatch between the intended and the actual movement); (2) high responsivity to low-intensity cutaneous stimuli applied passively, but unresponsive when their receptive fields came into contact with the floor during ongoing locomotion (see below); and (3) an enhanced discharge rate (of Purkinje cells), generally speaking, after permanent or temporary (cooling-probe) lesions in the IO.

The authors summarized the concept of the heterosynaptic action of climbing fibers – that is, that coincident (conjoint) activity in climbing fibers and in parallel fibers leaves a memory trace (engram) at the parallel-fiber Purkinje cell synapses – as a mechanism for which Ito (1989) proposed a long-term depression (LTD) of Purkinje cell excitability (Chapter 7).

However, as for function of the climbing fibers, Bloedel and Bracha (1998) concluded in their review that there is no generally accepted and well-substantiated viewpoint characterizing the precise function of the climbing fibers. The authors suggested that long-term changes in excitability can occur in Purkinje cells in association with learning, but these changes were not considered to be consistent with a role for LTD. Indeed, the authors suggested that the strongest data for learning-related plastic changes in the cerebellum implicated the target nuclei of the Purkinje cells (i.e., the cerebellar and vestibular nuclei), rather than the cerebellar cortex. In their own work, the authors had found a short-lasting enhancement of Purkinje cell simple spike (SS) output, rather than a LTD of Purkinje cell responsiveness, following climbing fiber activation.

Hypotheses concerning the function of the IO in relation to the overall function of the cerebellar system are also presented in Chapter 13.

5.15. Modulation of Sensory Impulses to the Inferior Olive

Starting from the known phenomenon that the sensory responsiveness of cells in the IO of waking animals is suppressed during certain phases of active movements, Weiss, Houk, and Gibson (1990) found a decreased responsivity of inferior olivary cells to light touch after a brief delay following stimulation of the rubrospinal tract in pentobarbital-anesthetized cats. The inhibition of impulses from the forelimb was blocked by transection of the reticulospinal tract and was assumed to probably occur at multiple levels along the neuraxis as a consequence of a corollary discharge from the rubrospinal tract. It was noted that the delay would allow peak inhibition to occur at the approximate time of contact with an object at the end of a goal-directed limb movement. The authors considered that such an inhibitory effect may help to explain the very low level of climbing fiber activity observed during motor behavior in awake animals (Weiss, Houk, and Gibson 1990).

In a subsequent anatomical study (McCurdy, Gibson, and Houk 1992), a direct connection between branches of the descending rubrospinal tract (and also for fibers descending from the sensorimotor cortex) and relay cells of the ascending sensory tract was found in the cuneate nucleus. This question was reviewed by Keifer and Houk (1994).

In an attempt to determine the pathways for inhibition of the rostral dorsal accessory olive (rDAO) from the red nucleus (there being no direct pathway in the cat), McCurdy, Houk, and Gibson (1998) studied the ascending pathways for the forelimb area of the rDAO. From their investigation, the authors suggested that there are two types of input to the rDAO – namely, one that is responsible for somatosensory sensitivity, and one that is most likely modulatory and inhibitory.

5.15.1. Sensory Avoidance as Input to Climbing Fibers: Microzones and Microcomplexes

Summarizing their results from electrophysiological studies on the intermediate cerebellum of barbiturate-anesthetized cats, Ekerot, Garwicz, and Jörntell (1997) found that climbing fibers with similar receptive fields terminated within narrow, sagittally oriented cortical strips, thus forming microzones. (To reiterate, a microzone, as specified by Ito [1984], is composed of a set of Purkinje cells projecting to a distinct group of nuclear neurons, and a microcomplex is the combination of the group of Purkinje cells and the associated nuclear neurons. Both mossy fibers and climbing fibers supply collaterals to the cerebellar nuclear cell groups, as well as project onto the corresponding microzone of cerebellar cortex.) Ekerot, Garwicz, and Jörntell (1997) suggested that climbing fibers carry information related to simple movements and that the receptive field of a microzone reflects the movement controlled. In particular, the movement controlled often acts to withdraw the climbing fiber receptive field from a stimulus (e.g., nociceptive) presented to the skin.

Thus, based on analyses of (1) cutaneous and muscle afferent climbing fiber input, (2) corticonuclear connections, and (3) the corresponding limb movements controlled, Ekerot, Garwicz, and Jörntell (1997) found that the cutaneous receptive fields have spatial characteristics suggestive of a relation to elemental movements. For example, for most climbing fibers, the spatial relationship is such that the muscle afferent input originates from muscles that, if activated, would tend to move the cutaneous receptive field of the climbing fiber toward a stimulus applied to the skin. In contrast, the limb movement controlled by the respective (cerebellar cortical) module (an ensemble of functionally coupled microzones) often has the opposite direction, and would thus tend to move the cutaneous receptive field away from a stimulus applied to the skin. The authors considered these findings to be consistent with the concept of a "braking action" and also the "error signal" hypothesis of climbing fiber function. Thus, unintended skin contact during the extension phase of reaching movements would give rise to climbing fiber discharges in microzones in the cerebellar cortex having receptive fields overlapping the affected skin area and, in turn, to a long-lasting reduction in transmission between parallel fibers active during the movement and their target Purkinje cells. The reduced inhibition of the corresponding nuclear output would act to avoid the skin contact when the movement is next performed.

As functional implications of their study on the gating of transmission in climbing fiber paths to the cerebellar cortex during locomotion in the cat, Apps and Lee (1999) suggested that different rostrocaudal regions of the same cortical zones may sample climbing fiber inputs at different times so that, collectively, they monitor activity during all phases of the step cycle. Thus, increased pathway excitability during the swing phase of the step cycle was interpreted as a "temporally tuned transcerebellar mechanism designed to intervene in the execution of the current step when an obstacle is contacted as the limb is manoeuvred towards footfall." (Apps and Lee 1999) This formulation was taken to be consistent with the widely held view that climbing fibers signal errors to the cerebellum whenever there is a mismatch between intended and actual movements (Oscarsson 1979).

Ekerot (1999), in a commentary on the above-cited paper of Apps and Lee (1999), drew attention to (1) the close relationship of climbing fiber cutaneous receptive field of a module to the associated controlled movement, and (2) the observation that climbing fibers easily activated by stimuli in a passive animal are not activated when similar stimuli result from active movement (i.e., during locomotion) but may discharge in response to unexpected stimuli. Thus, the gating of climbing fiber pathways during locomotion could be an efficient way to eliminate self-generated activation of climbing fibers during normal locomotion and to facilitate responses to inputs occurring during movement phases when no peripheral input is expected. Ekerot (1999) concluded that the results of Apps and Lee (1999) suggested that different strategies, specifically adapted to the function of the controlled motor system, are used by climbing fibers to evaluate motor performance.

The concept that the cerebellar cortex is divided into a number of sagittally oriented zones, each defined by its specific afferent connections from the IO and its efferent connections to the cerebellar (or vestibular) nuclei (thus forming a series of olivo–cortico–nuclear compartments or "modules"), continues to be explored, including in the waking animal (Apps 2000; Garwicz 2000).

In a computer modeling approach to the problem of an apparent discrepancy between anatomical and physiological information concerning the zonal organization of climbing fibers in the rat cerebellar cortex, Lee and Bower (1990) reported that their results suggested that several unique features of the olivocerebellar circuit may contribute to the appearance of zonal organization using anatomical techniques, but that the detailed pattern of patchy tactile projections seen with physiological techniques provide a more accurate representation of the organization in the part modeled (crus IIA of the lateral hemisphere).

5.15.2. Climbing Fiber–Purkinje Cell Interactions

Normally, a Purkinje cell is innervated by a single climbing fiber, but Bravin, Rossi, and Strata (1995) found evidence that rats made hypogranular (i.e., with a partial loss of granule cells) by methylazoxymethanol (MAM) or by X-irradiation exhibited innervation by more than one climbing fiber, which was attributed to the loss of granule cells and their associated parallel fibers (see also Chapter 11).

Rossi and Strata (1995) summarized the reciprocal trophic interactions in the adult rodent climbing fiber–Purkinje cell system. They stated that climbing fiber deprivation induces profound functional and structural changes in the Purkinje cell, such as formation of spines on proximal Purkinje cell dendrites, some of which become innervated by parallel fibers. However, these changes were reversed if the Purkinje cell were reinnervated by another climbing fiber. The authors concluded that the olivocerebellar input inhibits spinogenesis on proximal Purkinje cell dendrites and prevents other afferents from invading its own target domain. It was proposed that the normal distribution of synapses on Purkinje cell dendritic tree is controlled by the interplay between climbing and parallel fiber influences on Purkinje cell dendrites.

Zagrebelsky et al. (1996) found adaptive recovery of collateral sprouting (i.e., restoration of topography of projection maps) following IO lesions in the adult rat, from which it was concluded that topographic cues are available in the adult during postlesion plasticity to guide the restoration of the olivocerebellar projection map.

SIX

The Cerebellar Nuclei and Their Efferent Pathways: Voluntary Motor Learning

6.1. The Cerebellar Nuclei

This chapter, which is largely based on Brodal (1981) and Chan-Palay (1977), is concerned mainly with the lateral (dentate) nucleus, as representative of the cerebellar nuclei, which also include the interpositi (emboliform and globose) and the medial (fastigial) nuclei, the terms in parentheses indicating those for the human cerebellum.

6.1.1. Anatomical Aspects

In humans, there are four distinct cellular masses or nuclei in the white matter of each half of the cerebellum (also termed the deep cerebellar nuclei). Most medial is the fastigial nucleus, followed more laterally by the small globose and emboliform nuclei and, most laterally, the dentate. The dentate nucleus appears in sections as a wrinkled band of gray matter (not unlike the inferior olive) with a medioanteriorly directed hilus. In the rat, cat, monkey, and most mammals, the usually accepted counterparts are the nucleus medialis, nucleus interpositus anterior and posterior, and nucleus lateralis, respectively.

The dentate nucleus is enormous in humans, both in comparison with the other nuclei and in comparison with other species; in fact, it has been estimated to contain some 284,000 cells (see also Heidary and Tomasch 1969). The principal afferent fibers to the cerebellar nuclei are the Purkinje cell axons from the cerebellar cortex, which are inhibitory. Other afferents include collaterals of the climbing and the mossy fibers, which are excitatory. Almost all efferent fibers from the cerebellum are axons of cells in the cerebellar nuclei. Their destinations include the vestibular nuclei, the red nucleus, the thalamus, the reticular formation, the inferior olive (Chapter 5), and the cerebellar cortex itself (as mossy fibers). In this connection, Oscarsson (1980) pointed out that each group of nuclear neurons receives monosynaptic excitation and disynaptic inhibition from the same group of olivary neurons, and the olivo–cortico–nuclear unit is further bound together by nucleo-olivary and nucleo-cortical paths. This organization is discussed further below.

The organization of all four cerebellar nuclei is essentially similar. After the Purkinje cell axons enter the nuclei, they branch profusely. However, each fiber supplies a roughly conical region, as originally described by Ramón y Cajal (1995) and reemphasized by others subsequently.

In the cat, Purkinje cells outnumber nuclear cells by about 26 to 1, and each Purkinje axon makes synapses (mainly axodendritic) with some 35 nuclear cells. The ratio of Purkinje cells to nuclear cells is 30:1 in the rat and 14:1 in the monkey (Chan-Palay 1977, p. 378). In the lateral nucleus, the nuclear cells number 5,500 in the rat and 56,000 in the monkey. In the human, on the basis of counts and estimates, a total of about 311,000 neurons were found in all cerebellar nuclei of one hemisphere, with 284,000 in the dentate, 10,300 in the emboliform, 16,100 in the globose, and 5,200 in the fastigial nucleus. (As noted previously, the corresponding nuclei in rat, cat, monkey, and most mammals are termed the lateral, the interpositi, and the medial, respectively.)

In the rat, six types of synapses have been described, presumably related to the different kinds of afferents (Chan-Palay 1977). The axons of the nuclear neurons give off recurrent collaterals to the nuclei, which have been found to synapse with small cells in the nuclei. Both larger and smaller nuclear neurons give off axons to distant points.

Cell Types. In the human dentate nucleus, Golgi preparations reveal the presence of two classes of nerve cells: relatively large projection cells, which predominate, and small local-circuit neurons, which are scattered throughout the nuclear gray (Braak and Braak 1984). There are also small GABAergic cells projecting to olivary cells (Chapter 5). De Zeeuw, Van Alphen, et al. (1997) found that olivary axon collaterals (i.e., collaterals of climbing fibers) innervate not only non-GABAergic neurons in the cerebellar nuclei but also GABAergic nucleo-olivary cells, thus establishing a direct feedback loop to the inferior olive.

For the large dentate neurons, most of their somata, proximal dendrites, and initial axonal segments are covered by the inhibitory terminals of Purkinje cell axons (Chan-Palay 1977). The distal receptive surfaces of these cells, however, have numerous appendages of presumably high and low resistance that participate in multiple glomerular arrangements with excitatory inputs. The small neurons, however, appear to have a less sharp spatial division (proximal vs. distal) of excitatory and inhibitory inputs.

The terminal arborization of a single Purkinje axon is approximately conical in shape (Fig. 6.1), a pattern that is not unlike that in the inferior olive (Fig. 5.4). The resulting relationship between Purkinje axon terminal field and cells and their dendrites is depicted in Figure 6.2. As drawn in Figure 6.3 and indicated diagrammatically in Figure 6.4, collaterals of mossy and climbing fibers (both of which are excitatory), on their radial path through the dentate nucleus, pass sequentially through the dendritic fields or territories of successive neurons, whereas the conical terminal fields of Purkinje axons enclose entire neurons and parts of many neurons.

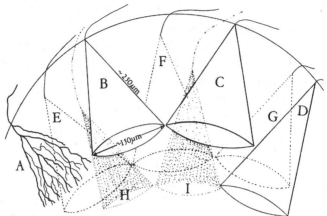

Figure 6.1. Diagram of the radial arrangement of Purkinje axon conical fields in the dentate (lateral) nucleus. Axonal plexus A shows the branchlets that define the conical field (of base diameter of about 100–150 mu) of one Purkinje cell. The remaining cones show variations of this basic pattern. In actuality, the cones overlap. (From Chan-Palay 1977; *Cerebellar Dentate Nucleus*, copyright 1977, Springer-Verlag, Heidelberg; reprinted by permission from publisher and author.)

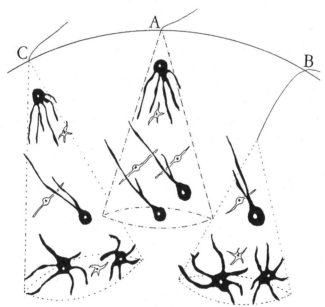

Figure 6.2. The relation between neurons (only samples are shown) of different types with their dendrites and the conical Purkinje axon field. Note that cones B and C (stippled) begin more deeply than cone A (dashed). Note also the trend to a particular orientation of specific types of neurons to the direction of the cones. (From Chan-Palay 1977; *Cerebellar Dentate Nucleus*, copyright 1977, Springer-Verlag, Heidelberg; reprinted by permission from publisher and author.)

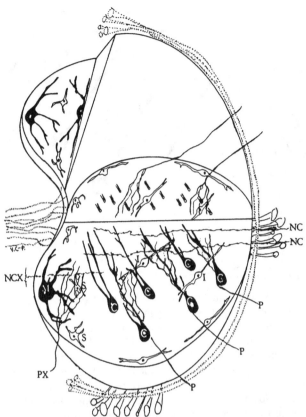

Figure 6.3. Diagram of organization of neurons and afferent axons in the lateral nucleus. The nucleus is encircled by packets of myelinated fibers (stippled). Parts of the nucleus have been cut away to show the arrangement of cells within. Note: (1) The columnar zone with its large columnar neurons (black, C) and bridging neurons (white, I); (2) the caudal pole with a large multipolar neuron (black, M) and small neurons (white, S). Purkinje axons (P) enter the central zone and may encompass whole columnar neurons. Extracerebellar afferents (NC) radiate across the nucleus, passing through columns of large neurons in succession. The small neurons are tilted at an angle and receive a large number of axonal contacts. In the noncolumnar zone, the Purkinje axon (PX) encompasses parts of the dendrites of several multipolar neurons, both large (M) and small (S). An extracerebellar axon (NCX) is shown. The relationships are represented diagrammatically in Figure 6.4. (From Chan-Palay 1977; *Cerebellar Dentate Nucleus*, copyright 1977, Springer-Verlag, Heidelberg; reprinted by permission from publisher and author.)

It is evident from Figure 6.4 that the large columnar neurons (C) and their dendritic fields tend to fall largely into the territory of one Purkinje axonal cone, whereas the large and small multipolar (swirl) neurons tend to share their well-spread dendritic fields into neighboring Purkinje axonal cones. It was suggested (Chan-Palay 1977) that such a restricted effect of the inhibitory field on single neurons could provide a means of preserving the specificity of the corticonuclear input, whereas the serial arrangement of the mossy and climbing fiber collaterals could provide a carefully timed sequence of excitatory stimuli to successive neurons, thus

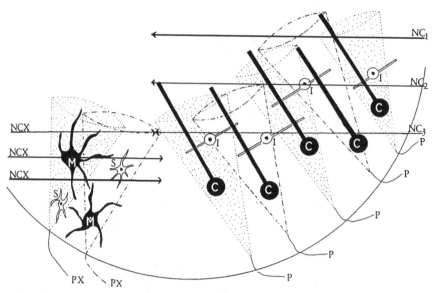

Figure 6.4. Diagram, based on Figure 6.3, of the relation between columnar neurons and swirls of neurons with their afferent inputs. On the right, the columns are presented; on the left, the swirls of multipolar neurons are shown. Because of their slender profile, individual columnar neurons (C) fall under the influence of single Purkinje axonal cones. The extracerebellar (NC$_1$–NC$_2$) axons cross the columns of several neurons in succession. The latter axons come in three thicknesses: thick (NC$_1$), medium (NC$_2$), and fine (NC$_3$). The small neurons (I) bridging the columns are tilted to receive a larger number of contacts with the noncortical afferent axons as well as the conical fields. In the swirled zones of multipolar cells, the Purkinje axons (PX) encompass portions of two (or more) large (M) and small (S) neurons. The extracerebellar axons (NCX) cross neurons in succession and various thicknesses of fibers are indicated. (From Chan-Palay 1977; *Cerebellar Dentate Nucleus*, copyright 1977, Springer-Verlag, Heidelberg; reprinted by permission from publisher and author.)

providing the basis of a delicate, modulated control of timing and intensity of a stimulus.

To reiterate, the fields of Purkinje axons in the dentate (lateral) nucleus can be considered as a series of radially arranged, overlapping cones that extend partially into the interior of the nuclear mass, each cone including a group of cells that it influences. In contrast, the non-Purkinje axons are radially arranged, simple fibers that enter the cell mass and course across successive neurons, making connections with them in passing. Thus, the Purkinje axonal fields are cones of inhibition for the nuclear cells under their influence, whereas the effect of noncortical axons (i.e., collaterals of mossy and climbing fibers) is one of varied rapid and slow (according to the diameter of the axon) excitatory influences to the successive nuclear cells in their paths (Chan-Palay 1977).

Purkinje Cell Axons Synapses onto Both Excitatory and Inhibitory Nuclear Neurons. De Zeeuw and Berrebi (1995, 1996) found that individual Purkinje cells can innervate both excitatory and inhibitory neurons in the cerebellar and vestibular nuclei, suggesting that the excitatory cerebellar and vestibular output system and the inhibitory feedback to the inferior olive are controlled simultaneously. The authors pointed out that Purkinje cells thus appear to simultaneously control the inhibitory feedback to the inferior olive (as part of a closed three-element anatomical pathway), and also the excitatory cerebellar output system, as part of an open anatomical pathway influencing motor commands. The authors also suggested that this finding could explain why olivary neurons appear to be unresponsive to stimuli generated during active movement (Teune et al. 1998; Chapter 5).

Serotonin and Cerebellar Nuclear Cells. Cerebellar nuclear cells are also subject to the influence of serotonin from serotoninergic fibers originating in the brain stem, suppressing amino acid (excitatory) synapses and enhancing GABAergic (inhibitory) synapses, so the net effect is a decrease in nuclear cell activity and consequently in cerebellar output (Kitzman and Bishop 1997).

6.1.2. Similarities Between Cerebellar Nuclei and the Inferior Olive

As mentioned in Chapter 5, several workers (e.g., Chan-Palay 1977) have been struck by a remarkable resemblance between the neurons of the nuclear border in the dentate nucleus and the neurons located at the periphery of the principal olivary nucleus, which delineate the margins of the nucleus by turning their dendritic arborizations internally (compare Fig. 6.3 with Fig. 5.3). The question has consequently arisen of whether such a similarity in the geometry and orientation of dendritic arborizations between the two structures may reflect their intimate relation in connectivity, structure, and function. Further, in the primate, both the dentate nucleus and the inferior olivary nucleus (as well as the thalamic neuropil) have a glomerular-type formation with the nuclear cell axon as the central presynaptic element, as a device of major importance (Chan-Palay 1977).

6.1.3. Functions of the Dentate Nucleus

From studies of recordings from monkeys trained to make rapid alternating flexion and extension movements at various joints of both upper and lower extremities, Thach, Perry, et al. (1993) concluded that the dentate nucleus controls muscle synergy and movement coordination more than the prime movers themselves. In this connection, Bastian and Thach (1995) evaluated the performance for reaching and for pinching movements in patients with lateral cerebellar lesions and also in patients with discrete lesions of the ventrolateral thalamus. It was found that lesions of the ventrolateral thalamus resulted in impaired pinching movements, but reaching movements were remarkably normal. In contrast, patients with cerebellar lesions involving the dentate showed a profound impairment of both pinching and reaching. It seemed probable to these authors (Bastian and Thach 1995) that the dentate influences fine finger movement (pinching) through the cerebellar–thalamo–cortical pathway, but affects elbow and shoulder movements (i.e., reaching) through descending pathways either via the parvocellular region of the (contralateral) red nucleus or, perhaps more likely, through the (contralateral) reticular tegmental nuclei. (See also Chapter 9, in relation to cognition.)

6.2. Efferent Cerebellar Nuclear Pathways

6.2.1. Destinations of Efferent Fibers from the Cerebellar Nuclei

Most of the efferents leave the cerebellum via the superior cerebellar peduncle, a minor portion via the middle and inferior peduncles. The efferents, in the human, will be considered in this brief survey by the individual nuclei, as detailed primarily by Brodal (1981).

Fastigial Nucleus. For the fastigial nucleus (the most medial nucleus), the main targets of the efferents are the pontine and medullary reticular formation and the vestibular nuclei, although there have also been some reports of terminations in the thalamus (nucleus ventralis posterior lateralis [VPL] and nucleus ventralis lateralis [VL]). Fibers passing directly to the spinal cord have been reported but questioned. The presence of some fibers to the following destinations have also been mentioned: pontine nuclei, nucleus reticularis tegmenti pontis, lateral reticular nucleus, paramedian reticular nucleus, and perihypoglossal nuclei.

Nuclei Interpositi (Anterior and Posterior) and Lateral (Dentate) Nucleus. These nuclei give off fibers that leave the cerebellum via the superior cerebellar peduncle. A considerable number of the fibers end in the thalamus, many in the red nucleus, and some in other destinations, particularly the brain stem. The *interpositus anterior* projects in a topical pattern to the caudal two thirds of the magnocellular part of the red nucleus. The large cells in the latter give rise to the relatively coarse fibers of the rubrospinal tract. The *dentate nucleus* (and also the interpositus posterior, to some extent), however, projects topically to the rostral one third of the red nucleus, the parvicellular part, the small cells of which give rise to the rather fine fibers of the rubro-olivary tract (see below).

In the monkey, Asanuma, Thach, and Jones (1983a) found that the thalamic termination zones for the dentate, interposed, and fastigial nuclei were identical and coincided with the cytoarchitectonically unique cell-sparse region of the thalamic ventral lateral complex. Asanuma, Thach, and Jones (1983b) also studied the brain stem and spinal projections of the cerebellar nuclei. The brain stem terminations of fibers arising in the dentate and interposed nuclei were similar – the red nucleus, the nucleus reticularis tegmenti pontis, and the inferior olivary complex – but there were some differences. Thus, the dentate nucleus projected only to the parvocellular red nucleus and the principal olivary nucleus, whereas the interposed nucleus projected only to the magnocellular red nucleus and to the two accessory olivary nuclei. There were extensive fastigial projections to the brain stem: nucleus reticularis tegmenti pontis, the lateral vestibular (Deiter's) nucleus, portions of the descending vestibular nucleus, the pontine nuclei, the pontine raphe, and parts of the reticular formation from the midbrain caudally. Projections to the spinal cord arose in the interposed and fastigial nuclei. No spinal projections were detected from the dentate nucleus.

Brodal (1981) pointed out that, from a functional point of view, it is of interest that the number of afferents to the red nucleus from the cerebral cortex is far smaller than the number of cerebellar nuclear afferents. In agreement with this fact, physiological studies have indicated that the cerebellar input to the red nucleus is more powerful than that from the cerebral cortex. Evidently little is known, however, about the corticorubral and rubrospinal tracts in humans.

Mention is made of a projection, in the monkey, passing from the dentate nucleus directly to the oculomotor nucleus, in a region known in the cat and monkey to receive primary vestibular fibers. These dentato-oculomotor fibers may therefore be a link in the vestibulo-ocular pathway.

Finally, the thalamic terminations of fibers from the nuclei interpositi and lateralis are not identical even if they overlap to some extent. In the cat, most fibers end in the lateral part of the nucleus ventralis lateralis, but some end laterally in the ventralis anterior and in the most medial part of the ventralis posterior lateralis.

6.2.2. Thalamic Ventrolateral Nucleus: Terminology

Pointing out that the nomenclature most commonly applied to the motor-related nuclei of the human thalamus differs substantially from that applied to the thalamus of other primates, from which most of the knowledge of input–output connections is derived, Macchi and Jones (1997) proposed a common nomenclature that reflects agreement about the equivalence of nuclei in the different species. As a result, according to them, it becomes possible to identify the nuclei of the human motor thalamus that transfers information from basal ganglia (substantia nigra and globus pallidus), cerebellum, and proprioceptive components of the medial lemniscus to prefrontal, premotor, motor, and somatosensory areas of the cerebral cortex. Correspondingly, stereotactic neurosurgical lesions that alleviate rigidity appear to have, as their thalamic target, the nuclei involved in pallidal circuits and now include the anterior part of the ventral lateral nucleus. The lesions that alleviate all types of tremor appear to have, as their targets, the nuclei involved in cerebellar circuits (i.e., the posterior part of the ventral lateral nucleus), possibly with extension into the proprioceptive lemniscal region of the ventral posterolateral nucleus. Destruction of the cerebellothalamic tract appears to be equally effective in alleviating tremor. Suppression of both rigidity and tremor may be obtained by a lesion in parts of both the cerebellar and pallidal terminal nuclei (i.e., posterior and anterior parts, respectively, of the ventral lateral nucleus), according to Macchi and Jones (1997).

6.2.3. Nucleocortical Projections within the Cerebellum (Recurrent Nucleocortical Feedback)

The existence of a projection from the cerebellar nuclei to the cerebellar cortex, the original report having been by Ramón y Cajal (1995), was for a time controversial.

A history of this question is given by Gould and Graybiel (1976); Tolbert, Bantli, and Bloedel (1976); Chan-Paley (1977, p. 352); Gould (1979); and Bloedel and Courville (1981). That there is an orderly nucleocortical projection within the cerebellum for each of the cerebellar nuclei, as well as for the vestibular complex, was demonstrated by neuroanatomical techniques in the cat by Gould and Graybiel (1976) and by Tolbert, Bantli, and Bloedel (1976) (see also Brodal and Kawamura 1980). The nucleocortical connection appeared to follow (in inverse direction) the plan of the inhibitory (Purkinje) pathway from the cerebellar cortex to the nuclei, thus providing an intrinsic feedback loop within the cerebellum.

The existence of a cerebellar nuclear-cortex projection was soon found in the dentate and interposed nuclei of a primate (Macaca mulatta), as in the cat, by Tolbert, Bantli, and Bloedel (1977), using electrophysiological and anatomical techniques. From their experiments, these authors concluded that the fibers of the nucleocortical projection arise at least in part as collaterals from nuclear neurons projecting to extracerebellar structures such as the inferior olive, the ventrolateral thalamic nucleus, or the red nucleus, depending on their site in the nuclei. In the cat, the fibers appeared to arise from all the different types of neurons in the cerebellar nuclei (Gould and Graybiel 1976; McCrea, Bishop, and Kitai 1978; Tolbert, Bantli, and Bloedel 1978), although in the monkey they appeared to arise principally from large multipolar neurons (Chan-Paley 1977; Tolbert, Bantli, and Bloedel 1978). Chan-Paley (1977) considered the neurons of the nuclear border, columnar neurons, and large asymmetrical neurons to be possible candidates for the nuclear cells of origin.

The nucleocortical projection was classified as a mossy fiber afferent system terminating in the granular layer of the cerebellar cortex, and thus using the indirect cortical route (i.e., via the granule cell–parallel fiber network) to the Purkinje cells. Thus, the typical repeated branching of mossy fibers was observed for the nucleocortical fibers along their course to the cerebellar cortex. As already mentioned, it was suggested that the nucleocortical and corticonuclear projections may be reciprocally organized (Tolbert, Bantli, and Bloedel 1978), although not completely so (Bloedel and Courville 1981; Chan-Paley 1977; Tolbert and Bantli 1979) (see Fig. 6.5).

Because the counterpart "nucleus" of the flocculus is the vestibular nuclear complex, it is reasonable to expect a corresponding feedback loop, comparable to that from the cerebellar nuclei to other parts of the cerebellar cortex. Such evidence of feedback from vestibular nuclei as mossy fibers to the granular layer in the flocculus was found by Miles et al. (1980).

The possibility of, in the main, a precise interaction between these two reciprocal fiber systems was suggested (Haines and Pearson 1979), although a strict one-to-one reciprocal was questioned (Dietrichs and Walberg 1979). In any case, it has been proposed that the nucleocortical system is a major component of the cerebellar cortical afferent system (Tolbert, Bantli, and Bloedel 1977).

Haines (1989) suggested that there are at least three, and possibly four, categories of nucleocortical (NC) cells: (1) ipsilateral reciprocal (found in, or in the periphery of, corticonuclear [CN] terminal fields formed by axons originating from the same cortical area to which the NC cells project); (2) ipsilateral nonreciprocal NC cells (located outside the CN terminal field); and (3) contralateral NC cells (found in the

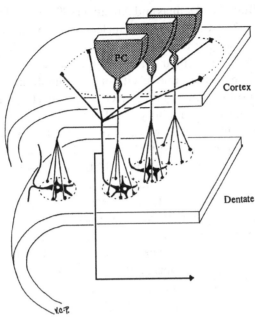

Figure 6.5. Comparison of the axonal fields of Purkinje cells and dentate nuclear neurons in the monkey. The Purkinje cells (PC) of the cerebellar cortex project single or multiple conical axon fields onto dentate neurons. Dentatocortical fibers are extended (perhaps as collaterals from extracerebellar projectional axons, as shown) and have extensive terminal fields in the overlying cortex. Although the two fields are basically reciprocal, the dentatocortical loop is more diffuse. (From Chan-Palay 1977; *Cerebellar Dentate Nucleus,* copyright 1977, Springer-Verlag, Heidelberg; reprinted by permission from publisher and author.)

opposite cerebellar nuclei). It seemed probable that the different types of NC cells have individualized functional characteristics (Haines 1989).

From their study of the topography of the nucleocortical projection in the cat, Trott, Apps, and Armstrong (1990), concluded that, at least for parts of the cerebellum, the nucleocortical projection and the corticonuclear (Purkinje cell) projection were not entirely reciprocal, a finding that could explain some earlier reports indicating a weak nucleocortical projection to the cortex. Further, confirming earlier reports, nucleocortical fibers were found to arise both from the small spindle-shaped (fusiform) cells and the larger, multipolar cell populations within the cerebellar nuclei (Fig. 6.3), indicating that both of these cell types can give off axon collaterals to the cerebellar cortex, thus providing a feedback pathway.

6.2.4. Nature of the Nucleocortical Projection: Excitatory vs. Inhibitory

At an early stage of the study of the nucleocortical projection, it was not clear whether it was excitatory or inhibitory (e.g., Chan-Palay, discussion of Tolbert 1982; Tolbert 1982; Tolbert, Kultas-Ilinsky, and Ilinsky 1980), but in the rat, Batini et al. (1989) reported that most of the nucleocortical fibers were GABAergic, but no GABAergic fibers projecting to the cerebellar cortex were found to originate from the lateral vestibular nucleus. Buisseret-Delmas and Angaut (1989) pointed out that the suggestion of Chan-Palay (1977), which is that the nucleocortical projection uses GABA as a neurotransmitter, may suggest that the projection includes both inhibitory (GABA) and excitatory fibers, because their termination as mossy fibers in the cerebellar cortex would imply non-GABAergic (excitatory) terminations.

However, in their study of cat granular layer glomeruli, Hámori and Takács (1989) found that, in addition to the inhibitory (GABAergic) axon terminals arising from Golgi cells (Type I terminals), there was a second type (Type II) GABAergic terminal (always accompanied by the first type), which arises from the cerebellar nuclei. The synapses of Type II terminals, although GABAergic, had some resemblance to excitatory terminals (i.e., large spheroidal vesicles). The authors indicated that, although the functional significance of the nucleocortical GABAergic terminals was unclear, this nucleocortical inhibitory innervation of the cerebellar cortex would have to be taken into account in future modeling of the cerebellum.

From their study of nucleocortical projections in the rat using immunohistochemical methods, Batini et al. (1992) concluded that both excitatory (glutaminergic) and inhibitory (GABAergic) fibers were present, and both terminate in the cerebellar cortex as mossy fibers some ipsilaterally ("reciprocally"), some contralaterally ("symmetrically"), to the mossy fiber-type rosettes in the granule cell layer. The authors characterized this feedback as a short-path, rapidly responding system contributing to fine control of Purkinje cell activity and functioning as a local microintegrator for the longer cerebellofugal pathways.

However, Kolston, Apps, and Trott (1995) did not find GABAergic nucleocortical fibers in their study using a combined retrograde tracer and GABA-immunochemical method, possibly for technical reasons, according to the authors.

Species Differences. Attention has also been drawn to species differences (Tolbert, Bantli, and Bloedel 1978). In the cat, nucleocortical fibers originating in the dentate nucleus project principally to the lateral hemisphere, whereas in primates, these fibers diverge over large areas of the ipsilateral cerebellar cortex including the vermis. The latter development appears to have emerged late in phylogenesis, reaching a significant development only in primates, which may be associated with the emergence of a neo- and paleodentate, in the ventrolateral (smaller-neuron), and dorsomedial (larger-neuron) parts, respectively, of the dentate nucleus (Tolbert, Bantli, and Bloedel 1978; for a review, see Tolbert 1982; see also Chapter 9). Umetani (1990) suggested that the marked differences in primary cortical targets of the interpositus and dentate nuclei among different species might represent the phylogenetic change in the development of coordination of more complicated and skilled fine movements.

As mentioned above, it initially appeared that the nucleocortical fibers terminate in the granular layer of the cortex, and hence are a part of the mossy fiber input system and are thus excitatory (Chan-Palay 1977; Tolbert, Bantli, and Bloedel 1977). Electronmicroscopic studies confirmed the excitatory nature of these synapses (Tolbert 1982). However, as mentioned, the possibility of an inhibitory nature for the nucleocortical fibers originating from the dentate nucleus was raised (Tolbert 1982).

Indeed, Hámori, Takács, and Petrusz (1990) found two classes of glutamate (excitatory) terminals in mossy fibers, with two somewhat differing sizes of synaptic vesicles – the larger ones being in fibers of extracerebellar origin, and the smaller ones being in fibers of intracerebellar origin (i.e., nucleocortical fibers). As mentioned above, these authors also found two classes of GABA terminals within cerebellar glomeruli of differing size of synaptic vesicles – the one of local cortical (i.e., Golgi cell), and the other originating from cerebellar nuclei. These findings suggested the existence of both inhibitory and excitatory feedback from cerebellar nuclei to cerebral cortex (Hámori, Takács, and Petrusz 1990).

6.2.5. Function of the Nucleocortical Fibers

Tolbert (1982), noting that many such fibers are collaterals of cerebellofugal projections to the brain stem, and that there is reciprocity to some degree of nucleocortical and corticonuclear pathways, suggested that the nucleocortical fibers, acting through Purkinje cell inhibition, result in a tempering of the output of the cerebellar nuclei.

Llinás (1982) raised the question of whether the nucleocortical pathway may serve the function of providing a certain amount of background activity in the mossy fiber system.

Ito (1984) suggested that, functionally, the nucleocortical fibers may serve as an internal feedback to the cerebellar cortex and, in conjunction with corticonuclear fibers, permit elaborate operations of microcomplexes (functional cortical-nuclear units).

In connection with the consideration of the nucleocortical fibers, it may be relevant to mention that, against a background of existing evidence that neurons projecting to the magnocellular part of the red nucleus are mainly found in the interposed nuclei, whereas those projecting to its parvocellular part are predominantly located in the lateral cerebellar nucleus, Teune, van der Burg, and Ruigrok (1995) concluded from a double labeling study in the rat that the nucleorubral (excitatory) projection and the nucleo-olivary projection (inhibitory) originate from separate populations in the cerebellar nuclei.

Also, Teune, Van Der Burg, De Zeeuw, Voogd, and Ruigrok (1998) recently reported that the same Purkinje cells can influence both inhibitory (GABAergic) cerebellar nuclear cells that project to the inferior olive and also excitatory (non-GABAergic) cells that project to premotor nuclei (e.g., the red nucleus, thalamus, and superior colliculus). The authors suggested that such an in-phase Purkinje cell modulation of nuclear inhibitory cells and nuclear excitatory cells could explain why olivary neurons appear to be unresponsive to stimuli generated during active movement.

6.2.6. The Nucleo-Olivary Fibers

The important topic of the nucleo-olivary (feedback) fibers is considered in Chapter 5.

6.3. Some Aspects of the Cerebellum and Motor Learning

Because, with the exception of the vestibulocerebellum, the outflow from the cerebellum is via the cerebellar nuclei, some aspects of the cerebellum and motor learning are considered here. Only a very small selection of the vast number of such studies are mentioned; other selected ones are considered in subsequent chapters.

6.3.1. The Cerebellum and Updating of Internal Models

In their review of voluntary motor learning, Ebner, Flament, and Shanbhag (1996) concluded that the cerebellum is closely linked to motor performance, being required for the production of smooth coordinated movements. The authors further suggested that the function of the cerebellum in updating internal models may be to provide needed neural processing, which itself needs precise definition.

6.3.2. Adaptation Learning vs. Skill Learning

Hallett, Pascual-Leone, and Topka (1996) made the distinction between adaptation learning and skill learning. Learning to throw a ball at a target while wearing prism spectacles would be an example of adaptation learning, whereas learning to play a piano would be an example of skill learning. In the authors' view, the cerebellum is principally responsible for adaptation learning, whereas in skill learning, the role of the cerebellum is smaller, and cerebral cortical structures, including the motor cortex, have a larger role. Donoghue, Hess, and Sanes (1996) considered adaptation as a reciprocal change of one behavior for another, as in exchanging speed for accuracy, or the reciprocal modification of motor output in response to gain changes in sensory input, as in the vestibulo-ocular reflex. Skill learning, as viewed by these authors, entails nonreciprocal modifications of output variables, such as speed and accuracy, and would include typing and playing a musical instrument.

Results from lesion, electrophysiological, imaging, and stimulation techniques suggest that the richly interconnected motor cortex (MI, Brodmann's area 4) is involved in both adaptive and skill learning, and several possible sites of activity-dependent plasticity (i.e., synapses) probably exist, of both long-term depression (LTD) and long-term potentiation (LTP) types (Chapter 7); the frequency or pattern of activation can determine whether a particular synapse increases or decreases its strength, in response to, for example, conjoint activation via two pathways (Donoghue, Hess, and Sanes 1996). These authors pointed out that there is also the possibility of formation of new synapses or removal of inactive ones. It should be kept in mind, of course, that the anatomical arrangement of the motor cortex is quite different from that of the "crystalline"-like structure of the cerebellum.

Asanuma (1996) pointed out that the projection from the somatosensory cortex (area 2) to the motor cortex is important in learning new motor skills, but not for their retention.

6.3.3. Purkinje Cell Encoding of Direction and Distance

In recordings in monkeys from Purkinje cells in the intermediate zone and adjacent hemispheric regions during a multijoint arm-reaching task under visual guidance with systematically varied movement direction and distance (Fu, Flament, et al. 1997), simple spike activity was found to be correlated with direction, distance, and target position. Comparison of these results with the behavior of motor cells of the cerebral cortex indicated that, among other differences, the correlations (with direction, distance, and target position) were weaker for simple spike discharges of Purkinje cells, and that for the majority of Purkinje cells, the simple spike discharge was significantly related to only a single movement parameter. It was also found that complex spike activity was correlated with distance and/or direction of the movement (Fu, Mason, et al. 1997). The authors concluded that the complex spike discharge of Purkinje cells is spatially tuned and strongly related to movement kinematics. Further, for both direction and distance tuning, the hemiregion of the workspace with the strongest complex spike modulation was generally opposite that of the strongest simple spike modulation, suggesting that the two systems operate in parallel to define spatial aspects of the task.

From recordings of the activity of Purkinje cells during short-lasting movements by trained monkeys, Kitazawa, Kimura, and Yin (1998) concluded that complex spikes occurring at the beginning of the reach movement encode the absolute destination of the reach, and the complex spikes occurring at the end of the movements encode the relative errors. The authors concluded that complex spikes convey multiple types of information, consistent with the idea that they contribute both to the generation of movements and to the gradual, long-term improvement of such movements.

6.3.4. Control of Limb Movement Velocity

Ebner (1998) suggested that mossy fiber afferents to the cerebellar cortex are a source of kinematic signals, providing information about movement direction and speed, which are integrated by the Purkinje cells such that the simple spike discharge of the latter (50–150 spikes/sec) generates a movement velocity signal (i.e., a vector). The author further suggested that the climbing fibers and, correspondingly, the Purkinje cell complex spikes (0.5–2.0 spikes/sec) may signal errors in movement velocity. It was thus proposed that the cerebellum uses the signals carried by the simple and complex spike discharges to control movement velocity for both step (reaching) and tracking arm movements.

6.3.5. Multiple Sites of Synaptic Plasticity in Addition to the Cerebellum

From a review of their own work and that of others, Bloedel et al. (1996) reiterated the view (Bloedel and Bracha 1995) that the plastic changes (Chapter 7) established during the acquisition of complex, volitional motor behaviors are distributed over multiple sites that participate in regulating the required movement, including, for example, nuclei onto which projections from specific regions of the cerebellum converge with other fiber systems involved in the behavior.

6.4. Organization of Reaching and Grasping

The organization of reaching and grasping movement in monkey cerebellar nuclei, as indicated by muscimol (a GABA agonist) injection, was explored by Mason et al. (1998). These authors found a prominent anteroposterior specialization within the forelimb zone such that the muscimol injection into the anterior interpositus impaired preshaping of the hand and manipulation of objects, whereas injections more posteriorly into the posterior interpositus and adjacent dentate produced deficits in the aiming of reach and the stability of the arm. From this organization into an anterior hand zone and a posterior reach zone, the authors concluded that distal and proximal musculature is coordinated by the adaptive influences of climbing fiber input to Purkinje cells, rather than by selection of Purkinje cells along beams of parallel fibers (Thach, Goodwin, and Keating 1992; see below and Fig. 13.6). In the authors' view (Mason et al. 1998), a relatively nonspecific recruitment of anterior and posterior nuclear cells occurs due to positive feedback in the limb premotor network, which is then shaped into an appropriate spatiotemporal pattern of discharge through the inhibitory input from Purkinje cells.

From a study in cats of the differential effects of inactivation (by means of the GABA agonist, muscimol) of the deep cerebellar nuclei on reaching and adaptive control, Martin et al. (2000) concluded that there are separate functional output channels from the anterior and posterior interpositus nuclei to the rostral motor cortex for distinct aspects of control, and from the anterior interpositus alone for trajectory adaptation.

To supplement the well-established features of the disynaptic excitatory projection to the primary motor cortex from the cerebellar nuclei (via the ventral thalamus) that had been obtained from the anesthetized cat and monkey, Holdefer et al. (2000) carried out experiments on monkeys during a reaching and button-pressing task. The authors reported that the results demonstrated a spatially specific, short-latency, primarily excitatory pathway from the cerebellar nuclei to the primary motor cortex in the awake monkey.

From a study to determine the effects of concurrent mucimol inactivation of the cerebellar interpositus and dentate nuclei on the capacity of cats to acquire and retain a complex, goal-directed forelimb movement, Wang et al. (1998) found that the animals could learn to execute the more difficult maneuvers during the inactivation of these nuclei. The authors concluded that the intermediate and lateral cerebellum are not required either for learning the type of complex voluntary movement used or for regaining the capacity to perform the task once it is learned. Nevertheless, when the cerebellum became available for executing a task learned in the absence of this structure, reacquisition of the behavior was usually necessary. Wang et al. (1998) hypothesized that the relearning observed after acquisition during muscimol inactivation reflects the tendency of the system to incorporate the cerebellum into the interactions responsible for the learning and performance of a motor sequence that is optimal for executing the task.

Complementarity of Cerebellar Cortex and Nuclei. Mauk (1997) suggested that the relative contributions of the cerebellar cortex and cerebellar nuclei are not constant but instead may depend on the amount and type of training experienced by the animal, and that such a complementarity could account for apparently differing results in motor learning, particularly adaptation of the vestibulo-ocular reflex (VOR) and blink conditioning.

6.5. Human Studies

6.5.1. Single vs. Multijoint Movements

From comparisons in normal control and cerebellar patients of touching a target object under conditions in which only flexion movement at the elbow (i.e., no movement at the shoulder) and motion of both elbow and shoulder were possible, Bastian, Zackowski, and Thach (2000) found that cerebellar patients performed better (less undershoot/overshoot) and exhibited less electromyographic (EMG) activity of shoulder muscles under the former conditions. In contrast, there was little difference of EMG activity for the two conditions in the control subjects. The authors suggested that the poorer control in the cerebellar patients when the shoulder could also move is due to an inability to generate muscle torques that predict and compensate for interaction torques in multijoint movements, rather than due to a general inability to generate sufficient levels of phasic torque, as suggested by Boose, Dichgans, and Topka (1999). (See also Topka, Konczak, and Dichgans 1998; Topka, Konczak, Schneider et al. 1998.) As a consequence, according to Bastian, Zackowski, and Thach (2000), reducing the number of muscles to be controlled appears to improve cerebellar ataxia.

Optimal Time-Varying Control of Joint Stiffness. Smith (1996) proposed that the cerebellum has an important role in motor learning by forming and storing associated muscle activation patterns for the time-varying control of limb mechanics (i.e., of agonist–antagonist muscle synergies or joint stiffness).

6.5.2. Comparative Imaging of Cerebellar Sensory Input and Motor Output

Using positron emission tomography (PET) for the measurement of regional cerebral blood flow (rCBF) to determine the extent to which the human cerebellum is activated during active movement (flexion and extension of the right elbow) in comparison with the same movement carried out passively with the aid of a motorized device, almost identical parts of the ipsilateral neocerebellar hemisphere and vermis of the posterior lobe were activated, in comparison to the rest position (Jueptner et al. 1997). In the same study, rather minimal differences (in the same cerebellar regions) were also found when the results for a joystick task were compared with merely imagining the same task. The authors considered their results to indicate that the neocerebellum may be much more concerned with sensory information processing than previously considered.

6.5.3. PET and Motor Practice Adaptation

Physiological adaptation during repeated performance of a simple motor task (brisk right-handed sequential finger-to-thumb opposition), in the form of a decrease in the physiological activation (i.e., decrease in regional blood flow during performance with practice), was reported by Friston et al. (1992) for the right cerebellar cortex and cerebellar nuclei. In contrast, the primary sensorimotor cortex did not show such an adaptation.

Dentate vs. Premotor Area. In a study of writing out unfamiliar nonsense characters, Seitz et al. (1994) found that during the early phase of learning there was a significant activation of the ipsilateral dentate nucleus. After overlearning, however, the dentate nucleus was no longer activated, whereas the premotor cerebral cortical areas were maximally activated. It was concluded that learning of new movement trajectories involves the cerebellum, whereas overlearned trajectorial movements are carried out by the premotor cortex.

6.5.4. Activation of Cerebellar Dentate Nucleus and Sensory Processing

Using imaging studies of the dentate nucleus in combination with tests of sensory stimulation and sensory discrimination with and without a motor component, Gao et al. (1996) found that the strengths of dentate activation were, in order, grasping objects, cutaneous stimulation, cutaneous discrimination, and discriminating grasped objects. The authors concluded that the lateral cerebellum (and dentate) is not activated by the control of movement per se, but rather during the acquisition and discrimination of sensory information.

6.5.5. Context Estimation by the Motor System

In view of the remarkably accurate and appropriate human motor behavior despite relative changes with time of the properties both of the body and of the objects in the environment (e.g., liquid being poured out of a bottle that thereby becomes lighter), Vetter and Wolpert (2000) drew attention to the point that the motor system has to estimate the context (i.e., the properties of objects in the world and the prevailing environmental conditions). On the basis of a series of pointing experiments, the authors showed that to determine the current context, the CNS uses information in a probabilistic way both from prior knowledge of how the context might evolve over time, and also from the comparison of predicted and actual sensory feedback.

6.5.6. Cerebellar Cortex and Cerebral Cortex as a Self-correcting Adaptive Control System

Parkins (1997) suggested that the cerebellar cortex and cerebral cortex facilitate two fundamentally different but complementary types of information representation and processing that reciprocally evaluate and correct each other, thereby providing the basis for a self-correcting adaptive control system. Thus, the cerebellum was considered to be characterized by parallel processing, polymodality, and low discrimination, whereas the cerebrum is assumed to be characterized by serial processing, unimodality, and high discrimination.

PART TWO

CEREBELLAR FUNCTIONS

SEVEN

Cerebellar Memory, Long-Term Depression, and Long-Term Potentiation

On a theoretical basis (as summarized in Chapter 13), both Marr (1969) and Albus (1971) invoked memory storage at the parallel fiber–Purkinje cell dendritic tree interface if the parallel fibers and the climbing fibers (both excitatory) were conjointly active. In Marr's theory, the efficacy of these synapses was postulated to become enhanced (facilitated) with such conjoint activation, whereas in Albus's theory, synaptic efficacy became diminished (depressed). Ekerot and Oscarsson (1981) found that impulses in climbing fibers resulted in a depolarization of Purkinje cell dendrites lasting about 100 milliseconds. The authors conjectured that this effect might induce plastic changes in the parallel fiber synapses onto Purkinje cell dendrites, as envisaged in theories of motor learning by the cerebellum.

The diminished synaptic efficacy predicted by Albus was soon discovered (Ito and Kano 1982; Ito, Sakurai, and Tongroach 1982) in the form of long-term depression (LTD; i.e., a significant diminution of the parallel fiber postsynaptic potentials induced in Purkinje cells and lasting for at least 1 hour).

That there is indeed a capability for plasticity is illustrated for a subject (Fig. 7.1) throwing darts at a target (Fig. 7.2) before wearing prism spectacles, while wearing the spectacles, and after removing them. It is the direction of throw of the dart (which is normally determined from the direction of gaze) that undergoes change followed by adaptation or recalibration, which is then followed by a rebound and reverse adaptation upon removal of the prism spectacles. However, if there is impairment of the inferior olive, as for a patient with hypertrophy of the inferior olive, there is no adaptation to wearing the prism glasses nor readaptation after their removal (Fig. 7.3).

Nonetheless, the question of memory for movements in the cerebellum and, in particular, of LTD as its basis, has continued to be somewhat controversial (see Lisberger 1995). Thus, there have been questions as to whether, in experimentally induced LTD, the climbing fiber stimulation rate is too fast in relation to the usual background firing rate of about 1 per second; whether LTD is sufficiently lasting to

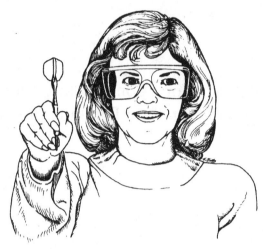

Figure 7.1. Throwing darts while wearing wedge prism spectacles (base to the right). The subject is looking directly at the target toward which she is pointing the dart, but because the prism bends the optic path 15 degrees to the right, her gaze is deviated 15 degrees to her left to see the target (she is looking at you). The portion of her face behind the lenses appears to the viewer to be displaced to her left because of the prism's bending of the optic path. The direction of throw is normally in the direction of gaze. The gaze direction has, however, been calibrated to the throw direction, and the aim of throw is true (at you). (From Thach, Goodkin, and Keating 1992; in *Annual Review of Neuroscience*, Volume 15, copyright 1992, Annual Reviews [www.AnnualReviews.org]; reprinted by permission from publisher and author.)

form the basis of memory; and whether the effect might actually be one of enhancement rather than of LTD (Bloedel, Bracha, and Larson 1993; Bloedel and Kelly 1992).

7.1. Nature, Mechanisms, and Function of LTD

An extensive early review of LTD in relation to the cerebellum was published by Ito (1989), with particular reference to its role as a memory element for cerebellar motor learning. Ito (1990, 1993c) also hypothesized that, regarding evidence that climbing fiber signals encode errors in motor performance of an animal, learning may proceed in cerebellar tissues in such a way that error signals of climbing fibers act to depress by LTD those parallel fiber synapses that are responsible for the errors. It is relevant to note that this hypothesis is in accord with the original Perceptron Rule of Rosenblatt (i.e., only those connections of the Perceptron that are in error are changed; Chapter 14).

Shibuki and Okada (1992) suggested that postsynaptic activity in Purkinje cells is negatively correlated with the direction of plastic changes (i.e., LTD vs. LTP) and that a different role is played in synaptic plasticity by cyclic guanosine monophosphate (cGMP).

From experiments on learning by rats in a complex maze, Seeds, Williams, and Bickford (1995) found that tissue plasminogen activator (tPA), which is associated

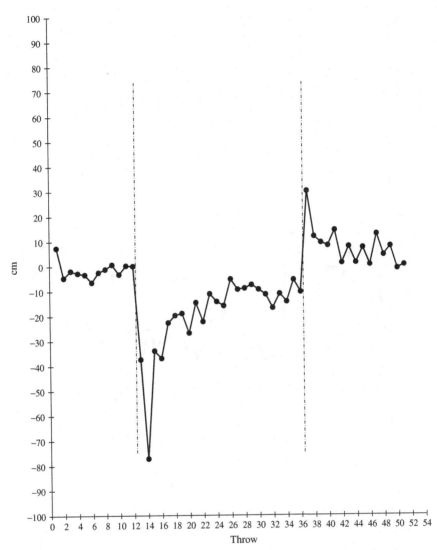

Figure 7.2. A plot of the horizontal location, relative to the target center, of each successive dart hit. Before introduction of the prism, the darts hit close to the center of the target. Introduction of the prism shifts the hits to the left (*down*), and with practice they normally return toward the center of the target as the recalibration of gaze direction–throw direction is made. After removal of the prism, the hits are normally shifted to the right (*up*), a result that shows that the throw direction is still calibrated 15 degrees off the gaze direction (in actuality, the error is never quite the whole 15 degrees). With practice, the gaze–throw directions readjust back to the original value. (From Thach, Goodkin, and Keating 1992; in *Annual Review of Neuroscience*, Volume 15, copyright 1992, Annual Reviews [www.AnnualReviews.org]; reprinted by permission of publisher and author.)

with developing and regenerating neurons, was increased in the Purkinje neurons following learning, thus indicating that the induction of tPA may play a role in activity-dependent synaptic plasticity.

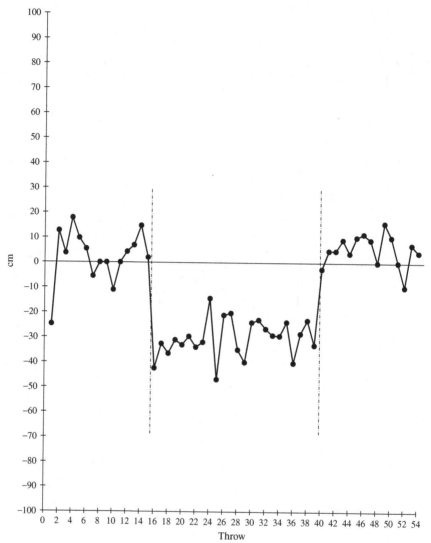

Figure 7.3. Patient with hypertrophy of the inferior olive, a degenerative disease of the inferior olive. After introduction of the prism, there is no recalibration of the gaze–throw directions, and the throws remain to the left of target center (*down*). After removal of the prisms, the hits land where they did before the introduction of the prisms, thus indicating no adaptation to the prisms in this subject. (From Thach, Goodkin, and Keating 1992; in *Annual Review of Neuroscience*, Volume 15, copyright 1992 Annual Reviews [www.AnnualReviews.org]; reprinted by permission of publisher and author.)

7.1.1. LTD as Level Setter Rather Than Role in Motor Learning

De Schutter (1995, 1997) suggested that cerebellar LTD, rather than functioning as an element of a memory trace (as in the Marr–Albus–Ito theories) by reducing the weight of most synaptic input to Purkinje cells, acts as a component of a local feedback mechanism that establishes and maintains the total excitation (i.e., the balance between excitation and inhibition) of the Purkinje cell at a level of depolarization such that the simple spike firing rhythm is maximally responsive to changes in parallel fiber input, all without participation by climbing fibers. (However, see Blond and Crépel 1996, De Schutter 1996, and Ito 1996.)

7.1.2. Transfer of Plasticity from Purkinje Cells to Stellate and Basket Cells

For more reliable function and more reliable long-term storage, Kenyon (1997) proposed plasticity at parallel fiber synapses onto stellate and basket neurons (which greatly outnumber Purkinje cells by 10–20 times) as a backup to the modification of synapses at parallel fiber–Purkinje cell synapses. The relatively short-term effect at the Purkinje cells would be transferred (after a threshold is exceeded) to the stellate and basket cells, which would then affect Purkinje cells via their inhibitory influence on the latter. For Purkinje cells, the model assumes a bidirectional form (about an equilibrium level) of climbing fiber-dependent LTD/long-term potentiation (LTP) – decrease in synaptic weight when active during elevated climbing fiber input, and increase when active during reduced climbing fiber input. Recurrent collaterals from Purkinje cells to both stellate and basket cells were also assumed.

7.1.3. Plasticity and Metaplasticity

As a possible basis for more efficient learning in the cerebellar cortex, Schweighofer and Arbib (1998) suggested that Cerebellar Adaptive Rate Learning (CARL), a mechanism that concentrates learning on those parallel-fiber–Purkinje cell synapses, the adaptation of which is most relevant to learning an overall pattern, and at the same time the contribution of those synapses that are not relevant to the overall pattern are assigned lower learning rates. The concept is based on making the learning rate at a given synapse dependent on an exponentially weighted cumulative sum of recent weight changes at the synapse. As a basis for the memory of the weight changes, second messenger concentrations or proteins were suggested. The authors termed this adaptation of learning rates among different synapses metaplasticity, in contrast to the term *plasticity*, which refers to changes at a given synapse. It was suggested that cerebellar metaplasticity would be especially relevant to execution of multijoint movements.

7.1.4. Plasticity at Climbing Fiber Synapses

On the basis of studies on olivocerebellar axons, Strata and Rossi (1998) suggested that plasticity may occur at the climbing fiber–Purkinje cell dendrite interface as well as at the parallel fiber–Purkinje cell dendrite interface, in such a way as to not only detect temporally coincident events, but also to select defined inputs impinging upon spatially restricted Purkinje cell dendritic domain. Thus, the climbing fiber would not be viewed as a fixed structure having a stereotyped effect on the Purkinje cell dendritic tree, but rather as a fine-tuning mechanism having its effect both in space and in time on synaptic plasticity, not unlike LTD.

7.1.5. Cellular Mechanisms of Cerebellar LTD

It is well accepted (Daniel, Levenes, and Crépel 1998) that induction of LTD of parallel fiber-mediated responses is triggered by the influx of Ca^{2+} into Purkinje cells through voltage-gated Ca^{2+} channels and by the activation of two groups of glutamate receptors: ionotropic alpha-amino-3-hydroxy-5-methyl-4-isoxazole proprionic acid (AMPA) receptors and type-1 G-protein-coupled metabotropic receptors (mGluR1). In addition, there is wide agreement that second messenger cascades occurring after the rise of intracellular Ca^{2+} concentrations involve protein kinase C (PKC) activation and nitric oxide (NO) production.

Further clarifying the nature of LTD (although not all questions have been answered; cf. Llinás 1995), it has been reported that blocking Purkinje cell PKC (which is a requirement for induction of LTD) by means of a protein kinase inhibitor blocks cerebellar LTD and the adaptation of the vestibulo-ocular reflex (De Zeeuw, Hansel, et al. 1998).

7.1.6. Intermediary Mechanisms in LTD

Generally speaking, LTD has become an active area of interest in relation to a number of aspects of synaptic plasticity. The following is only a partial listing of additional studies in relation to (1) ionic cellular mechanisms (Crépel et al. 1994; Konnerth, Dreessen, and Augustine 1992; Linden and Connor 1993; Linden, Smeyne, and Connor 1993); (2) desensitization or change of functional characteristics of postsynaptic receptors and second messengers (e.g., (a) nitric oxide (Boxall, Lancaster, and Garthwaite 1996; Hartel 1994; Hémart et al. 1994; Hémart et al. 1995; Linden, Dawson, and Dawson 1995) [see also below]; (b) mutations [Aiba et al. 1994; Kashiwabuchi et al. 1995]).

7.1.7. Nitric Oxide and LTD

Using an experimental arrangement to test motor learning in which one forelimb of a cat is exposed to a moving belt velocity higher than that of other limbs during locomotion, Yanagihara and Kondo (1996) found that the motor learning (i.e., adaptation to the higher belt velocity) was abolished by application of either an inhibitor of NO or of a scavenger of nitrous oxide to the cerebellar cortical locomotion area. It was concluded that NO in the cerebellum plays a key role in the induction of LTD.

It has been reported that LTD cannot be induced in Purkinje cells in mice that are genetically lacking the enzyme for synthesizing NO, namely, neuronal nitric oxide synthase (nNOS; Lev-Ram, Nebyelul, et al. 1997). Although the genetically defective animals exhibited normal behavior superficially, the authors had not yet tested for specific deficits (e.g., eye blink, vestibulo-ocular reflexes).

Lev-Ram, Jiang, et al. (1997) drew attention to the point that, of the two components of LTD, namely, presynaptic activity coincident with postsynaptic depolarization, the first can be replaced by NO (which arises from and mimics parallel fiber stimulation) and the second by calcium ion, thus indicating that these two messengers are sufficient for LTD induction.

A number of reviews concerning LTD have appeared (e.g., Crépel et al. 1996; Daniel, Levenes, and Crépel 1998; Kano 1966; Linden 1996a, 1996b; Linden and Connor 1995).

7.1.8. In vitro Classical Conditioning of LTD

Using rabbit cerebellar slices and intradendritic recordings, Schreurs, Oh, and Alkon (1996) reported classical conditioning in the form of LTD by parallel fiber stimulation (100 Hertz for 80 milliseconds) followed immediately by climbing fiber stimulation (20 Hertz for 100 milliseconds) with an intertrial interval of 30 seconds. Control slices received unpaired stimulation. The slices subjected to paired stimulation showed substantial and persisting depression (LTD) of Purkinje neuron excitatory postsynaptic potentials to parallel fiber stimulation relative to unpaired controls.

7.2. Long-Term Potentiation

In contrast to the long-term potentiation (LTP) of parallel fiber–Purkinje cell synapses that results from conjunctive stimulation of climbing fibers and parallel fibers, stimulation of parallel fibers alone can result in the parallel fiber-mediated excitatory postsynaptic potentials (EPSPs) being potentiated (LTP) (Hirano 1990a, 1990b; Sakurai 1987, 1989; Salin, Malenka, and Nicoll 1996; Schreurs and Alkon 1993).

7.3. Combined LTD and LTP

7.3.1. Self-Regulating Equilibrium (LTD/LTP) of the Cerebellar-Inferior Olivary System

Kenyon, Medina, and Mauk (1998a) advanced a mathematical model of the cerebellar olivary system in which cerebello-olivary negative feedback enables an equilibrium level of spontaneous climbing fiber activity (i.e., of LTD and LTP), leading to self-regulation in which there is a balance of LTD and LTP. Their mathematical model assumes that parallel fiber–Purkinje cell synapses decrease in strength when the parallel fiber is active during a climbing fiber input (LTD) and increase in strength when the parallel fiber is active without a climbing fiber input (LTP), thus enabling a bidirectional change in synaptic weight. In turn, a disruption of the above-mentioned equilibrium followed by its restoration accompanies cerebellar motor learning (Kenyon, Medina, and Mauk 1998b).

A formulation similar to that of Kenyon, Medina, and Mauk (1998a, 1998b) was advanced by Miall et al. (1998), who examined the question of the function of the irregular background firing rate (of about 1 Hz) of climbing fibers (and therefore of Purkinje cell complex spikes) in relation to the LTD at parallel fiber–Purkinje cell synapses arising from conjoint climbing fiber–parallel fiber firing, on the one hand, and LTP arising from tonic firing of the parallel fibers alone, on the other hand. The hypothesis being explored was whether the low background firing rate of climbing fibers (in the absence of movement) represented a mechanism for generating an amount of LTD that would just balance the LTP induced by parallel fiber firing alone (see also Kenyon, Medina, and Mauk 1998a, 1998b; Mauk and Donegan 1997). The hypothesis was tested by analysis of existing recordings of Purkinje cell simple spikes and complex spikes to search for the predicted increase in simple spike firing rate prior to complex spikes, the presumed mechanism for which would be the inhibitory feedback to the inferior olive from the deep cerebellar nuclei. Thus, an increase in the Purkinje cell simple spike rate would result in greater inhibition of excitatory and inhibitory deep cerebellar nuclear cells, the effect of the latter being to disinhibit olivary cells, resulting in turn in an increase in the frequency of climbing fibers (the possible effect of the olivonuclear collaterals being ignored in the formulation), thereby completing the feedback loop, so Purkinje cells would neither fall silent due to LTD of their inputs nor be driven into excessive activity through LTP.

Miall et al. (1998) found a small but statistically significant increase in simple spike activity about 150 msec before apparently random complex spikes recorded during a pause between visually guided movements. This interval was not only much longer than expected on the basis of axonal and synaptic delays from the Purkinje cells to the inferior olive and back again, but also close to the estimated visuomotor feedback delay. Thus, if the Purkinje cell simple spike increased rate represents a predictive signal and the complex spike represents an error-correcting mechanism, then the interval between the increased rate of simple spikes and the complex spike would be expected to depend on the delay between the movement and the feedback it causes; hence, the observed interval would be appropriate. As for the function of such a corrective mechanism in the absence of movement, it was suggested that the predictive nature of the Purkinje cell discharge may act as a feedforward (Chapter 16) motor correction, fine-tuning ongoing processes in higher motor centers.

7.3.2. Adaptive Sensory Processing, LTD, and LTP in Cerebellum-Like Structures of Mormyrid Electric Fish

As described more extensively in Chapter 12, certain mormyrid electric fish have a cerebellum-like structure, the electrosensory lobe, which includes Purkinje-like cells, a granule layer, and parallel fibers, and appears to act as an adaptive sensory processor. Thus, learned predictions about sensory input are generated and subtracted from actual sensory input so unpredicted inputs stand out. The sensory input is relayed to the basal region of the Purkinje-like cells, and the predictive signals are relayed by parallel fibers to the apical dendrites of the same cells (Bell et al. 1997). These authors found that excitatory postsynaptic potentials were enhanced (LTP) or depressed (LTD) after pairing with a postsynaptic spike to the cell, depending on the timing relation between the two stimuli. Depression occurred only if the imposed postsynaptic spike followed the excitatory postsynaptic potential within 60 msec.

In this connection, the decrease in synaptic effectiveness (i.e., plasticity) in the cerebellum-like electrosensory lateral line lobe (ELL) of a mormyid electric fish (Chapter 12) was found by Bell et al. (1997) to occur only if a postsynaptic spike in the Purkinje-like cell followed the parallel fiber-induced EPSP within 60 msec.

7.3.3. Temporal Aspects and Sites of LTD and LTP

Linden (1996a) found that three different manipulations that interfere with protein synthesis (i.e., a translation-inhibiting drug, transcription-inhibiting drugs, and physical isolation of the synaptic zone from the Purkinje-cell nucleus) all produced an attenuation of the late phase of cerebellar LTD in culture. Because none of these preparations depend on stimulation of presynaptic elements for induction or monitoring, the results suggested that protein synthesis in the postsynaptic compartment of Purkinje cells contributes to expression of a late phase of cerebellar LTD, thereby influencing dendritic function. In contrast, Linden (1998) concluded that the expression of LTP in the cerebellum in culture is presynaptic, at least in part.

In relation to induction of LTP by parallel fiber–Purkinje cell dendrite activity alone, Kistler and van Hemmen (2000) developed a mathematical and computer model – the "spike-response" model – for synaptic long-term plasticity that relies on the relative timing of pre- and postsynaptic action potentials (APs). The learning process does not rely on an external teacher signal; it is unsupervised. The authors stressed that, of particular importance for any kind of information processing based on spiking neurons and temporal coding, was the finding that such a mechanism of synaptic plasticity is able to strengthen those input synapses that convey precisely timed spikes at the expense of synapses that deliver spikes with a broad temporal distribution.

7.3.4. Cortical and Nuclear LTP/LTD and Self-Regulating Equilibrium of Climbing Fiber Activity

In questioning whether a molecular mechanism for long-term expression of synaptic plasticity alone can suffice for explaining the persistence of memories, Medina and Mauk (1999) concluded that learning and memory require that these cellular mechanisms be integrated within the architecture of the neural circuit. To illustrate the point, the authors examined by computer simulation the ability of three forms of plasticity at mossy fiber synapses in the (deep) cerebellar nucleus to contribute to learning and memory storage. The results suggested that, in the presence of reasonable patterns of "background" cerebellar activity, only one form of plasticity allowed for the retention of memories, namely, plasticity controlled by the activity of the Purkinje cell, which was resistant to ongoing activity in the circuit. For plasticity at the synapses of mossy fiber collaterals controlled by the nucleus or by collaterals of climbing fibers, the circuit was unable to retain memories because of interactions within the network that produced spontaneous drift of synaptic strength. The results further suggested that the stability of synaptic weights derives from a self-regulating equilibrium of climbing fiber activity controlling LTP/LTD in the cerebellar cortex and a similar equilibrium of Purkinje cell activity controlling LTP/LTD in the nucleus. For climbing fibers, this equilibrium was considered to depend on circuitry that allowed the Purkinje cell to regulate the activity of its single climbing fiber input.

7.3.5. Regulation of Synaptic Efficacy by Coincidence of Postsynaptic APs and Unitary EPSPs

Markram et al. (1997) reported that the coincidence of postsynaptic APs and unitary EPSPs in cerebral cortical pyramidal cells induced changes in EPSPs. Their average amplitudes were differentially up- or downregulated, depending on the precise timing of the postsynaptic APs relative to EPSPs. The authors concluded that these observations suggest that APs propagating back into dendrites serve to modify single active synaptic connections, depending on the pattern of electrical activity in the pre- and postsynaptic neurons.

7.3.6. Number of Climbing Fibers and Receptors on Purkinje Cells in Relation to Number of Parallel Fibers

In connection with parallel fiber–Purkinje cell dendrite synapses, Takács et al. (1997) found that, despite an induced decrease in the number of parallel fibers (to the extent that many postsynaptic Purkinje cell dendritic spines were devoid of parallel fiber input), a decrease in the number of the corresponding Purkinje cell receptors did not occur (i.e., metabotropic glutamate receptor type 1a [mGluR1a]). This result indicated that the expression and subcellular distribution of these receptors are inherent, genetically determined properties of Purkinje cells. These authors reiterated the difference in the sites of termination of climbing fibers (i.e., onto the "stubby" spines on the primary and secondary dendritic branches of Purkinje cells) and the sites of termination of the parallel fibers (i.e., onto the tertiary "spiny branchlets"), which account for more than 95% of the axonal input to the Purkinje cells.

A reciprocal trophic interaction between climbing fiber terminal arborizations and Purkinje cells was found by Strata et al. (1997), such that when the climbing fiber is missing, the Purkinje cell undergoes a hyperspiny transformation and becomes hyperinnervated by parallel fibers. However, this change was found to be reversible. The climbing fiber-deprived Purkinje cell is able to elicit sprouting of nearby intact climbing fibers, and the new arbor is able to restore synaptic connections fully.

7.3.7. Rebound Potentiation of Inhibitory Synapses on Purkinje Cells

Kano et al. (1992) reported a new form of Purkinje cell plasticity (in addition to LTD) in which stimulation of the (excitatory) climbing fiber synapses is followed by a long-lasting (up to 75 min) potentiation of inhibitory synapses on the Purkinje cells, a postsynaptic phenomenon that the authors termed *rebound potentiation*. Normally, the authors suggested, spontaneous climbing fiber activity maintains the inhibitory (GABA$_A$) receptor sensitivity at a high level, but in the absence of climbing fiber activity, the GABA$_A$ receptor sensitivity and, therefore, the efficacy of inhibitory synapses decreases, causing the observed increase in excitability of Purkinje cells. The authors pointed out that the phenomenon of rebound potentiation of inhibitory synaptic currents itself, as well as LTD, may have an important role for learning in the cerebellum.

7.4. LTD Induced by Climbing Fibers Alone

In the classic Marr–Albus–Ito models of cerebellar function (Chapter 13), conjoint activation of the climbing fiber (inducing a massive, unvarying response) and parallel fiber synapses (inducing graded responses) onto Purkinje cells result in LTD (i.e., decreased efficacy of the parallel fiber synapses). Hansel and Linden (2000) reported that the climbing fiber synapse itself can also express LTD following brief tetanic stimulation at 5 Hz. As possible consequences of such climbing fiber LTD, the authors mentioned the following: (1) an alteration of Purkinje neuron throughput, as evidenced in its firing probability and/or in the subsequent pause; (2) modification of the cerebellar network function through modulation of dendritic integration and heterosynaptic (climbing fiber, parallel fiber) processes; and (3) modification of the process of pruning of multiple climbing fibers to each Purkinje neuron.

7.5. LTP at Mossy Fiber–Granule Cell Synapses

D'Angelo et al. (1999) reported that high-frequency mossy fiber (MF) stimulation paired with granule cell (GrC) membrane depolarization induces a stable N-methyl-D-aspartate (NMDA) receptor-dependent enhancement of synaptic transmission (i.e., MF–GrC LTP). The authors indicated that LTP at the MF–GrC synapse, previously assumed to be unmodifiable, provides the cerebellar network with a large additional reservoir for memory storage, in view of the 10^{11} granule cells and four times as many MF–GrC synapses, which may be necessary to optimize pattern recognition and, ultimately, cerebellar learning and computation.

EIGHT

The Vestibulocerebellum and the Oculomotor System

8.1. The Flocculonodular Lobe (the Vestibulocerebellum)

The flocculonodular lobe is the oldest part of the cerebellum (i.e., the archicerebellum). It occupies the major portion of the primitive cerebellum (e.g., in the lamprey and urodele amphibia; Nieuwenhuys 1967), as indicated in Chapter 2. Further, it is with the flocculonodular (posterior) lobe of the cerebellum that the vestibular nuclei of the brain stem are most closely associated (Brodal and Jansen 1954). Correspondingly, among the afferent fibers to the flocculonodular lobe, the vestibular ones are the most significant. Primary or direct vestibular fibers (i.e., from the end-organ, the vestibular organ) reach the flocculus, nodulus, and the adjoining part of the uvula, as well as the fastigial nucleus and the lingula. Of these, the nodulus is a later phylogenetic development than the flocculus. It appears that, whereas primary vestibular fibers decrease in phylogenesis, secondary fibers undergo an increase.

In a study of the climbing fiber projection to the rat flocculus and adjacent ventral paraflocculus, Ruigrok, Osse, and Voogd (1992) found that two parts of the inferior olive (the dorsal cap of Kooy and the ventrolateral outgrowth) are both connected with a set of two alternating zones of floccular/ventral parafloccular Purkinje cells, suggesting that these zones reflect functionally distinct and discrete units related to specific aspects of visuomotor control. As is the case for the newer part of the cerebellum, the flocculus also exhibits a zonal organization into longitudinal strips (or, more exactly, orthogonal to the long axis of the folia) of its input climbing fibers and its output Purkinje fibers to vestibular nuclei (Graf, Simpson, and Leonard 1989; Simpson, Van der Steen, and Tan, 1992; Tan, Epema, and Voogd 1995; Tan, Gerrits, et al. 1995; Tan, Simpson, and Voogd 1995).

Efferent fibers from the flocculus terminate only in vestibular nuclei, whereas those from the nodulus terminate in the reticular formation, the fastigial nucleus, and the vestibular nuclear complex.

In their extensive review of the anatomical organization of the vestibulocerebellum (Fig. 3.1), Voogd, Gerrits, and Ruigrok (1996) stressed its modular organization, which makes the prefix "vestibulo" something of a misnomer, derived as it was from one particular mossy fiber input and from the anatomical designation for one of its main output stations.

8.2. The Vestibulo-Ocular Reflex

The vestibulo-ocular reflex (VOR) serves to reduce the movement of visual images on the retina (i.e., retinal or visual slip) during head movement. According to Ito's (1970) original flocculus hypothesis of the VOR control (see below), it is the H zone (of the flocculus) that adaptively controls the gain of the horizontal VOR, by reference to retinal errors.

8.2.1. The VOR as a Potential Model for Cerebellar Function

The VOR, in providing the reflexive compensatory eye movements induced by head movements, is based primarily on a three-neuron arc composed of primary vestibular neurons, secondary vestibular neurons, and oculomotor neurons (see Ito 1982a, for a brief history and an early review). However, the reflex also involves the cerebellum, and it is not only the oldest but also the simplest of the neuronal systems in which the cerebellum is involved. The VOR does not entail the additional complexities of input either from the limbs or from the cerebral cortex. It is for this reason that it is selected for more detailed consideration than are the functions of the spinocerebellum and the cerebrocerebellum.

In view of the above-mentioned relative simplicity, a detailed examination of the VOR may provide clues to the basic function of the cerebellum in its more complex functions in the control of voluntary movements (e.g., of the limbs; Graf, Simpson, and Leonard 1989; Stone and Lisberger 1989). Thus, Ito (1972) proposed that the cerebellar theories of Marr (1969) and Albus (1971; see Chapter 11) be tested with the VOR. Ito (1998) remarked that the VOR, because of its close relationship with the cerebellum and its marked adaptiveness, has become a model system for studying the functions of the cerebellum. Raymond and Lisberger (2000) pointed out that motor learning in the VOR is a simple form of learning, but it has many parallels at the behavioral and circuit level with other forms of cerebellum-dependent learning (see, e.g., Raymond, Lisberger, and Mauk 1996). In view of these parallels, and in view of the highly uniform architecture of the cerebellum, the authors suggested that by studying a simple and tractable system like the VOR, general principles may be uncovered that apply to the cerebellum as a whole, and that such principles may in time be applied to understanding the role of the cerebellum in more complex behaviors, perhaps even in nonmotor functions. In this text, this well-established tradition, of primary emphasis on the vestibulocerebellum for the reasons just cited, is followed.

8.2.2. Mechanisms of the VOR and Its Gain Change (Plasticity)

It has been found that the simple spike firing rate of the majority of Purkinje cells in the monkey flocculus is a neural analog of eye velocity relative to the world (i.e., gaze velocity; Lisberger and Fuchs 1978a, 1978b; Miles et al. 1980). Two mossy fiber signals affecting the firing of these Purkinje cells were found: the one encoding eye velocity with respect to the head, and the other the head velocity with respect to the world, so the output of these Purkinje cells encodes the linear (vector) addition of these two signals (i.e., gaze velocity).

8.2.3. Effects of Cerebellectomy

Grossly, the VOR appears to be unaffected in the cat and monkey after total cerebellectomy (Robinson 1981). Both slow and quick phases of eye movements seem superficially normal; however, on attempted sustained lateral gaze, a slow drift back to the primary position occurs. There is also a deficit in the ability to use vision to modify eye velocity during the VOR. But the most dramatic change after cerebellectomy or a lesion of the vestibulocerebellum (primarily the flocculi and nodulus) is the complete loss of adaptive plasticity of the gain of the VOR. Accordingly, one function of the vestibulocerebellum is evidently to use vision to effect corrections of irregular vestibulo-ocular movements as well as to make long-term plastic adjustments of the reflex. These adjustments are normally made by several reciprocal, vestibulocerebellar connections (Fig. 3.1). Thus, the primary vestibular afferents send collaterals to the vestibulocerebellum, and there are reciprocal connections between this structure and the vestibular nuclei and the prepositus (hypoglossi) nucleus.

8.2.4. Plasticity of the VOR, Its Site(s), and Mechanisms

The gain of the VOR for monkeys and cats is normally close to 1.0 in its operating range, so that eye velocity compensates rather closely for head velocity. (For rodents (rabbits), the vestibulocollic (neck) reflex also contributes substantially to the ocular compensation for head movement. In the latter, the VOR itself has a gain as low as 0.3–0.5, whereas the sum of the VOR gain and the vestibulocollic (head-stabilizing) reflex gain reaches a level of 1.0. However, the reflex operates basically in open-loop fashion, and there is no immediate corrective feedback path. The result is that the image on the retina shifts its position in the absence of correct compensation (retinal slip). Correction does take place, however, via vision: the gaze error resulting from wearing telescope glasses is corrected for in about 5 days. The reversal of vision resulting from reversing (Dove) prisms results in a reversal of the reflex (i.e., the direction of gaze becomes the opposite of normal).

8.2.5. The Flocculus Hypothesis

Ito (1972, 1982a) suggested the cerebellum as the neural substrate for this plasticity, and a chain of pathways was soon discovered from the retina through the dorsolateral

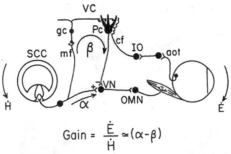

$$\text{Gain} = \frac{\dot{E}}{\dot{H}} \approx (\alpha - \beta)$$

Figure 8.1. Simplified version according to Robinson (1976) for Ito's (1972) hypothesed basis of adaptability of gain of the VOR. Output of semicircular canal (SCC) projects directly to vestibular nucleus (VN) with gain α and indirectly via mossy fibers (mf), to granule cells (gc), parallel fibers, and Purkinje cells (Pc) in the vestibulocerebellum (VC) with gain β. Retinal image slip signal is conveyed from retina via accessory optic tract (aot) through nucleus of optic tract (not labeled) and inferior olive (IO) to Purkinje cells via climbing fibers (cf). If cf activity could change mf-Pc synaptic gain β, the gain of the entire reflex could be changed to eliminate retinal slip during head movements. $\dot{E}$, eye velocity; $\dot{H}$, head velocity; (gain $\alpha = \dot{E}/\dot{H}$), OMN, oculomotor nucleus. (From Robinson 1976; in *Journal of Neurophysiology,* Vol. 39, copyright 1976, American Physiological Society; reprinted by permission of the publisher and author.)

part of the accessory optic tract to the tectal nucleus of the optic tract, thence via the central tegmental tract to the inferior olive, and thence to the flocculus via climbing fibers (Maekawa and Simpson 1973). This pathway conveys direction-specific information about movement of large parts of the visual world (Simpson and Alley 1974). (In a subsequent report, Maekawa and Takeda [1975] found that impulses from the optic nerve also activated the dorso-rostral portion of the flocculus via mossy fibers. Thus, it was suggested that the mossy fiber pathway from retina to flocculus acts as a visual feedback pathway to the VOR system.) Balaban, Kawaguchi, and Watanabe (1981) reported that neurons in the dorsal cap of Kooy of the inferior olive, which receive retinal input and project (as climbing fibers) to the flocculus, also send collaterals to the vestibular nuclei.

8.2.6. Long-Term Depression as a Mechanism for Adaptation of the VOR

Ito's flocculus hypothesis of VOR control proposed that retinal error signals induce long-term depression (LTD; Chapter 7) and associated processes within the flocculus, leading to improved performance of the VOR by minimization of retinal error (Ito, 1982a, 1984, 1993b). The retinal image movement is reported to the flocculus in three dimensions, the preferred axes of which parallel rather closely those of the semicircular canals (Simpson, Graf, and Leonard 1989; Simpson, Van der Steen, and Tan 1992).

Corroborative evidence for Ito's hypothesis was originally adduced by Robinson (1976), who provided a simplified version (Fig. 8.1) of Ito's original diagram. Evidence for a mechanism for the plasticity that permitted bidirectional changes was described by Ito (1976b, 1984), as shown in Figure 8.2. Ito (1984) considered that the flocculus hypothesis for plasticity of the VOR is of general applicability among different species.

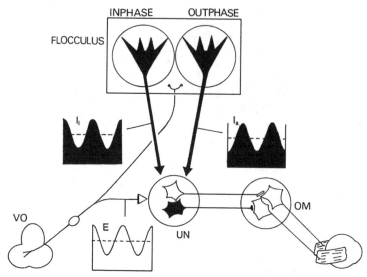

Figure 8.2. Modification of the VOR by in-phase and out-of-phase responses of flocculus Purkinje cells. E, spike density histogram for the primary vestibular afferent impulses; I_i and I_a [I_o], same but for in-phase and out-of-phase Purkinje cell discharges, respectively. Note that when superimposed in second-order vestibular neurons (UN [VN]), I_i cancels E, whereas I_a [I_o] reinforces E. VO, vestibular organ; OM, oculomotor nucleus. (From Ito 1984, *The Cerebellum and Neural Control*, copyright 1984, Lippincott Williams and Wilkins; reprinted by permission of publisher and author.)

8.2.7. Alternatives to the Floccular Hypothesis

A view different from that of Ito's flocculus hypothesis of the VOR was proposed by Miles and Lisberger (1981), who concluded that the available evidence indicated that the modifiable elements underlying the long-term adjustments in the VOR are located in brain stem vestibular pathways rather than in the floccular lobes. These authors did, however, conclude that the flocculus does appear to have an important, inductive role in the adaptive process, providing at least part of the error signal that guides the long-term adjustments in the brain stem.

Ito (1993a) reviewed the evidence supporting the floccular hypothesis of VOR control, and commented on opposing views particularly in relation to the anatomy of the flocculus and paraflocculus and the relative predominance of eye velocity signals and vestibular signals in mossy fiber input to the flocculus. (These questions are considered further below.)

Also as an alternative to Ito's (1970) original view that the flocculus acts as a variable gain element to regulate brain stem neuronal activity producing the VOR was the suggestion of Pastor, De la Cruz, and Baker (1997). From recordings of Purkinje cells during short-term adaptive changes of the VOR induced by oscillating goldfish in a moving visual surround that modified the ratio of eye to head velocity (gain), these authors concluded that the actual site of adaptive plasticity lies in brain stem VOR and optokinetic nystagmus (OKN) sites rather than in the cerebellum itself, but under the influence of Purkinje cells. It was proposed that the latter cells

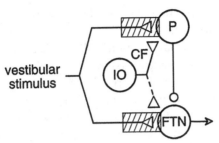

Figure 8.3. Simplified circuit diagram for the VOR according to Raymond and Lisberger (1997). The putative sites of plasticity are indicated by the shaded regions. Three neural signals converge at each site: the activity of inputs driven by the vestibular stimulus, the activity of climbing fibers (CFs) from the inferior olive (IO), and the simple spike activity of Purkinje cells (P). (FTN), flocculus target neuron in the vestibular nucleus. The dashed climbing fiber collateral to the FTN indicates that this connection may exist but is not well described. (From Raymond and Lisberger (1997); in: *Learning and Memory*, Vol. 3, copyright 1997, Cold Spring Laboratory Press; reprinted by permission of publisher and author.)

integrate corollary head and eye velocity signals to continuously adjust the setpoint in the brain stem sites.

In an analysis of recordings from neurons in monkeys concerning the neural basis for motor learning in the VOR (Lisberger, Pavelko, Bronte-Stewart, and Stone 1994; Lisberger, Pavelko, and Broussard 1994), which was supplemented by behavioral studies in monkeys wearing spectacles to vary the gain of the VOR, Lisberger (1994) concluded that the hypotheses of both Miles and Lisberger (1981; i.e., that the primary site of learning is in the brain stem) and Ito (1972; i.e., that learning occurs in the flocculus and is guided by the conjunction of vestibular mossy fiber inputs and visual climbing fiber inputs) were incomplete. A new hypothesis was proposed in which sites of motor learning in the VOR may lie both in the brain stem VOR pathways and in the vestibular inputs to the flocculus and ventral paraflocculus of the cerebellum.

In relation to the critiques offered by du Lac et al. (1995) of Ito's flocculus hypothesis (and of other models) of the VOR, and of long-term depression (LTD) as a mechanism for modification of the VOR, a series of experiments were suggested toward clarification of questions that the authors had raised in this controversial area (Ito 1993a; Lisberger and Seijnowski 1993).

8.2.8. Multiple Sites and Mechanisms of Plasticity of the VOR

In an overview of learning in the VOR, Raymond and Lisberger (1997) indicated the existence of two sites of plasticity: the first in the vestibular pathway to Purkinje cells in the floccular complex (flocculus and ventral paraflocculus) of the cerebellar cortex, and the second being at the vestibular inputs to neurons in the vestibular nucleus that are targets of inhibition from the floccular complex (floccular target neurons or FTNs; Fig. 8.3). The authors reiterate that it is the conjunction of head turns and image motion that causes motor learning. If image motion is in the same direction as head motion, then the learned change is a decrease in the gain of the VOR. If image motion is in the opposite direction from head motion, then the learned change is an increase in the gain of the VOR.

In examining different subclassifications of Purkinje cells in the floccular complex, such as "eye contraversive," "eye ipsiversive," "vestibular ipsiversive," and "vestibular contraversive," Raymond and Lisberger (1997) concluded that each subclass of Purkinje cells, which receive inputs from mossy fibers carrying vestibular, eye movement (efference copy or corollary discharge), and visual (image motion) signals, carried essentially the same information about required changes in the gain of the VOR. (The authors noted that the latency of the visual signal to the cerebellar cortex is about 100 milliseconds longer than the latency of the vestibular inputs, in contrast to about 20 milliseconds for the vestibular inputs themselves.)

Ito (1998) suggested that it is unlikely that VOR adaptation is retained in the rapidly transmitting (5–15 milliseconds) three-neuron arc, but the question of whether the late (20–45 milliseconds), modifiable responses are mediated in the flocculus, the brain stem, or both (as suggested by Raymond, Lisberger, and Mauk 1996) still remained unsolved.

In relation to mechanisms and models of the VOR, Lisberger (1996) listed several questions (none of which had straightforward answers). These were as follows: is it appropriate to model the memory mechanism as a change in the strength of synaptic transmission; is retinal slip required for learning the VOR; are there sites of learning for the VOR that are not sites of memory (i.e., Purkinje cells and brain stem cells, respectively); and can mechanisms of plasticity such as LTD function in the intact brain as well as in slices of brain tissue.

Raymond and Lisberger (2000) summarized their studies in the last few years on mechanisms of gain change in the VOR as follows. The VOR stabilizes images on the retina by using vestibular signals to generate compensatory smooth eye movements in the opposite direction from head motion. When image motion on the retina (retinal slip – an error signal) is present during head turns, motor learning adjusts the VOR to reduce image motion during subsequent head turns. The learning depends on the cerebellar–floccular complex, comprising the flocculus and ventral paraflocculus. The gain of the VOR is defined as the ratio of eye movement amplitude to head movement amplitude during head turns in total darkness (i.e., in the absence of visually driven, tracking eye movements that can occur in the light). For rhesus monkeys, VOR-driven eye movements are normally opposite in direction and approximately equal in amplitude to head movements, so the VOR gain is close to 1.0.

Learned changes in the gain of the VOR can be induced by pairing particular movements of the head with particular movements of a visual stimulus. In general, paired head and visual stimuli moving in the same direction induce a decrease in gain, whereas movement of the two stimuli in opposite directions result in an increase in gain. In this way, gains of 0 and 2.0, for example, can be induced in principle.

Raymond and Lisberger (2000) pointed out that previous hypotheses had proposed two different bases of plasticity during motor learning in the VOR: (1) the flocculus hypothesis (Ito 1972, 1982a), which suggested that plasticity in the circuit for the VOR was based on coincident activity in climbing fibers carrying visual signals and parallel fibers carrying vestibular signals (actually a combination of vestibular, visual, and eye-movement signals); and (2) the coincidence of activity in Purkinje cells and brain stem vestibular pathways (Miles and Lisberger 1981). Both hypotheses were based on results obtained with 5 Hertz or less sinusoidal oscillations (velocity profiles) for the visual and vestibular stimuli.

Extending the frequencies of the velocity profiles upward to 10 Hertz yielded results that were not in accord with either of the previous hypotheses. Two alternative new hypotheses were therefore proposed (Raymond and Lisberger 2000): (1) motor learning (i.e., a gain change) in the VOR is mediated by a single form of plasticity in which climbing fiber activity induces a change in the strength of the vestibular parallel fiber synapses about 100 milliseconds earlier (a timing constraint that appeared to be inconsistent with LTD but perhaps not other cerebellar cortical such as inhibitory mechanisms); and (2) multiple mechanisms of motor learning occur in the VOR.

In a detailed review, Ito (1998) summarized cerebellar learning in the VOR, including the history of the VOR going back to about 1930, when the VOR attracted the attention of anatomists and physiologists, including Magnus, Lorente de Nó, and Szentágothai, as a simple neural system mediated by a three-neuron arc. The VOR evokes eye movements in the direction opposite to head movement, thus serving to stabilize vision automatically relative to space. The complexity of eye movement directions in the VOR is matched by the complexity of the 12 muscles in the two eyes and of the 10 vestibular receptors (three semicircular canals and two otolith organs in each of the two labyrinths). Ito's review primarily considered the horizontal VOR.

More recently, the VOR arc has been reexamined, Ito (1998) indicated, because of its close relationship with the cerebellum, in particular, with the flocculus, an evolutionarily older part of the cerebellum. The VOR, therefore, provides a simple model system for studying the functions of the cerebellum. In about 1970, Ito proposed the flocculus to be a center of learning for changes in the VOR gain (Ito 1982a).

There are species differences: in rabbits and cats, the flocculus has 5 to 6 major folia, and in rats, usually only 1 folium (Ito 1998). In the classic anatomy of the monkey cerebellum, 10 folia have been described for the flocculus, but recent studies on neuronal connectivity have revealed that the rostral 5 belong to the ventral paraflocculus rather than to the flocculus itself. Thus, from study of the course of mossy fibers and climbing fibers to the cerebellar cortex in monkeys, Nagao et al. (1997) concluded that Purkinje cells in the ventral paraflocculus behave differently from those in the flocculus and are related to ocular movements following movement of the visual field and smooth pursuit (see below) of a moving target, but not to the VOR. Ito (1998) stressed the importance of identifying (e.g., by local electrical stimulation) a narrow zone of Purkinje cells of the flocculus, the H (for ipsilateral horizontal canal) zone, in relating data, obtained from the flocculus, to the horizontal VOR.

At the conclusion of his review of cerebellar learning in the VOR, Ito (1998) appended a series of three outstanding questions. First, does LTD account for long-term or even permanent memory? This question has not been answered because of technical difficulties that currently do not allow the time course of LTD to be followed for more than 3 hours. But this question is central to the cerebellar learning theories and, to answer it, new technologies for marking LTD are required. Second, is the memory in VOR adaptation controlled by the flocculus alone, by brain stem pathways, or both? Although the available evidence consistently indicates that the flocculus, with LTD mechanisms, plays a crucial role in induction of the VOR adaptation, a role of the flocculus in its retention still remains to be verified. If a brain stem pathway is involved, how can the adaptation induced in the flocculus be transferred to the brain stem pathway? Third, how can the functional role of oculomotor signals in the VOR be determined? The eye velocity and position signals in Purkinje cells in the flocculus might reflect feedback from the oculomotor system to the flocculus, or it might encode the inverse dynamics of the eyeballs. How might these two alternative possibilities be distinguished experimentally?

It is evident that, even for the relatively simple VOR, questions still remain; all the more so for trunk and limb movements, not to mention the question of cognition.

8.2.9. Roles of Mossy and Climbing Fibers in the Plasticity of the VOR

Given that the plasticity of the gain of the VOR is dependent on the vestibulocerebellum and on both mossy fiber and climbing fiber input, the question arises as to whether this control mechanism (for which the term *"recalibration"* has been used by some authors) sheds light generally on cerebellar cortical mechanisms (Ito 1984). The two fiber systems, mossy and climbing, convey distinctly different information from distinctly different sources to the cerebellar cortex. Mossy fibers convey information about head movement (actually, head velocity), and climbing fibers convey visual information about retinal slip.

For eye movement, Stone and Lisberger (1989) proposed a synergistic combination of visual input to the flocculus both via climbing fiber and via mossy fiber pathways to the flocculus. In this formulation, the high-gain mossy fiber pathways would respond to and act on large errors such as those encountered during the initiation of movement or during the response to sudden changes in trajectory, whereas the low-gain climbing fiber pathways would respond to and minimize the small errors encountered during steady-state motor performance. These authors considered that such a role for climbing fiber pathways did not exclude the possibility of a role for climbing fibers in long-term changes in mossy fiber–Purkinje cell synapses.

In other systems involving the cerebellum, the distinction between the origins of mossy fiber input and climbing fiber input are less clear, particularly when the diverse and overlapping origins of the two are taken into account, as is apparent from the listing of their respective sources (Chapters 4 and 5). Ito (1984, pp. 335–336) made the distinction between a feedforward (open-loop) system (e.g, the VOR), in which the climbing fiber system should have a signal source separate from that of the mossy fiber system, and a feedback (closed-loop) control system (e.g., optokinetic nystagmus), in which both climbing fiber and mossy fiber systems could have the same (retinal-slip) signal source, although the two could have separate transfer characteristics appropriate to their own roles.

In relation to the role of climbing fibers, Ito (1984, p. 338) viewed the inferior olive not so much as a comparator for generating an error signal from two different inputs, but rather as an encoder for error signals generated further downstream or upstream so as to generate irregular, low-rate climbing fiber discharges.

Against the background of a tentative general hypothesis that the principal role of the cerebellum, through its influence on motor systems, is to monitor and optimize the quality of sensory information entering the brain, Paulin, Nelson, and Bower (1989) considered the VOR to be a specific case in point, and suggested that the transfer function for the VOR should be capable of continuous and rapid change during head movements.

Finally, in relation to the question of "motor learning" (plasticity), Ito (1984) pointed out that this term implies both "adaptation" and "learning," which are not always clearly distinguished from one another. He also emphasized that "learning" implies more than "adaptation" and, borrowing from control theory terminology (in which both terms imply self-optimization of parameters), suggested that "learning" indicated an accelerating process with repetition of trials that is not implied by "adaptation" (compare the section on adaptation vs. skill learning in Chapter 6).

8.2.10. "Functional Flocculectomy"

Luebke and Robinson (1992, 1994) explored the effect in the cat of "functional flocculectomy" (i.e., the effect of repetitive stimulation of climbing fibers on "motor learning" in the VOR), on the basis that such learning should be abolished if the Purkinje cells are prevented from sending any meaningful signal to the motor target. It was found that, if the normal gain of 0.7 were doubled to 1.4, or halved to 0.35, no trend of a return to normal gain occurred as long as the flocculus was functionally disabled, but a return to a gain of 0.7 occurred in its usual time course upon termination of the functional flocculectomy. Thus, the functional flocculectomy blocked "motor learning." However, after 3-day adaptation to an altered VOR gain, blocking floccular output by 7-Hertz stimulation did not change the gain of the VOR, irrespective of initial values of 0, 0.7, or 1.4. The latter finding appeared inconsistent with storing of any kind of synaptic changes in the cerebellum (i.e., in the contribution of Purkinje cells to the VOR), and the authors were puzzled by this result, unless it was assumed that the changes occurred in the deep cerebellar nuclei (i.e., in this case, in the vestibular nuclei), as had been postulated by Miles et al. (1980).

Recently, Ito (1998) pointed out that there is an important technical problem concerning the exact site of stimulation to be kept in mind with the technique of "functional flocculectomy."

8.2.11. Oculomotor Neural Integrators

The conversion of eye-velocity commands, from the semicircular canals, for example, to eye-position commands for the motor neurons of the extraocular muscles necessitates a neural integrator. Arnold and Robinson (1997) described a neural network model that learns to simulate the integration process, to change its gain (by minimization of retinal slip), and at the same time to compensate for orbital mechanics

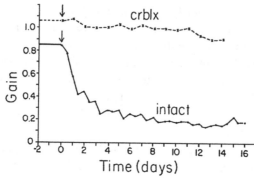

Figure 8.4. Time course of VO gain after cats begin to wear reversing prisms (arrows) without (lower curve) and with (upper curve) vestibulocerebellectomy. Note, in the latter, the lack of change of gain, which is also higher. (From Robinson 1981; in Brooks (ed.), *Handbook of Physiology, Vol. II, Motor Control, Part 2*, 1981, copyright American Physiological Society, Bethesda; reprinted by permission of the publisher.)

(see also Robinson 1989). The model includes an equal number (14) of excitatory and inhibitory neurons. The integration employs positive feedback through lateral inhibition conveyed by an inhibitory commissure.

The integrator action of the semicircular canals themselves, however, is imperfect, forming a leaky integrator with a relatively short time constant (Ito 1984). Thus, if a steplike increment of angular velocity is applied to the head, the discharge rate in primary vestibular afferents rises rapidly to a level determined by the magnitude of the velocity step. The discharge rate then begins to fall, returning to the baseline level after 10 to 12 seconds, thus signaling to the brain that the head is stationary even though it is still in motion. Another neural integrator (a velocity-storage integrator) thus becomes necessary, having an output lasting 30–60 seconds, which would result in sustained compensatory eye movements (Ito 1984), thus compensating for the leaky integrator action of the semicircular canals.

8.2.12. Climbing Fibers, Plasticity, and LTD

Climbing fibers are essential for the plastic changes in the VOR to occur. Either flocculectomy or olivary lesions abolished the plastic adaptation of the reflex in the rabbit or cat. The loss of the plasticity is illustrated in Figure 8.4 (see also Fig. 7.3).

In relation to the question of LTD and bidirectional (two-way) adaptation (i.e., increase and also decrease of the VOR gain), Ito (1993b) pointed out that the bilateral labyrinths each give rise to sets of parallel fibers that can independently undergo LTD out of phase.

Using the VOR as a model, Lisberger and Seijnowski (1992) demonstrated that changes in the transient component of a neuron's responses can be transformed into changes in the steady-state output of a neural network by the use of recurrent (feedback) connections (compare Robinson 1989).

A question related to that of plasticity of the gain of VOR is that of the nature and site of compensation for unilateral loss of vestibular nerve function, the nystagmus from which can disappear in about 3 days (Robinson 1981). A role of the vestibulocerebellum (although not necessarily of the fastigial nucleus), as opposed to purely brain stem mechanisms, was not clearly established.

8.3. The Optokinetic Reflex and Optokinetic Nystagmus

Fuchs et al. (1992) concluded that the then available evidence strongly suggested that the nucleus of the optic tract in primates, as in lower species, is the origin of the visual pathway for horizontal OKN. Cohen et al. (1992) reached a similar conclusion, noting that the activity of the nucleus is related to the slow component of optokinetic nystagmus, perhaps via a direct (but not demonstrated) or indirect projection to the eye-movement velocity storage mechanism (or more precisely, velocity-storage integrator [Raphan, Dai, and Cohen 1992]) in the vestibular system. The velocity-storage integrator itself (see also Arnold and Robinson 1997) is considered responsible for the dominant time constant of the VOR, the slow phase of the OKN, and for that of optokinetic after-nystagmus (OKAN, see below). It was considered that OKN can be viewed as the visual concomitant of angular head movement for stabilization of gaze in a lighted stationary environment, particularly in instances in which the gain of the VOR is not unity, or in instances in which it is inadequate for gaze stabilization because of rectilinear motion or vergence (Cohen et al. 1992). (Possible mechanisms underlying the gain changes of the optokinetic reflex [OKR] are discussed by Frens, Mathoera, and Van der Steen [2000].)

In a review, du Lac et al. (1995) stressed the importance of including the OKR and smooth-pursuit eye movements in discussions of the VOR because the former two visual tracking systems share circuitry with the latter. These authors proposed that modification ("memory") of the VOR is based not only on changes in the vestibular inputs via mossy fibers to Purkinje cells in the flocculus-paraflocculus, but also on changes in the vestibular inputs onto flocculus target neurons in the brain stem, especially for the earliest modified component of the VOR (see also Lisberger and Seijnowski 1992).

A series of lumped-system models for combined VOR and OKR extrapolated to the case of locomotor coordination by the cat's cerebellum (intermediate zone) was proposed by Boylls (1980).

8.4. Plasticity of Postrotatory Nystagmus and Optokinetic After-Nystagmus

There is also evidence of plasticity of the time constant of decay of the slow-phase velocity of postrotatory nystagmus or OKAN during exposure to a stationary visual surround (visual suppression); this plasticity is lost in monkeys after lesions of the nodulus and uvula (Waespe, Cohen, and Raphan 1985). It seems probable that there is a cerebellar flocculus sidepath for the brain stem OKR pathway and also for the cervico-ocular reflex, thus providing a basis for adaptation of these reflexes as well as for the VOR. The existence of such sidepaths would constitute a generalized "flocculus hypothesis of the coordinated ocular reflex control" (Ito 1984). In this connection, synchronous firing (i.e., within 2 milliseconds) of Purkinje cells in the

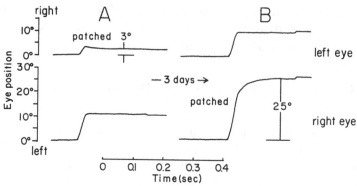

Figure 8.5. Saccadic plasticity. A monkey is trained to follow a spot that jumps by 10 degrees. (A) Its left eye is weakened by tenectomy and patched. That eye subsequently makes hypometric saccades one-third as large as those of the normal eye and with a backward postsaccadic slip (top left). (B) Three days after switching the patch, the weakened eye has regained ability to make correct (orthometric) saccades, whereas the good eye, under cover, makes hypermetric saccades with postsaccadic slip in the opposite direction (bottom right). This demonstrates that the central nervous system can repair dysmetria (created by a peripheral lesion) in this case by increasing gain (saccade size/retinal error) of the central part of saccadic system. (From Robinson 1981; in Brooks (ed.), *Handbook of Physiology, Vol. II, Motor Control Part, 2, 1981*, copyright American Physiological Society, Bethesda; reprinted by permission of the publisher. Modified after Optican and Robinson 1980; *Journal of Neurophysiology*, Vol. 44, 1980.)

vestibulocerebellum during rotational optokinetic stimulation of (ketamine-anesthetized) rabbits was reported by Wylie, De Zeeuw, and Simpson (1995).

8.5. Plasticity of Saccades

In addition to that for the VOR, there is also evidence for a cerebellar side loop for saccadic eye movements (Optican and Robinson 1980; Robinson 1981; Strata, Rossi, and Tempia 1995), as indicated in Figure 8.5. In that study (Optican and Robinson 1980), the tendons of both horizontal recti of one eye of monkeys were incised and then a patch placed over that eye. The muscles became reattached but the eye was permanently weakened; it only moved, for example, one-third as far as the normal eye. When the patch was switched to cover the normal eye, the saccades of the seeing (weak) eye were initially hypometric. Over the course of 3 days, however, the saccades of the weakened eye increased to the correct size. The eye under cover (the normal eye) now made excursions almost three times normal. After switching the patch back to the operated eye, the seeing (normal) eye initially made grossly hypermetric saccades, but they returned to normal in 1.5 days. It was found that the adaptive response to switching the patch was lost after total cerebellectomy or after large lesions of the midline cerebellum, including the vermis and paravermis of lobes V–VII and most of the fastigial nuclei. Optican and Robinson (1980) concluded that the principal contribution of the cerebellum to saccadic eye movement is the adjustment of the gains of the cerebellum for the eye movement during the saccades (i.e., the pulse-generating mechanism) and for the positioning of the eyes after a saccade (i.e., the stepgenerating mechanism).

Using a different experimental paradigm, Goldberg et al. (1993) also obtained failure of saccadic adaptation as a result of a lesion in the cerebellar nuclei (primarily the fastigius). It was concluded that the cerebellum provided the basis of the adaptation.

Kawano and Shidara (1993) concluded from several lines of evidence that the Purkinje cells in the ventral paraflocculus of the monkey play a role in the short-latency (of the order of 50 milliseconds), ocular-following response induced by constant-velocity motion of a random dot pattern on a backlit screen.

Starting from the point that damage to the cerebellar vermis results in permanent loss of accuracy of saccades, and also from the proposal that the vermis adjusts the gain of the saccadic internal feedback loop in response to information about the amplitude of the intended saccade, Dean, Mayhew, and Langdon (1994) and Dean (1995) described a model for producing fast and accurate saccades that includes burst firing in the fastigial nuclei (the output nuclei for the vermis) in conjunction with brain stem mechanisms. It was suggested that the same principle may underlie the cerebellum in generating fast movements of other parts of the body.

Their et al. (2000) reported, on the basis of single-unit recordings from saccade-related Purkinje cells in the cerebellar vermis in monkeys, that unlike individual Purkinje cells, the population response of large groups of Purkinje cells gives a precise temporal signature of saccade onset and offset, thus helping to determine saccade duration. In turn, modifying the time course of the population response by changing the weights of the contributing individual Purkinje cells, discharging at different times relative to the saccade, would directly translate into changes in saccade amplitude.

8.5.1. Site of Saccadic Adaptation in Humans

By use of positron emission tomography (PET), Desmurget et al. (1998) investigated the neurophysiological substrate of human saccadic adaptation, finding that metabolic changes attributable to the process of saccadic adaptation were localized to the medioposterior cerebellar cortex (i.e., in an oculomotor region of the cerebellar vermis from which Purkinje cells project to the fastigial nuclei). The authors concluded that plasticity in saccadic adaptation occurs in these Purkinje neurons.

8.6. Smooth (Predictive) Pursuit Eye Movements

Stone and Lisberger (1990) concluded that the gaze-velocity Purkinje cells (GVP-cells) of the monkey flocculus have two important roles in pursuit eye movements: (1) they contribute to the initiation of pursuit by relaying visual-motion inputs from extrastriate visual cortex to brain stem oculomotor structures, and (2) they appear to provide a positive eye-velocity signal that aids in maintaining steady-state pursuit.

A biologically based neural-network cerebellar model for predictive smooth pursuit eye movements using complex two-dimensional trajectories was described by

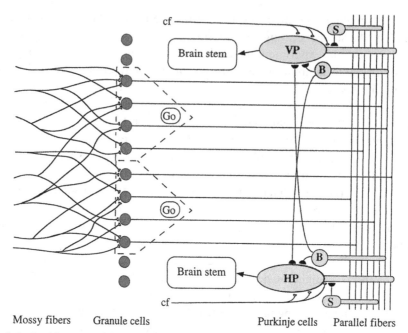

Figure 8.6. Architecture of the cerebellar model for predictive smooth pursuit eye movements. Mossy fibers are randomly connected to granule units. Dotted lines: hypothesized influence of Golgi (Go) cell receptive fields that allow only those granule cells with the highest activity to generate outputs. Axons from granule cells bifurcate into two parallel fibers that excite horizontal (HP) and vertical (VP) Purkinje units. Basket (B) and stellate (S) units receive excitatory parallel fiber input and inhibit Purkinje cells. The action of these unit types is collapsed into "Purkinje units" that allow both positive and negative "parallel fiber" weights. Climbing fiber (cf) inputs are used to train the network. (From Kettner et al. 1997; in *Journal of Neurophysiology*, Vol. 77, 1997, copyright American Physiological Society; reprinted by permission of the publisher.)

Kettner et al. (1997). The architecture of the model is shown in Figure 8.6, a block diagram in Figure 8.7, and results in Figure 8.8. Prediction was made possible by the inclusion of a temporary storage mechanism ("eligibility trace") at the site of alteration of synaptic weights (i.e., at the parallel fiber–Purkinje–dendrite interface) of the order of 100 milliseconds, which in effect compensated for the delay in arrival (via the climbing fibers) of the error signals arising from retinal slip, relative to the arrival times of the mossy fiber signals. Two Purkinje cells (in the flocculus/paraflocculus) were modeled, one each for horizontal and for vertical eye movements (Fig. 8.7). Results from testing the model, including with unperturbed (superimposed sinusoids) and perturbed (abrupt changes in direction) trajectories, were compared with results from monkeys using the same test trajectories, with close correspondence between the two. Tracking time lags of 8 milliseconds (model) and 20 milliseconds (monkey), increasing to 80 and 90 milliseconds, respectively, after perturbations of the trajectories. For computational simplicity, the parallel fiber-to-Purkinje unit weights were allowed to assume both positive and negative values, to simulate the combined direct positive activation via parallel fiber input and indirect negative activation via basket and stellate cells. The authors pointed out some similarities to other models.

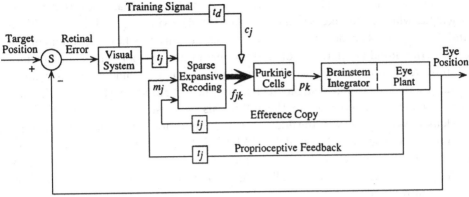

Figure 8.7. Block diagram of the cerebellar model for predictive smooth pursuit eye movements. (Although the brain stem integrator and the eye plant are modeled by the same set of equations in the model, these two functions are distinguished in the diagram to emphasize their different neural substrates and the idea that both proprioceptive and efference copy signals may provide eye position and velocity position.) All lines indicate the flow of multivariate information, with the heavier arrow indicating the wider bandwidth associated with the expansive recoding of mossy fiber inputs. Smaller boxes: pure delays. Open arrowhead: indirect action that climbing fiber training signals have on information throughput by the climbing fiber training signals as a result of the alteration of network weights via the learning rule. Visual input to the system is assumed to take the form of retinal error signals that are obtained by a subtraction at the node labeled S of target and eye position signals. (From Kettner et al. 1997; in *Journal of Neurophysiology*, Vol. 77, 1997, copyright American Physiological Society; reprinted by permission of the publisher.)

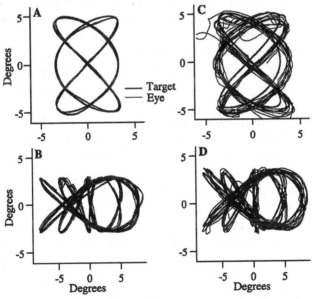

Figure 8.8. Comparison between tracking by the predictive smooth pursuit cerebellar model for eye tracking (A, B) and monkey eye tracking (C, D) along complex trajectories. Further details of the trajectories (Lissajous figures) are given in the original paper. (From Kettner et al. 1997; in *Journal of Neurophysiology*, Vol. 77, 1997, copyright American Physiological Society; reprinted by permission of the publisher.)

From recordings of single-unit activity from the fastigial nucleus of rhesus macaques while the monkeys visually tracked small moving targets, Fuchs, Robinson, and Straube (1994) concluded that the fastigial nucleus may have a prominent role both in the initial acceleration of smooth pursuit and possibly in its maintenance. Moreover, the presence of saccade-related neurons in this same area was believed to suggest that the caudal fastigial nucleus may have a global role in the acceleration of all conjugate eye movements. The authors also suggested that the caudal fastigial nucleus may cooperate with the flocculus in the generation of pursuit eye movements.

From inactivation studies with the GABA-agonist, muscimol, Robinson, Straube, and Fuchs (1997) concluded that the caudal fastigial nucleus of monkeys, like the flocculus-paraflocculus, is a cerebellar region involved in the control of smooth pursuit eye movements.

8.7. Ocular Following Responses

Kawano, Takemura, et al. (1996) reported that, in alert monkeys during ocular following responses (OFR) induced by sudden movements of a large-field visual stimulus of different velocities and durations, not only is visual information (i.e., concerning retinal slip) reported to Purkinje cells of the ventral paraflocculus (VPFL) by the pretectal nucleus of the optic tract (NOT) as a climbing fiber/complex spike input, but also by the dorsolateral pontine nucleus (DLPN) as a mossy fiber/simple spike input.

Yamamoto et al. (1997) described a mathematical model that reproduces ocular following responses and incorporates intermediate neural signals. The model consists of two systems: a nonlinear system relating retinal slip to simple spike firing frequency of Purkinje cells in the ventral paraflocculus (VPFL), and a linear system that relates VPFL simple spike firing frequency to eye movement. The authors reported that the model accurately reproduced the firing frequency of Purkinje cells and ocular following responses from visual stimulation paradigms used in physiological experiments.

To analyze quantitatively the relationship between ocular following responses and Purkinje cell simple spike firing frequency in monkeys, Gomi et al. (1998) employed an inverse dynamics representation of the eye movement for reconstructing the temporal waveform of simple spike firing of Purkinje cells of the ventral paraflocculus. It was concluded that the latter cells could not alone provide the necessary final motor command because, although acceleration and velocity were properly enclosed, the positional component correlated with eye movement in the opposite direction.

The same technique of inverse dynamics representation was also used to examine Purkinje cell complex spikes in the ventral paraflocculus (Kobayashi et al. 1998) during ocular following responses. Findings included that the spatial coordinates of the complex spikes were aligned with those of simple spikes, and the speed-tuning properties of complex spikes and simple spikes were more linear for eye movement than retinal slip velocity, indicating that the complex spikes contain a motor component in addition to the previously identified sensory component. It was concluded that complex spikes may contribute to long-term interactions between parallel and climbing fiber inputs, such as LTD and/or potentiation.

8.8. Maintenance of the Body Scheme

The vestibular nuclei receive visual and proprioceptive as well as vestibular information about head motion, and it is now clear that these nuclei are involved in spatiotemporal transformation allowing the measurement of head motion in space (Wiener and Berthoz 1993). Droulez and Cornilleau-Pérèz (1993, p. 491) drew attention to the relevance of Kalman filtering (Chapter 14) to the problem of multisensory fusion in the moving organism.

From study of a patient with a progressive lesion of the superior parietal lobe, Wolpert, Goodbody, and Husain (1998) advanced the hypothesis that an internal estimate of the state of both the world and of the body itself, based on sensorimotor integration, is optimally carried out as a recursive process of successive updating of the internal estimate, and that loss of such an internal estimate between successive updates (e.g., visual) results in symptoms such as failure of memory for the position of a limb.

NINE

The Cerebellum and Cognition

The importance of the cerebellum in relation to movement control has long been established, but in recent years, the question has been raised as to whether the cerebellum may also have a role in cognition or thought processes. In this chapter, this question, which has been at once intriguing and controversial (Barinaga 1996), will be considered, especially in view of the uniformity of cerebellar anatomy. From this uniformity, it would follow that the same basic type of computation that is performed in the vestibulocerebellum and the spinocerebellum would also be carried out in the neocerebellum (lateral cerebellum, cerebellar hemispheres). Assuming that the neocerebellum does participate in cognitive phenomena or is essential for such mental activities, interfacing the cerebellum with the cerebrum (cerebral cortex), and the specific nature of their joint transactions, is formidable. It is far beyond the reach of this text to venture solutions to these questions. Rather, this chapter summarizes some of the history and findings in relation to the question of the cerebellum and cognition. If signal adaptive control is indeed an appropriate model for the vestibulocerebellum and the spinocerebellum, and for the evidently motor functions of the cerebrocerebellum, then because cerebellar anatomy is essentially uniform throughout the "cognitive cerebellum," there would seem to be a high probability that those parts of the lateral cerebellum that appear to be involved with cognition are also functioning as adaptive controllers.

An extensive review of the field is provided in the text edited by Schmahmann (1997), comprising 28 papers by some 60 contributors. In this collection, cognition is understood to include thought processes such as executive function, learning, memory, visual analysis, and language. The topics of emotion, personality, and behavior are also included.

9.1. Some History: Earlier Reports

Leiner, Leiner, and Dow (1986) came to the conclusion that the cerebellum is involved not only with motor dexterity but also with mental dexterity or mental skills (i.e., cognitive processes). They based their conclusions on phylogenetic data (the parallel enlargement of the dentate nucleus and the frontal association areas of the neocortex), ontogenetic data (the parallel maturation of the cerebellum [at age 15–20 years] and mental capabilities), and clinical data (subtle deficits that escape routine examination upon testing patients with cerebellar lesions). The authors suggested tomographic brain scans on humans as a method for testing these new concepts. (For further elaboration on this theme by these authors and for additional references, see Leiner, Leiner, and Dow 1991.)

In this connection, Leiner, Leiner, and Dow (1991) drew attention to two parts of the dentate nucleus in humans and to a lesser extent in monkeys: a dorsal part, which sends projections to motor areas of the frontal cortex, and a ventral part (the "neodentate"), which sends projections to cognitive areas of the prefrontal cortex (Middleton and Strick 1994), the "cortex of cognition" (Goldman-Rakic 1995).

It is the ventral part of the dentate, the neodentate, that the authors attribute participation in cognitive operations such as counting, timing, sequencing, predicting, anticipatory planning, error detecting and correcting, shifting of attention, adaptation, and learning, all in the scope of a general computational function of the cerebellum (Leiner, Leiner, and Dow 1991). (In a commentary, Bower [1995] suggested that the latter formulation was too broad and, at the same time, reemphasized the view of the cerebellum as coordinating the acquisition of sensory data [see Chapter 13], rather than coordinating movement as such.)

In addition to the appreciably enlarged cerebellum and association areas of the cerebral cortex in humans as compared with the higher apes, Leiner, Leiner, and Dow (1987) drew attention to the relative decrease in the size of the magnocellular part of the red nucleus, in relation to adaptive mechanisms in manipulation of symbols in cognitive functions.

9.2. Anatomical and Physiological Studies

The sources of anatomical projections to the pontine nuclei from neocortical association areas that have been demonstrated in rhesus monkeys include posterior parietal (Schmahmann and Pandya 1989), superior temporal sulcus and superior temporal (Schmahmann and Pandya 1991), and prefrontal (Schmahmann and Pandya 1997a) regions. It was suggested by these authors that the cerebellum may be an essential node in the distributed corticosubcortical neural circuits for cognitive operations.

On the basis of combined anatomical and physiological studies in monkeys, and using a new technique of transneuronal transport of herpes simplex virus (e.g., from prefrontal cortex retrogradely to the dentate nucleus via the thalamus), Middleton and Strick (1997) concluded that cerebellar output influences skeletomotor, oculomotor, and prefrontal regions of the cerebral cortex, and that each cortical field receives input from a distinct region of the respective cerebellar nucleus (i.e., the dentate). It was suggested that cerebellar output channels to the prefrontal cortex may be involved in cognitive aspects of behavior such as working memory. Such a view would challenge the traditional one that the cerebellum is confined to the coordination of motor activities, the authors concluded.

According to Middleton and Strick (1998), the cerebellum, via its nuclei, projects not only to the primary motor cortex, but also to the premotor and prefrontal cortex. Further, there is evidence for reciprocal projections from neocortical areas to the cerebellum. These authors have given the name "output channels" to the distinct clusters of neurons in the cerebellar nuclei from which the projections to the cerebral cortex originate. In addition, it was considered that the neuroanatomical substrate exists for cerebellar dysfunction to contribute to some of the cognitive deficits in neuropsychiatric disorders (Middleton and Strick 1998).

In a review challenging the view that basal ganglia and cerebellum are solely concerned with motor control, Middleton and Strick (2000) concluded that it is now apparent (from anatomical studies in animals and from imaging studies in humans) that there are multiple cortical areas that are the target of basal ganglia and cerebellar output, including not only the primary motor cortex but also subdivisions of premotor (assumed to be cognitive in function), oculomotor, and inferotemporal areas. For the cerebellum, the prefrontal areas, including areas 9 (planning, working memory) and 46 (spatial working memory, but not the inferotemporal cortex), were considered by the authors to receive projections from the ventromedial dentate nucleus.

Concerning the question of possible cerebellar learning mechanisms in cognitive activity, Schmahmann (1996) pointed out a problem related to the origins of mossy fibers and climbing fibers, the ultimate interaction of which is presumed to lie at the basis of synaptic plasticity according to the Marr–Albus–Ito theory (Chapter 13). Thus, the input from the cerebrum to the red nucleus–inferior olive system (and hence, to the climbing fibers) appears to be predominantly motor in origin, whereas the pontine system (and thus the mossy fibers) receives motor and sensory, as well as associative and paralimbic, information from the cerebrum. The question therefore arises as to whether the red nucleus–olivary system can be involved in cognitive processing or whether additional pathways from the cerebrum to the red nucleus in humans will be demonstrated (Schmahmann 1996).

9.2.1. Clinical Studies

Schmahmann (1991) extensively reviewed clinical and laboratory data concerning possible involvement of parts of the cerebellum in higher activities, such as the cerebellar hemispheres (lateral cerebellum) in cognitive function or thinking. For future clarification of this area, special emphasis on more extensive neurobehavioral studies on patients with cerebellar lesions was emphasized. (In response, the importance of critical evaluations was stressed by Botez [1992]; see also the reply by Schmahmann [1992].)

An increase in the time interval required for voluntary shifts of selective attention (i.e., between auditory and visual stimuli) was found by Akshoomoff and Courchesne (1992) in patients with damage to the cerebellum, in comparison with a control group of normal subjects. The authors theorized that this function of the cerebellum may operate via its previously described sensory modulation properties (e.g., Crispino and Bullock 1984). The increased time required for voluntary attention shifts was compared with the increased reaction times to voluntary movement responses to sensory cues in patients with neocerebellar damage.

Silveri, Leggio, and Molinari (1994) reported a case of a right cerebellar infarct with right hemicerebellar syndrome and agrammatic speech consisting of production of infinitive forms instead of inflected forms, and omission of free-standing grammatic morphemes. The authors suggested that the cerebellum provides the temporal interplay among neural structures responsible for production of sentences.

The Cerebellar Cognitive Affective Syndrome: "Dysmetria of Thought." Schmahmann (1998) provided an overview of the cerebellum in relation to cognition and emotion, including (by analogy with dysmetria or incoordination of the limbs) "dysmetria of thought" (i.e., impairments of higher-order behavior) and such findings as difficulties with concept formation and visual-spatial disturbances.

Based on clinical and laboratory studies of 20 cerebellar patients, Schmahmann and Sherman (1998) characterized a "cerebellar cognitive affective syndrome," a constellation of behavioral findings that were clinically prominent in patients with lesions involving the posterior lobe of the cerebellum and the vermis. The changes included impairment of executive functions such as planning, set-shifting, verbal fluency, abstract reasoning, and working memory; difficulties with spatial cognition including visual-spatial organization and memory; personality change with blunting of affect or disinhibited and inappropriate behavior; and language deficits such as agrammatism and dysprosodia. The authors concluded that the constellation of deficits implicates disruption of cerebellar modulation of neural circuits linking prefrontal, posterior parietal, superior temporal, and limbic cortices with the cerebellum, and are engaged in motor, sensory, cognitive, affective, and autonomic activity.

9.3. Visuomotor Transformations

Stein and Glickstein (1992), in their extensive review of the role of the cerebellum in the visual guidance of movement, reiterated that, in the coordinate transformation required for converting the retinotopic array arriving at the occipital cortex to the myotopic (muscle-oriented) array of the ventral horn cells of the spinal cord, the posterior parietal cortex performs the first stage by associating the retinotopic visual signals with eye and head position, thus yielding an output denoting the location of targets with respect to the observer. This information, which is conveyed to the cerebellum, appears to indicate where a target is in terms of what eye or limb movement would be acquired to acquire it. The task for the cerebellum would then be to complete the transformation into the necessary coordinated contractions of the muscles that would be employed to execute it, the details of which are unclear (Stein and Glickstein 1992).

In the conclusion to their review of the role of the cerebellum in visual guidance of movement, Stein and Glickstein (1992) remarked that the basic processing function of the cerebellar cortex is to set up a plastic internal representation of the sensory-motor system under the benevolent instruction of the climbing fiber input.

From study of a patient with massive ipsilateral cerebellar stroke, Bloedel, Bracha, and Larson (1993) found that the data supported the notion that the cerebellum is essential, not for the initial learning of a tracing movement, but rather for performing the learned movement with the required rotation of the original image.

Jeannerod et al. (1995) pointed out the complexities entailed in the grasping part of reaching and grasping for an object. Its size and shape must be coded and transformed into a pattern of distal (wrist and finger) movements, a visuomotor transformation that in monkeys is carried out conjointly by the inferior parietal lobule (more globally) and by the inferior premotor area (in greater detail). The latter contains a basic "vocabulary" from which many dexterous movements can be constructed as coordinated-control programs. Correct execution of grasping, the authors pointed out, requires an intact (downstream) primary motor cortex (area 4). In primates, lesions of this area, as well as of the pyramidal tract, result in a profound deficit in the control of individual fingers, in contrast to lesions of the inferior parietal lobule, which typically result in misreaching with an awkward grasp that fails to take on the correct shape.

Timmann et al. (1996) reported that patients with cerebellar lesions are capable of substantially improving their performance of a complex motor task involving the recall of memorized shapes and the visuomotor control of a tracing movement. The authors concluded that it is highly feasible that the cerebellum plays a critical role during the acquisition of a task, but that this role is not necessarily linked with the exclusive storage of the critical memory engram within the cerebellum itself.

There is evidence (e.g., Wang et al. 1999) indicating the existence of two cerebral visual pathways in humans (i.e., a dorsal stream for spatial and motion vision, and a ventral stream for object and form vision). In this connection, Schmahmann and Pandya (1997a, 1997b) pointed out that primary or associative visual cortical areas concerned with the peripheral visual field, visual spatial parameters, and visual motion project to the pontine nuclei (and thence to the cerebellar hemispheres), whereas regions concerned with the central visual field and visual object identification do not. These differences may suggest that the former type of visual information requires some type of processing or transformation (e.g., of coordinates; see below) by the cerebellar hemispheres whereas the latter type of visual information does not.

Glickstein (1997) emphasized that damage to the massive dorsal stream of extrastriate visual areas projecting to the pontine nuclei, either at a neocortical level or en route, produces profound disturbance in visuomotor guidance. It was concluded that the visual guidance of the limb that survives occipitofrontal disconnection is evidently mediated via the cerebellum.

From a series of experiments with monkeys designed to clarify the putative role of the cerebellum in cognition (e.g., in relation to working memory), Nixon and Passingham (1999) concluded that, unlike the dorsal prefrontal cortex (area 46), the cerebellum is not essential for working memory or for the executive processes necessary for correct performance, although it may contribute to the preparation of responses.

In this connection, Eskandar and Assad (1999) reported on the dissociation of visual, motor, and predictive signals in the parietal cortex in monkeys trained to use a joystick to guide a spot to a target. Neurons in the medial superior temporal (MST) area were selectively modulated by the direction of visible moving stimuli, whereas neurons in the medial intraparietal (MIP) area were selectively modulated by the direction of hand movement. In contrast, the selectivity of cells in the lateral intraparietal (LIP) area did not directly depend on either visual input or motor output; instead, these cells appeared to encode a predictive representation of stimulus movement.

9.4. Somatosensory Stimuli: Self-Produced vs. Externally Produced

Blakemore, Frith, and Wolpert (1999) proposed that the extent to which a self-produced tactile sensation is attenuated (e.g., its tickliness) is proportional to the error between the sensory feedback predicted by an internal forward model (Chapter 16) of the motor system (from the "efference copy" or "corollary discharge" of the motor command) and the actual sensory feedback produced by the movement (i.e., the "reafferenz").

9.5. Imaging Studies

Particularly in view of the drawbacks of earlier atlases of the cerebellum, a significant advance has been made by Schmahmann et al. (2000) in the form of the recently published magnetic resonance imaging (MRI) atlas of the cerebellum. In compiling the atlas, the authors paid particular attention to the difficult problem of terminology.

In a survey of 275 positron emission tomography (PET) and MRI studies of imaging of cortical and subcortical structures of a large variety of different cognitive tests (e.g., attention and working memory, language and semantic memory retrieval, episodic memory encoding/retrieval, priming, and procedural memory), Cabeza and Nyberg (2000) found that, among subcortical structures, the cerebellum was consistently activated in several different types of cognitive processes (in contrast to the basal ganglia, for which activations were common only during motor-skill learning).

A diversity of imaging studies on the cerebellum and cognition have been carried out, as indicated by the following.

PET Study of Cerebellar Timing Functions. Jueptner et al. (1995), using PET to examine regional cerebral blood flow (rCBF) in a cerebellar timing function, found that during simple finger movements there was increased activation of the inferior parts of the ipsilateral cerebellar hemisphere in comparison with the resting condition, but that during similar finger movements carried out to signal lengths of time intervals, additional activations of the cerebellar vermis and both cerebellar hemispheres, indicating to the authors that the cerebellum is involved in timing tasks separable from motor tasks (finger movement). (See also Chapter 10.)

Finger Movement Rate and rCBF. Evidence of a relation between rCBF and the frequency of timed repetitive flexion of the right index finger against the right thumb was reported by Sadato et al. (1996). It was found that the left primary sensory cortex and the right (superior) cerebellum showed no significant activation at very slow rates (0.25 and 0.5 Hertz), a rapid increase of rCBF with increasing rates up to 2 and 2.25 Hertz), but no further increase at 3 and 4 Hertz. In contrast, the posterior supplementary motor area (SMA) shows a reverse trend – highest activation at very slow rates but no significant activation at the very fast rates. In a related study using rCBF with PET, resting activation levels were compared with those for increasingly complex sequential finger movements at 0.5 Hertz (Catalan et al. 1998). A large increase in activation from rest to simple repetitive movements was found, with the shortest sequence found in the contralateral primary sensory and premotor cortex, supplementary motor area, and ipsilateral cerebellar cortex, suggesting an executive role by these areas in running sequences. In particular, it was concluded that for voluntary limb movements, the cerebellum is clearly important for the temporal order of and precision in the execution of motor programs.

Motor Sequence Learning. In a PET study of motor sequence learning in which subjects learned sequences of key presses by trial and error, Jenkins et al. (1994) found that the cerebellum was activated both during learning of an unfamiliar sequence and while a well-practiced sequence was being executed.

Tactile-Stimulus–Generating Movements vs. Nontactile-Stimulus–Generating Movements. Using functional MRI (fMRI), Blakemore, Wolpert, and Frith (1999) found that the somatosensory cortex showed increased levels of activity when subjects were presented with tactile stimuli that were delivered externally as compared with stimuli that were self-produced. In the cerebellum, there was less activity associated with a movement that generated a tactile stimulus than with a movement that did not, a difference that suggested that the cerebellum is involved in predicting the specific sensory consequences of movements and in providing the signal that is used to attenuate the sensory response to self-generated stimulation. The hypothesis that activity in the cerebellum contributes to the decrease in somatosensory cortex activity during self-produced tactile stimulation received confirmation from results indicating that activity in the thalamus and in primary and secondary somatosensory cortices correlates with activity in the cerebellum when tactile stimuli were self-produced but not when they were externally produced. This result was considered to support the proposal that the cerebellum is involved in predicting the sensory consequences of movements, which in this study results in attenuation of the somatosensory response as a consequence of matching between the presumptive cerebellar-predicted and the actual sensory feedback for self-produced tactile stimuli. (See also Chapter 5, and Gellman, Gibson, and Houk 1985.)

MRI During Cognitive Processing with Pegboards. Kim, Ugurbil, and Strick (1994) employed MRI, with its greater resolution than PET, to explore activation of the dentate nucleus in normal subjects while carrying out a visually controlled task of simple shifting of a line of pegs, and while carrying out the task of solving a difficult pegboard puzzle. A large bilateral activation of the dentate was found during attempts to solve the pegboard puzzle, several times greater in area than that activated during simple movement of the pegs. The authors concluded that these results provided support for the concept that the computational power of the cerebellum is applied to cognitive functions as well as to the control of movement.

SPECT During Counting vs. Imagined Tennis Movements. A significant cerebellar activation (in addition to cerebral changes) during silent counting and during imagined tennis movements by normal subjects, employing rCBF (a measure of neuronal metabolism) using single photon emission computerized tomography (SPECT) was reported by Decety et al. (1990). The results suggested to these authors that the cerebellum may participate in pure mental activity and play a further role in the temporal organization of neuronal events related to cognition.

fMRI and Verbal Fluency. With fMRI of the human brain during tests of verbal fluency (nonvocal generation of words starting with a given initial letter) in right-handed normal subjects, Schlösser et al. (1998) found activation in the right cerebellum (and left prefrontal cortex) in comparison with a baseline task of simple counting.

PET During Processing of Single Words. In a study using PET for the processing of single words, Peterson et al. (1989) found activation in the right lateral inferior cerebellum, a region distinct from those associated with motor tasks, suggesting to the authors an involvement with a "cognitive" rather than sensory or motor computation.

PET and Cerebellar Pathology. In study of a patient with a PET-confirmed extensive damage to the right cerebral hemisphere with a variety of tasks involving complex nonmotor processing (e.g., rule-based word-generation tasks), Fiez et al. (1992) found that the patient's performance on standard tests of memory, intelligence, "frontal function," and language skills was excellent, but there were profound deficits in practice-related learning (e.g., in repetitive trials of verbs generated in response to presented nouns) and in the detection of errors. The authors concluded that the results suggest some cerebellar functions may be generalized beyond the purely motor domain.

9.6. Reservations Concerning the Role of the Cerebellum in Cognition

As indicated above, the question of cognitive functions of the lateral cerebellum, in conjunction with the neodentate in humans, has been controversial (e.g., Bloedel 1993; Glickstein 1993; Ito 1993c; Leiner and Leiner 1997; Leiner, Leiner, and Dow 1993a, 1993b; Thach 1996b, 1997).

An overview of imaging studies of language, learning, and memory (Desmond and Fiez 1998) included a discussion of the problems (e.g., the question of increased vs. decreased cerebellar activation after learning) and the limitations faced by those who use neuroimaging to investigate cerebellar function.

9.6.1. Failure To Find Cognitive Performance Deficits in Cerebellar Patients

A cautionary note on the interpretation of the results of cognitive function tests in cerebellar patients was raised by Helmuth, Ivry, and Shimizu (1997), who failed to find support for a role of the cerebellum in verbal learning or attention. However, these authors reiterated the view that the cerebellum has a special role in the internal representation of temporal information in cognitive functions. Thus, Ivry (1993) indicated that several lines of evidence (including that in healthy subjects there was a correlation between performance on movement and on perception tasks that required precise timing) implicated cerebellar involvement in the explicit representation of temporal information, although not necessarily in all timing tasks, or in more than some limited range.

9.6.2. The Need for Additional Data

Thach (1996b) indicated the need for caution in interpretations of PET studies concerning the cerebellum. Because PET activity is correlated with blood flow, and in turn with neural activity mostly in presynaptic terminals, activity at these afferent terminals could result in excitation, inhibition, or no change in activity of output nuclei. Thus, an increase in blood flow does not necessarily mean that the cerebellar output is active.

In relation to the cerebellum and cognitive activities, Thach (1996b) expressed the view that demonstration of pathways from the cerebellum to the relevant neocortical areas, or evidence that cognitive activity is impaired by cerebellar lesions, was still needed.

In relation to the question of nonmotor functions of the cerebellum, it should be pointed out that in humans the neocerebellum comprises about 90% of the cerebellar volume and is interconnected primarily with the cerebral cortex, most prominently with the central region and the posterior parietal cortex (Brodal and Bjaalie 1997; i.e., after removal of these regions, approximately two thirds of the nuclei are filled with heavy terminal degeneration). It was concluded that the major part of the corticopontine projection probably concerns limb and eye movements, especially movements under visual guidance. Other cortical areas projecting to the pontine nuclei and of possible cognitive significance, as summarized by Brodal and Bjaalie (1997), include the cingulate gyrus (e.g., initiation, motivation, goal-directed behavior, visuospatial and memory functions), the polysensory areas within the superior temporal sulcus, parts of the parahippocampal gyrus, auditory association cortex, and prefrontal area 9. However, these authors stated that projections to the pontine nuclei from most parts of the temporal lobe and the prefrontal cortex are either absent or minimal. Further, there is considerable divergence in the corticopontine system, so even very small volumes of cerebral cortex project to widespread parts of the pontine nuclei, terminating almost exclusively on dendrites. Yet, there is considerable convergence from the pontine nuclei to the cerebellar cortex, so axons from neurons in many parts of the pontine nuclei (totaling some 800,000 neurons in the cat) converge to a small volume of cerebellar cortex (e.g., a fraction of a folium).

To reiterate, Brodal and Bjaalie (1997) indicated that a particular cortical region has access to widely separated parts of the cerebellum (i.e., the neocerebellum), and that a particular part of the cerebellar cortex would receive convergent inputs from different parts of the cortex. These authors concluded that more precise determination of the amounts of corticopontine projections concerned with cognitive tasks, relative to those of more clearly motor-related tasks, is needed.

Ivry and Fiez (2000) presented a detailed critical discussion of hypotheses and experimental studies (including neuroimaging) relating cognition to the cerebellum. In their discussion, the authors noted that "No explicit models have been developed to explain how error-correction would be implemented in a cognitive task." They concluded as follows:

> In general, we have adopted a somewhat skeptical perspective, seeking convergence from anatomical, neuropsychological, and neuroimaging studies for the proper evaluation of the various functional hypotheses that have been developed over the past decade. We do not intend this skepticism to be taken as an attempt to dismiss these hypotheses. It is essential to maintain an open mind as researchers develop experiments that will allow strong inference and seek theoretical accounts that may integrate various hypotheses. At the same time, the conservative nature of evolutionary processes leads us to expect that there will be some continuity between the contributions of the cerebellum to motor control and the contribution of this structure to language and thought.

9.7. Theories of the Cerebellum and Cognition

9.7.1. Cognition, Context, and Cerebellum

By analogy with the concept that the motor cerebellum might combine simple movement elements and link them together to a novel stimulus or context, Thach (1998c) suggested that the "cognitive cerebellum" might also combine simple cerebral "cognitive units" into larger complexes, linking them by trial-and-error learning to a triggering context. This proposal could then be the basis for mental subroutines forming "background" to the "foreground of conscious thought." The operations in playing chess were given as an example.

9.7.2. Cognition and Adaptive Control

Parkins (1997) suggested that the concept of adaptive control, already applied to the cerebellum, be extended to the cerebrum, thus permitting a complementary interaction between the two in relation to cognitive processes.

9.7.3. Additional Theories

Additional theories concerning the cerebellum and cognition are considered in the latter part of Chapter 16, following the consideration of internal models. These theories include Wolpert and Kawato's multiple paired forward-inverse model and Kawato's bidirectional theory approach to consciousness.

TEN

Timing Functions, Classical Conditioning, and Instrumental Conditioning

10.1. Timing Functions

In a comparative study of normal controls and patients with cerebellar lesions, Ivry and Keele (1989) found a deficit both in the production and perception of timing tasks (i.e., an increase in the variability of performing rhythmic tapping) and increased difficulty in making perceptual discriminations concerning small differences in durations of a standard tone.

Based on consideration of results from experimental animals and normal subjects and from patients with cerebellar lesions in studies of classical conditioning, temporal conditioning to different time intervals, of rhythmic movements of fingers, judgments of the duration of brief tones, comparisons of the velocities of moving objects, and the like, Keele and Ivry (1990) raised the question of whether the cerebellum (or the cerebellum together with closely related structures) provides a common computation for diverse tasks, in particular, for time. The authors termed the concept an adaptive timing hypothesis.

Impaired perceptual judgments of the velocity of moving stimuli, but not of their position, were reported by Ivry and Diener (1991) by patients with cerebellar lesions; the difference was not attributable to eye movements. It was concluded that the results confirm the role of the cerebellum in perceptual functions requiring precise timing.

According to Ivry (1993) several lines of evidence, including that from healthy subjects, indicate there is a correlation between performance on movement and on perception that requires precise timing, which implicates cerebellar involvement in the explicit representation of temporal information. However, such evidence was not necessarily found in all timing tasks, or in more than some limited range.

In a review of the representation of temporal information in perception and motor control, Ivry (1996) suggested the possibility that both the cerebellum and the basal ganglia have a role in internal timing: the cerebellum operating over a relatively short temporal window and the timing functions of the basal ganglia being used in tasks spanning longer durations. As for mechanisms, the author mentioned the emphasis on network models, in which time is distributed across a set of neural elements the different elements of which provide an interval-based representation, as compared with the older concept that temporal codes rely on endogenous oscillatory processes.

In their review of the biological basis of time estimation and temporal order, Lalonde and Hannequin (1999) considered that it had been established, on the basis of tests of normal subjects and patients with brain lesions, that the cerebellum, the basal ganglia, and the prefrontal cortex are involved in time estimation (as evaluated by temporal discrimination, verbal estimation, temporal production, and temporal reproduction). In particular, the authors cited the hypothesis that the central timer is located in the cerebellum, while the planning abilities subserving the estimation of longer intervals are mediated by the prefrontal cortex.

Possible mechanisms underlying time perception and temporal processing were reviewed by Wittmann (1999), who associated temporal processing of intervals of a fraction of a second up to a few seconds with the cerebellum, and temporal processing of intervals from seconds to minutes with the basal ganglia. Correspondingly, an interval-based timing mechanism would apply to the cerebellum, and a clock-plus-counter system to the basal ganglia.

In contrast to the preceding reports, Harrington and Haarland (1999) concluded from a review of focal lesion, pharmacological, and functional imaging studies that there was less evidence for the proposal that timekeeping operations are supported by the cerebellum than for the basal ganglia.

In a review of the basis of movement initiation (e.g., in relation to reaction time [RT] determinations), Lalonde and Botez-Marquard (1997) suggested that the dentate nucleus triggers the onset of movement through the dentate-ventroanterior and ventrolateral (VA-VL) thalamic-motor cortex pathway. However, when this pathway is inactivated (e.g., by cooling), or perhaps even in intact animals under some conditions, alternate pathways, such as dentato-intralaminar thalamo-cortical, dentato–reticulo–spinal, and interposito–rubro–spinal pathways may take over.

To investigate possible differences between cerebellum and prefrontal cortex in temporal processing tasks, Casini and Ivry (1999) tested control participants and patients with either prefrontal or cerebellar lesions on temporal and nontemporal perceptual tasks under two levels of attentional load. Each trial involved a comparison between a standard tone and a subsequent comparison tone that varied in frequency, duration, or both. When participants had to make concurrent judgments on both dimensions, patients with frontal lobe lesions were significantly impaired on both tasks, whereas the variability of cerebellar patients increased in the duration task only. The authors concluded that the difference suggests that deficits in temporal processing tasks observed in frontal patients can be related to the attention demands of such tasks, whereas cerebellar patients have a more specific problem related to timing.

10.2. Classical and Instrumental Conditioning

In the paradigm of classical conditioning of the eyeblink conditioned response using a tone as the conditional stimulus (CS), followed by a puff of air as the unconditional stimulus (US), Mauk, Steinmetz, and Thompson (1986) obtained conditioned responses by replacing the unconditional stimulus with electrical stimulation of the dorsal accessory olive.

In an extensive review, Gluck, Reifsnider, and Thompson (1990) drew attention to the mutual relevance of neural-network (connectionist) models and adaptive signal processing (Chapter 14), on the one hand, and models for classical (Pavlovian) conditioning (including the eyeblink or nicticating membrane response) and adaptation to the vestibulo-ocular reflex (VOR) on the other hand, as well as the relevance of the cerebellum in such learning processes.

Lalonde (1994), reviewing evidence concerning instrumental (i.e., by reward or punishment, as opposed to classical or Pavlovian conditioning of reflexes) learning or conditioning in mice with genetic defects (i.e., lurcher, staggerer, nervous, Purkinje-cell degeneration mutants) and with stereotaxic lesions, and relating this evidence to findings in humans with heredodegenerative ataxias, concluded that there was emerging evidence that the cerebellum is involved in spatial and nonspatial instrumental learning tasks (e.g., water maze learning), an indication that the cerebellum has a role in spatial orientation.

From a series of conditioning experiments on forelimb reflex systems in cats in which the GABA agonist, muscimol, was used to inactivate the intermediate cerebellum temporarily, Kolb et al. (1997) concluded that classically conditioned reflexes elicited by aversive stimuli involve the cerebellum more globally rather than just the intermediate part.

Schreurs et al. (1997) reported localized learning-specific changes in dendritic membrane and synaptic excitability of Purkinje cells in rabbits that could be detected in slices 24 hours after classical conditioning (paired presentations of tone and periorbital electrical stimulation) in the intact animal. The authors suggested that long-term changes within Purkinje cells that effect such enhanced excitability may occlude pairing-specific long-term depression.

A review of the cerebellum and conditioned reflexes, with particular reference to the eyeblink/nictitating membrane response, appeared in Yeo and Hesslow (1998).

10.3. Conditioned Eyeblink Reflex: Learning in Cerebellar Cortex and Nuclei

The question of whether the cerebellar cortex is essential to eyeblink conditioning has been a much explored topic (e.g., Yeo and Hardiman 1992, who came to the conclusion that cerebellar cortical mechanisms are important for the learning and execution of the eyeblink reflex). Welsh and Harvey (1989) concluded that the results of their study reaffirmed the role in the cerebellum in regulating the sensorimotor processes necessary for conditioning. It was believed that deficits in learned responses observed after cerebellar lesions are secondary to a broader deficit in performance, including a sensory component and a motor component.

Based on a comparison of behavioral and physiological data on classical conditioning of the eyelid (eyeblink) response, and of motor learning in the VOR, Raymond, Lisberger, and Mauk (1996) suggested a three-element hypothesis: (1) Learning occurs in both the cerebellar cortex and the deep cerebellar nuclei; memories can be stored at both sites. (2) The component of learning that occurs in the cerebellar cortex is critical for regulating the timing of movements. (3) The output from the cerebellar cortex guides learning in the deep cerebellar nucleus; hence, learning that occurs in the cerebellar cortex can be transferred in part or completely to the respective cerebellar nucleus. One possibility suggested for the guiding mechanism was that of the simple spike output of Purkinje cells. A corollary of the hypothesis was that some sites of learning and short-term memory may not be sites of long-term memory.

From recordings from the cerebellar nuclei in cats during a complex operantly (instrumentally) conditioned forelimb movement in cats, Milak, Bracha, and Bloedel (1995) found that the task-related modulation of firing rates reached a peak at the time the task was first performed successfully, and then progressively decreased (but did not disappear) as the task became well practiced. The authors believed such a trend in the amplitude of modulation of firing rates is consistent with the view that the cerebellum participates in establishing and reinforcing a set or pattern of neural interactions required for effectively executing the desired task.

In further experiments, these authors (Milak et al. 1997) found that inactivation of the cerebellar nuclei (by means of the GABA antagonist, muscimol, particularly the interposed nuclei) resulted in appreciable impairment of, but not total loss of, cats' ability to execute the task. It was concluded that it is improbable that any single cerebellar nucleus is likely to be a critical storage site for the engram (memory) established during learning of the task.

In view of some earlier reports to the contrary, Krupa and Thompson (1997) reexplored in rabbits the question of whether reversible inactivation of the cerebellar interpositus nucleus completely prevents acquisition of the classically conditioned eyeblink response. It was found that learning was completely blocked by low doses of muscimol, and the animals subsequently acquired the conditioned response normally.

Svensson, Ivarsson, and Hesslow (2000) reported that an abrupt increase in intensity of the conditioned stimulus (CS) decreases the eyeblink conditioned response (CR) latency, but when the high CS intensity was maintained over several trials, the short CR latency gradually increased until the CR was again elicited at the unconditioned stimulus (US) onset. Investigation revealed that prerubral and precerebellar structures were not involved in the change of timing of the CR, indicating that cerebellum and/or postcerebellum structures are responsible.

10.4. Cerebellar Timing Mechanisms and Conditioned Eyeblink Response

In view of the apparent lack of delay lines of sufficient length in the cerebellar cortex for the necessary delays of up to 4 seconds required for modeling the classically conditioned eyeblink response, and considering that a slow neuron response seemed to be the most likely candidate, Fiala, Grossberg, and Bullock (1996) constructed a mathematical model based on activation of a metabotropic glutamate receptor second messenger system in Purkinje cells as a substrate for adaptive timing. In this way, the interstimulus interval between the onset of parallel fiber activity associated with the CS and climbing fiber activity associated with the US onset could be bridged.

Moore, Desmond, and Berthier (1989) employed a tapped delay line in conjunction with variable weights (at parallel fiber–Purkinje cell synapses, and also at parallel fiber–Golgi cell synapses) in their neural network model for the conditioned nictitating membrane (eyeblink) response in rabbits. The site of the delay line was assumed to be the pontine nuclei.

From their study of conditioned eyeblink responses in ferrets, Svensson, Ivarsson, and Hesslow (1997) concluded that the CS is transmitted through the mossy fibers and that the mechanism for timing the CR is situated in the cerebellum.

Considering the mechanism of eyelid conditioning (in which a neutral stimulus such as a tone is repeatedly paired with a reinforcing or US to promote the acquisition of a CR; the eyelids close in response to the tone alone), and saccadic eye movements (the rapid eye movements used to shift gaze from one direction to another), Mauk et al. (2000) concluded that the cerebellum influences movement execution by feedforward use of sensory information via temporally specific learning.

10.5. Conditioned Eye-Blink Response after Lesions of the Interpositus Nucleus

Lesions in the interpositus nucleus in rabbits have been reported to result in alteration (i.e., more poorly organized) of, but not elimination of, the eyeblink response in rabbits, suggesting that this nucleus may be involved in the production of important features of conditioned responding such as system timing function (Katz and Steinmetz 1997).

Poldrack and Gabrieli (1997), in a review of sites of long-term memory, cited the deep cerebellar nuclei (the interpositus nucleus, in particular) as being the site for the memory trace of the conditioned eyeblink response in both animals and humans.

Kim and Thompson (1997) provided evidence indicating that the cerebellum is essential for eyeblink (nictitating membrane) conditioning: lesioning, recording, stimulation, reversible inactivation, and brain-imaging studies. In particular, the authors cited evidence that reversible inactivation of the anterior interpositus nucleus and overlying cerebellar cortex by cooling, or by application of the GABA-receptor agonist, muscimol, or lidocaine (a local anesthetic), during training completely prevents learning of the CR, whereas inactivation of the efferents (superior cerebellar peduncle, red nucleus) does not prevent learning. The authors concluded that, in the absence of Purkinje cells, eyeblink conditioning is reduced significantly, and lesions of the interpositus nucleus block eyeblink conditioning completely in mice and other animals. Thus, it appeared that there might be a parallel or distributed learning system that can support eyeblink conditioning (i.e., that memory traces for eyeblink conditioning might occur in both the cerebellar cortex and the interpositus nucleus).

Thompson et al. (1998) concluded that the reinforcement or "instructive" or "teaching" pathway for eyeblink (nictitating membrane) conditioning is the inferior olive–climbing fiber projection system to the cerebellar cortex. (The authors determined that this conclusion applied in general to classical conditioning of behavioral responses learned with aversive US and was relevant to any behavioral response so learned [e.g., limb flexion, eyeblink, head turn] for all mammals, including humans.) This view was considered by the authors to be consonant with the classic theories of the cerebellum as a learning machine (e.g., Albus 1971; Brindley 1964; Ito 1972; Marr 1969), in which theories information about movement errors and aversive US were provided by the inferior olive–climbing fiber system, and information about movements, contexts, and other types of sensory information was held to be projected to the cerebellum via the mossy fibers, coming from the pontine nuclei and other sources that synapse onto granule cells in the cerebellar cortex, giving rise to parallel fibers. Blocking in eyeblink conditioning was considered by the authors (Thompson et al. 1998) to result from inhibitory feedback to the inferior olive from the interpositus nucleus.

Green and Woodruff-Pak (2000) concluded that the cerebellum – in particular, the ipsilateral interpositus nucleus in rabbits (and also apparently in humans) – is essential for the formation of the simple association between the CS and the US necessary in all eyeblink classical conditioning paradigms.

10.6. Models of Conditioned Eyeblink Reflex

Bullock, Fiala, and Grossberg (1994) proposed a spectral timing model of how the cerebellum learns adaptively timed responses (i.e., for variable interstimulus intervals for CS and US) during conditioned nictitating membrane (eyeblink) response (NMR) in rabbits. The spectrum, or range, of time intervals is based on the assumption that there is a range of rates of response of granule cells to the mossy fiber input. The granule cells in turn are inhibited after a correspondingly variable time via the Golgi cell–granule cell negative feedback loop. The ensemble of partially timed responses summate to generate an accurately timed population response. Long-term potentiation (LTP) of mossy fibers collaterals to interpositus nucleus cells are presumed to allow conditioned excitation of the adaptive gain of the response, whereas long-term depression (LTD) of parallel fiber–Purkinje cell synapses allows learning of adaptively timed reduction in Purkinje cell inhibition of interpositus nuclear cells and hence the conditioned NMR.

Mauk and Donegan (1997) proposed a model of classical eyeblink conditioning within the general framework of the Marr (1969)–Albus (1971) hypothesis and based on four primary hypotheses: (1) There are two cerebellar sites of plasticity. The first is at the cerebellar cortex among granule cell synapses onto Purkinje cells and at the climbing fibers, at which there is LTD (when there is a conjunction of granule cell axon and climbing fiber activation) and LTP (when granule cell axons alone are activated). The CS activates mossy fibers, the US activates climbing fibers. The second site of plasticity is at the interpositus nucleus, among collaterals of mossy fibers, Purkinje cell axons, and nuclear cells, at which LTD occurs when synapses of collaterals of mossy fibers decrease in strength (LTD_{nuc}) when active in the presence of strong inhibitory Purkinje cell input, whereas LTP occurs when the Purkinje cell input decreases transiently (LTP_{nuc}). The plasticity both at the cortex and at the interpositus nucleus is thus bidirectional. (2) Climbing fiber activity is self-regulated to an equilibrium level. (3) A time-varying representation of the CS in the cerebellar cortex permits the temporal discrimination for CR timing. (4) The ability of a particular segment of the CS to be represented consistently across trials varies as a function of time after the CS.

Mauk and Donegan (1997) reported that results obtained with the model indicate success based on (1) its ability to explain acquisition and extinction and the apparent distribution of plasticity between cortex and interpositus nucleus suggested by lesion studies, (2) its ability to explain both response timing and the inter–stimulus–interval (ISI) function without hypothetical parameters that are specifically related to the ISI (such as arrays of time constants or time-varying eligibility periods for plasticity, (3) its ability to explain apparently contradictory results of reversible lesions of the interpositus nucleus, and (4) the many specific and empirically testable predictions suggested by the underlying assumptions.

10.7. Adaptive Modification of Reflex Blinks

In a study by Pellegrini and Evinger (1997) of the involvement of the cerebellar cortex in the adaptive modification of corneal reflex blinks and spontaneous blinks, both acute and chronic lesions of the cerebellar cortex containing blink-related Purkinje cells blocked adaptive increases in ipsilateral, but not contralateral, obicularis oculi activity. The results were considered to be consistent with the hypothesis that the cerebellum is part of a trigeminal reflex blink circuit.

To investigate how the cerebellum generates and makes use of temporal information, Medina et al. (2000) used large-scale computer simulations of eyelid conditioning. The adaptive timing displayed by the simulated CRs was mediated by two factors: (1) different sets of granule were active at different times during the CS (i.e., the tone CS [delivered via mossy fibers; the unconditioned air-puff stimulus being delivered via climbing fibers] was emulated by activation of tonic- and phasic-firing mossy fiber inputs), and (2) responding was not only amplified at reinforced times but was also suppressed at nonreinforced times during the CS. The authors found that the prediction from the simulations that partial lesions of the cerebellar cortex should unmask short latency responses (i.e., at nonreinforced times) as well as leave intact a timed component was confirmed by observations on eyelid responses from a rabbit that had received a small electrolytic lesion in the anterior lobe of the cerebellar cortex.

10.8. Conditioned Reflexes in Humans with Cerebellar Pathology

In a comparative study of conditioned eyeblink reflexes in normal humans and in patients with cerebellar lesions, in which a delay classical conditioning paradigm using a tone (conditioned stimulus) and a midline forehead tap (unconditioned stimulus) were paired, Bracha et al. (1997) found that the normal subjects developed anticipatory eyeblinks to the tone in one session, whereas the patients failed to do so in four consecutive training sessions. In contrast, both patients and normal subjects exhibited a high level of eyeblinks to visual threat, probably a naturally acquired CR. The authors concluded that patients with cerebellar lesions cannot acquire, but can retain, conditioned eyeblink reflexes.

ELEVEN

Cerebellar Pathology in Humans and Animals: Genetic Alterations

11.1. Synopsis of Principal Findings in Human Cerebellar Disease

To provide the elements of a clinical perspective, this chapter includes limited information about symptoms and signs of cerebellar disease in humans. From the wealth of available sources on clinical neurology, the material here has been adapted primarily from Victor and Ropper (2001), with additional material from the classical paper by Holmes (1939).

Lesions of the cerebellum in humans give rise to basically three types of abnormalities: (1) decrease of muscle tone (hypotonia), (2) incoordination (ataxia) of volitional movement, and (3) disorders of equilibrium and gait. Extensive lesions of one cerebellar hemisphere can give rise to all three types of abnormalities, on the same side as the lesion, as can lesions of the cerebellar nuclei and/or cerebellar peduncles. Lesions of the dentate nucleus or of the superior cerebellar peduncle result in the most severe and lasting symptoms.

Hypotonia, which refers to a decrease in passive resistance of muscles to movement (e.g., extension of a limb) is ascribed to a depression of gamma and alpha motor neuron activity, and tends to disappear with time.

The most prominent manifestation of cerebellar disease (i.e., abnormalities of volitional or intended movement) are included under the general heading of cerebellar incoordination or ataxia. These terms include dyssynergia, dysmetria, and dysdiadochokinesis (impaired or slowed repetitive reversals motion [e.g., of alternation or pronation-supination of the forearm; Fig. 11.1], or successive touching of each finger to the thumb). Complete impairment of such alternation maneuvers is termed adiadochokinesis. Holmes (1939) characterized these disturbances as abnormalities in rate, range, and force of movement. The finger-to-target (e.g., the examiner's finger) test particularly brings out dyssynergia and dysmetria, especially at the end of the movement. The velocity and force of the movement are not checked in the normal manner, and a series of jerky movements may terminate the maneuver. Or, the limb

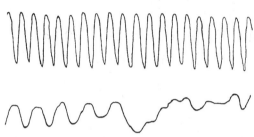

Figure 11.1. Tracings of rapid pronation-supination of the forearm from a patient with uni-lateral cerebellar symptoms. The movements of the affected arm (lower trace) were initially regular though slower and of smaller amplitude than the normal side (top trace), but became irregular and the arm became more or less fixed in supination. Muscular contractions appeared to spread aimlessly over the whole of the affected limb, including unwanted shoulder and finger movements. (From Holmes, 1939, in *Brain* Vol. 62, 1939, copyright by Oxford University Press; reprinted by permission; modified by Rothwell, 1994; *Control of Human Voluntary Movement (2nd ed.)* copyright 1994; reprinted by permission of the copyright holders.)

may overshoot the mark (hypermetria), followed by a series of secondary corrective movements in which the finger (or toe) sways around the target or moves from side to side a few times on the target itself. Such a side-to-side movement of the wrist and finger as it approaches its target has traditionally been termed intention tremor, and arises from the instability of the shoulder and elbow, and is due in part but not entirely to hypotonia. Lack of proper stabilization of a proximal joint (shoulder, hip) interferes with and impairs the accuracy of movement of the more distal segments of a limb.

Decomposition of a movement into its constituent parts is seen particularly in multijoint movements, (e.g., bringing finger to nose or heel to shin), during which there is a tendency to complete the movement at one joint (e.g., the shoulder or elbow) before the initiation of the movement at another joint (e.g., the elbow or shoulder), instead of the smooth execution of both movements conjointly. The more components there are to a movement, the more irregular the movement. One pa-tient characterized his difficulty as follows: "The movements of my left arm are done subconsciously, but I have to think out each movement of the right (affected) arm. I come to a dead stop in turning and have to think before I start again" (Holmes 1939).

Dysequilibrium or disorder of stance, with normal movements of the limbs, typi-cally results from disease of the midline cerebellum or vermis.

Eye movements may become impaired. For saccadic (stepwise) movements, upon attempted fixation of an eccentric target, the eyes may overshoot the target (saccadic dysmetria) and then undergo a succession of smaller terminal fixations. Smooth pur-suit movements (e.g., following the examiner's moving finger) are slower than nor-mal, so that catchup saccades (fast eye movements) occur. Attempted lateral gaze,

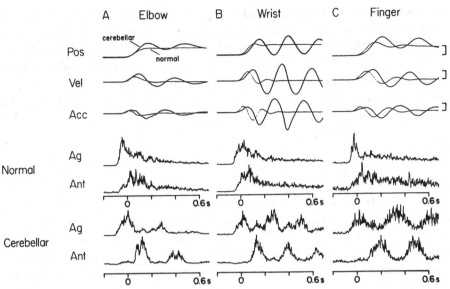

Figure 11.3. Delayed anatagonist EMG activity (bottommost of lower set of traces) associated with hypermetria (upper set of traces) in a patient tested for ballistic flexion movements 3 years after infarction of the left cerebellar hemisphere. Averaged records of 15–20 flexions on the normal side and on the cerebellar affected side made about the elbow (A), wrist (B), and finger (C). Records synchronized to start of movement (time 0 milliseconds). EMG (Ag, agonist; Ant., antagonist) records from the two sides were scaled to give approximately the same magnitudes. Target distance, 30 degrees. Calibrations: position, 30 degrees; velocity, 300 degrees per second; acceleration, 2,000 degrees per second^2. (From Hore, Wild, and Diener 1991; in *Journal of Neurophysiology*, Vol. 65, 1991, copyright American Physiological Society; reprinted by permission of the publisher.)

the inadequacy of temporal sequencing of motor preparation and execution. The authors concluded that the cerebellum appears to coordinate the relative timing between motor preparation and execution; in contrast, the basal ganglia appeared to have a minor role in motor preparation.

From mathematical analysis (using inverse dynamics equations) of motion studies during reaching by patients with cerebellar lesions, Bastian et al. (1996) concluded that a major role of the cerebellum is to generate muscle torques at a given joint that will predict the interaction torques being generated by other moving joints and compensate for them as they occur. For this purpose, the authors suggested that the cerebellum would make use of multiple sources of information (from neocortex and the periphery) to scale muscle activity in such a way as to overcome inertial characteristics of the limb and compensate for the interaction torques caused by other moving linked segments.

11.5. Vision and Cerebellar Reaching Ataxia

From a study of upper limb reaching movements in patients with cerebellar ataxia, Day et al. (1998) found that there were prolonged reaction times; the movements were more variable, less accurate, and performed more slowly; the paths (of finger tips) were more circuitous and longer than normal irrespective of whether visual cues were available; and there were large constant errors at the end of movement, but only in darkness (Fig. 11.4). The authors concluded that the spatial errors arise because the cerebellum contributes to preparatory motor processes that, based on limb proprioceptive and visual information, compute the pattern of muscle activity required to launch the limb accurately toward a target.

11.5.1. Figure Tracing and Impaired Temporal Integration

In a group of cerebellar patients and normal subjects, the cerebellar patients were found to be substantially impaired in their capacity to perceive two-dimensional irregular shapes that were to be traced out, reproduced with sight, and blindfolded (i.e., using only kinesthetic cues; Shimansky et al. 1997), findings that confirmed earlier studies. The authors indicated that there was also evidence that the deficit relates in part to a reduced capacity to integrate temporal sequences of sensory cues.

Timmann et al. (1996) reported that patients with cerebellar lesions are capable of substantially improving their performance of a complex motor task involving the recall of memorized shapes and the visuomotor control of a tracing movement. The authors concluded that it is highly feasible that the cerebellum plays a critical role during the acquisition of a task, but that this role is not necessarily linked with the exclusive storage of the critical memory engram within the cerebellum itself.

11.6. Effects of Lesions in Animals

11.6.1. Cerebellar Tremor Produced by Limb Perturbations

Vilis and Hore (1980) studied the tremor that followed limb perturbation in monkeys before and after cryoprobe cooling in the region of the dentate and interpositus nuclei. During cooling, there was no delay in the reflex response of the agonist (stretched) muscle that contributed to the return of the arm following the perturbation. However, the onset of the subsequent antagonist activity was delayed, which resulted in overshooting the target during the corrective return. The antagonist activity was also prolonged, resulting in a second cycle of oscillation. A similar delay and prolonged burst then occurred in the agonist, and then again in the antagonist, resulting in continued oscillations (3 to 5 Hertz). The authors suggested that, normally, the motor cortex generates a command to the antagonist muscle to terminate the return on the basis of predictive information provided by the cerebellum. During cooling, however, the motor cortex does not receive this predictive information, but instead receives the delayed information resulting from stretch of the antagonist muscle, which arrives too late to stop the corrective return, resulting in the overshoot. It also prolongs the antagonist EMG activity, thus initiating a second cycle of oscillation and so on.

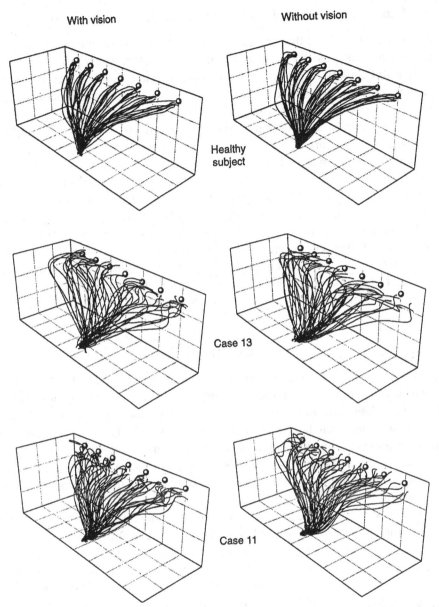

Figure 11.4. Perspective view of movement paths of one healthy subject (top) and two patients with Friedreich's ataxia. All movements within a block of trials have been superimposed. Panels on the left show movements performed with vision of target and finger. Panels on the right show movements performed in darkness. The circles indicate the position of the targets. The dotted grid projected onto each of the three planes consists of squares with 10 centimeter sides. (From Day et al. 1998; *Brain* 121, copyright 1998, Oxford University Press; reprinted by permission of publisher and author.)

11.6.2. Impairment of Movement of Single vs. Multiple Joints

Thach et al. (1993) found that transient neural activity recorded from the cerebellar dentate nucleus preceded activity in the motor cortex, which in turn preceded the first EMG activity associated with movement onset. However, inactivation of the dentate nucleus delayed the onset of activity in motor cortex and of movement. The cerebellum projects (via the thalamus) to areas of cerebral cortex anterior to the primary motor cortex (area 4), that is, to premotor (area 6), frontal eye fields (area 8), and possibly to the prefrontal region (areas 9 and 10; Thach et al. 1993).

In contrast to the minor deficits in the monkeys during execution of learned single joint movements resulting from temporary inactivation of individual cerebellar nuclei by muscimol injection, dramatic deficits of multijoint movements resulted from such injections. Fastigial inactivation led to inability of the animal to sit, stand, or walk. Injection into the interposed nuclei caused a gross action tremor in reaching movements; and after dentate injection, overshoot on reaching resulted together with an inability to pinch. Independent movement of wrist, thumb, and index finger was preserved. The authors concluded that cerebellar activity covaries with and controls compound movements, not (directly) simple movements (Thach et al. 1993).

11.7. Genetic Defects

Applications of gene transfer technology in neurobiology (van der Neut 1997; Verhaagen and Schrama 1997) offer promise of understanding of function through induced pathology (e.g., in behavioral studies). Approaches include the following: transgenic mice, in which there is overexpression of a specific gene product; antisense techniques and homologous recombination, which enable the study of physiological consequences of the absence of a specific gene product; and gene targeting, the mutation of a gene by means of homologous recombination in embryonic stem cells, leading to knockout mice.

In a review of transgenic mouse technology and the harnessing of homologous recombination to eliminate genes in living animals, Morgan and Smeyne (1997) illustrated several examples of the use of these technologies (transgenesis) to investigate the development of the mouse cerebellum, ranging from using inert marker transgenes to follow the organization strategy of the cerebellum, to eliminating specific cell populations and modifying the function and fate of Purkinje cells. The authors pointed out that the cerebellum is a particularly attractive neural structure for studies involving transgenesis. It is composed of relatively few neuronal types; its cytoarchitecture, synaptic connections, physiology and development have been extensively documented; and the loss of cerebellar function leads to a readily observed non-lethal behavioral phenotype.

In relation to the cerebellum, consequences of gene disruption include the following: effects on granule cell migration (Caroni 1997); modification of properties of granule cells (Jones et al. 2000); loss of granule cells, with resulting severe cerebellar impairment (Pennacchio et al. 1998; Shmerling et al. 1998), thus offering possible avenues of exploration of the functional role of granule cells; Purkinje cell degeneration (Ross 1997); impaired LTD and motor coordination (Funabiki, Mishina, and Hirano 1995); blockade of LTD and of adaptation of the VOR (De Zeeuw et al. 1998).

An example of interfacing of genetics with the cerebellum is the modeling, in transgenic mice, of the pathogenesis of the human disease spinocerebellar ataxia type 1 (SCA1), in which the most frequently seen and most severe alterations are loss of Purkinje cells and neurons in the inferior olive (Clark and Orr 2000; Cummings, Orr, and Zoghbi 1999).

11.7.1. Persistence of Multiple Climbing Fiber Innervation of Purkinje Cells

In PKCγ (Purkinje cellγ) mutant mice, which exhibit impaired motor coordination, the normal developmental transition from multiple to single climbing fiber innervation of each Purkinje cell is defective, so that in adult mutant mice, almost one half of Purkinje cells are still innervated by multiple climbing fibers, whereas other aspects of cerebellar anatomy and physiology appeared normal (Chen et al. 1995; Kano et al. 1995). The same failure to eliminate the normal synapse of multiple climbing fibers onto a single Purkinje cell can be induced by postnatal irradiation (Fuhrman et al. 1995).

According to Kano et al. (1997), the premature cessation of regression of supernumerary climbing fibers in mice is associated with a genetically determined deficiency in type 1 metabotropic glutamate receptors (mGluR1). The animals, whose Purkinje cells remain multiply instead of singly innervated, are viable but show symptoms of cerebellar dysfunction, such as ataxic gait, intention tremor, and dysmetria, and have impaired motor coordination and motor learning.

In the case of PLCβ4 mutant mice, the animals were viable and fertile, but as a consequence of impaired climbing fiber synapse elimination during postnatal development, they exhibited various signs of ataxia that became evident some 2 to 3 weeks after birth: general uncoordinated movements, body swaying while moving, ataxic gait, and intention tremors (Hashimoto et al. 2000).

11.7.2. Possible Cerebellar Nuclear Compensatory Mechanism for Purkinje Cell Loss

However, there is evidence of a possible compensatory mechanism in the loss of Purkinje cells associated with the genetic defect in Purkinje cell degeneration. Thus, Bäurle, Helmchen, and Grüsser-Cornehls (1997) reported that in Purkinje cell degeneration (PCD) mutant mouse, in contrast to the expected decrease in gamma-amino butyric acid (GABA) in cerebellar and vestibular nuclei and the subsequent increase in neuronal activity in these nuclei, there was actually a decrease. The authors concluded that the cells in these nuclei undergo a structural reorganization and develop diverse physiological and biochemical responses in the course of genetically determined PCD, which would account for the phenotypically mild motor disturbances observed in PCD mutant mice. The authors further suggest that such functional compensation, leading to only moderate motor impairment, could help explain the apparent discrepancy between clinical signs of ataxia in humans and the histopathological changes.

In mutant mice lacking the glutamate receptor $\delta 2$ subunit (GluR$\delta 2$) in Purkinje cells, there is impaired parallel fiber–Purkinje cell synapse stabilization during cerebellar development, which results in fewer parallel fiber synapses (Kurihara et al. 1997).

11.7.3. Genetic Alterations of Divisions of the Cerebellum

It is clear that other neurological mutants can be useful tools for studying abnormal development with, in some cases, abnormal function (Eisenman 2000). Examples include (1) the *meander tail* mutant mouse, which exhibits a phenotype consisting of a crooked tail and a cerebellum having an abnormal anterior part in which there is no layer of granular cells (but the number of Purkinje cells is increased), and a behavioral ataxia most probably associated with the cerebellar malformation. (2) The *Lurcher* mutant mouse, in which, in the heterozygote, there is premature death of all the Purkinje cells in the cerebellum. Subsequent to the Purkinje cell loss, there is a secondary loss of cerebellar granule cells and inferior olive cells. Despite these losses, the normal topographic organization of the cerebellum is retained. During this process, the normally projecting olivocerebellar climbing fibers contact the Purkinje cell somas in a normal fashion, but as development proceeds, they never enter the molecular layer to entwine the developing Purkinje cell dendritic trees in the normal fashion. (3) The *Weaver* mutant, which in the cerebellum shows a graded degree of decrease of granular cells, much more so in the medial than in the lateral cerebellum. The cerebellum is much reduced in size but retains a semblance of normal foliation. The granule cells and Purkinje cells (PC) are the primary targets of the *Weaver* gene.

11.7.4. Learning of Treadmill and Equilibrium Behavior Before and After Cerebellectomy in Lurcher Mutant Mice

Le Marec and Lalonde (2000) examined the sensorimotor skills of the spontaneous mouse mutant, *Lurcher* (with cerebellar cortical atrophy), while the animals were on either a fast or a slow treadmill. The treadmills were inclined at one of three slopes and required forward movements to avoid footshocks. The authors concluded that cerebellar cortical degeneration (including both Purkinje cells and granule cells during developmental stages and of the inferior olive in adult *Lurcher* mutants) impaired the time course of acquisition, but not the long-term retention, of the treadmill task.

Caston et al. (1995) carried out studies before and after cerebellectomy concerning the maintenance of equilibrium on a rotating rod by normal controls and lurcher mice (which exhibit a massive loss of neurons in the cerebellar cortex and in the inferior olivary nucleus, but whose deep cerebellar nuclei are essentially intact). It was found that the deep cerebellar nuclei sufficed for motor learning, provided the task was not too difficult (rate of rotation of the rod: 20 rpm). However, the cerebellar cortex was required when the task was more difficult (30 rpm). The authors concluded that the adaptive motor capabilities of lurcher mice are more limited than those of control animals.

TWELVE

Specialized Cerebellum-Like Structures

There are cerebellum-like structures, including the valvula and the electroreceptive lateral line lobe (ELL), that are found in certain species of fish, as well as the mammalian dorsal cochlear nucleus, the architecture and molecular biology of which in some respects strikingly resemble that of the cerebellum of vertebrates. These merit separate discussion from the topics in Chapter 2 on comparative anatomy of the cerebellum.

12.1. The Valvula

In addition to a true cerebellum (corpus cerebelli), there are several structures in electroreceptive fish (particularly the mormyrids), including the valvula, that are recognizably cerebellar or cerebellar-like. This resemblance suggests that a comparative study of them could yield some general rules concerning the cerebellum (Bell and Szabo 1986). Thus, among the bony fishes (teleosts), the mormyrids, which comprise certain African fresh-water fish, possess a cerebellum that is divided into the usual parts, that is, the body (corpus cerebelli), and a part arranged quite differently, the valvula. This highly unusual structure is considered in some detail.

The valvula, which is actually unique to the mormyrids, can grow to relatively large dimensions, covering all other parts of the brain (Fig. 12.1). This enlargement has been considered to be related to the high degree of differentiation of the lateral line system in these fish, which have a weak electric organ in the tail. They also have electroreceptors, which to a large extent are constituted of lateral line organs distributed over the body, and which have become modified to be sensitive to electric fields in the water (Nieuwenhuys and Nicholson 1969a). This combination of an electric organ and electroreceptors constitutes an electrosensory system with which the fish, by sensing distortions resulting from objects in the electric field, can gain information about its environment.

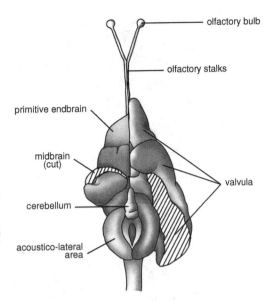

Figure 12.1. Dorsal view of a dissection of the brain of *Mormyrus kannume*. Most of the valvula cerebelli has been removed on the left side and the posteriomedial part of it on the right, exposing the underlying structures, including the very small body of the cerebellum. On the left side, the roof of the midbrain has been removed, exposing a portion of the valvula within its ventricle. (From Herrick 1924a; *Neurological Foundations of Animal Behavior*, copyright 1924 Holt, Rinehart, and Winston; reprinted by permission of Harcourt, Inc.)

The cerebellum in mormyrid fish is not only larger than any other among vertebrates in relative size, but the extraordinary valvula cerebelli is also almost certainly histologically the most regular, geometrically ordered (crystalline) structure in the central nervous system in vertebrates. The valvula in mormyrid fish consists of a repeatedly folded, continuous single ribbon of 300 mu width and an estimated 1 meter in length (i.e., about the same length as the unfolded Purkinje cell layer of the human cerebellum but far narrower in width; Bell and Szabo 1986; Braitenberg and Atwood 1958).

Of particular interest concerning the valvula is the fact that its ridges or corrugations (Figs. 12.2, 12.3) are made up of only the molecular layer (i.e., the layer of parallel fibers and the dendritic trees of the Purkinje cells) and the bodies of the Purkinje cells, but not the layer of granule cells. Such folds are absent in the body of the cerebellum (Fig. 12.4). Further, because the granular layer does not participate in the superimposed folds of the valvula, the axons of the granule cells do not bifurcate as in the body of the cerebellum, and the horizontal fibers arise directly from the granule cells. As a result, successive Purkinje cell dendritic trees are activated in a strict temporal sequence.

The intersections of parallel fibers with Purkinje dendrites are strictly ordered (Fig. 12.5), forming an almost crystal-like array (Kaiserman-Abramof and Palay 1969), which is indicative of a precise processing of the input data arriving on the parallel fibers, perhaps providing the capability for evaluating brief time differences. The overall arrangement in the valvula has some resemblance to an adaptive phased-array arrangement for a spatiotemporal (or temporospatial) transformation (Widrow and Stearns 1985; c.f., also Braitenberg 1967), which, to be adaptive or modifiable, would likely require a climbing fiber input to the Purkinje cells. It appears that

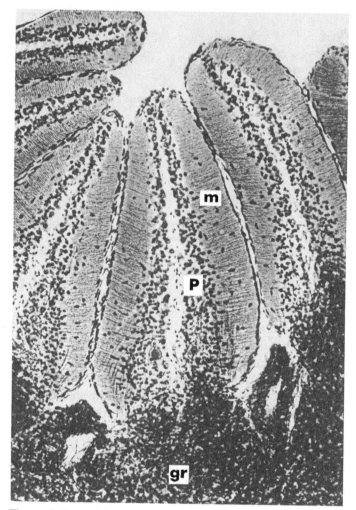

Figure 12.2. The cerebellum of the mormyrid, *Petrocephalus bovei*: section from valvula of the cerebellum. Key: gr, granular layer; P, Purkinje layer; m, molecular layer. (From Nieuwenhuys 1967; reprinted by permission of the author.)

climbing fibers are not apparent in the valvula by light microscopy (Nieuwenhuys and Nicholson 1969b) but are identifiable by electron microscopy (Kaiserman-Abramof and Palay 1969).

It has been suggested that both the anatomy and the physiology of a part of the valvula (i.e., having mormyromast-ampullary connections) indicates that its major role relates to the electrosensory system in modulating the sensory input of the latter, particularly in view of its large relative size and histological specialization, but the existence and the nature of such a role have remained unsettled (Bell 1986; Bell and Szabo 1986; Bullock 1986; Nieuwenhuys, ten Donkelaar, and Nicholson 1998, p. 839; Russell and Bell 1978). Thus, other electrosensitive species do not have such a large valvula, and hence such an association has been questioned; nonetheless, at

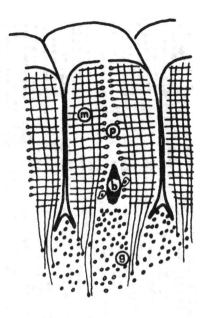

Figure 12.3. Diagram of the structure of a valvular ridge. m, Molecular layer; P, Purkinje cell area; b, basal bundle of fibers; g, granular layer. (From Russell and Bell 1978; in *Journal of Neurophysiology*, Vol. 41, copyright 1978, American Physiological Society; reprinted by permission of the publisher.)

least part of the valvula (in mormyrids at least) appears to be involved in processing electrosensory information (Finger, Bell, and Russell 1981).

Wullimann and Northcutt (1990) pointed out that, whereas electroreception evolved anew in mormyrids, vision was reduced concomitantly in this group of fishes, because primary visual projections are less extensive in mormyrids than in most other teleosts.

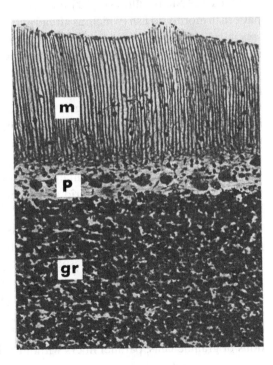

Figure 12.4. The cerebellum of the mormyrid, *Petrocephalus bovei*: section from body of the cerebellum. Note the typical three layers (granular, Purkinje, molecular) in the cerebellum proper. (From Nieuwenhuys 1967; reproduced by permission of the author.)

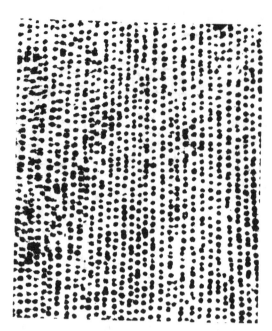

Figure 12.5. Section through a valvular ridge. The molecular layer has been cut parallel to the surface. The rows of dots represent transversely cut dendrites of Purkinje cells. The spaces between the rows of dots correspond to the traversing parallel fibers, which would thus lie in the plane of the page. The dendritic trees of the Purkinje cells spread in a plane perpendicular to the rows of dots, perpendicular to the plane of the page. *Petrocephalus bovei*, × 1360. (From Nieuwenhuys and Nicholson 1969b; *Neurobiology of Cerebellar Evolution and Development*, copyright 1969, American Medical Association; reprinted by permission of the publisher.)

12.1.1. Function of the Valvula

As noted above, the mormyrid valvula is believed to receive input from the transformed lateral line organs that function as electric sensors in these specialized fish (Altman and Bayer 1997, p. 5).

Meek and Nieuwenhuys (1991) suggested that the Purkinje cell dendritic palisade pattern in mormyrid fish (which, as already noted, have electric receptors) is probably specialized for optimal interactions with the spatiotemporal patterns in parallel fibers, in contrast to the mammalian configuration, which these authors suggested is probably specialized for optimal interactions with climbing fibers. It was further suggested that palisade orientation of the dendrites of mormyrid Purkinje cells (Fig. 12.6, middle) might increase the tuning of Purkinje cells for specific input waves not only in the transverse, but also in the apicobasal and rostrocaudal direction, probably an ultimate optimization for coincidence detection by the cerebellum. In contrast, the mammalian Purkinje cell configuration was suggested as being optimal for integration of parallel fiber and climbing fiber inputs, possibly for gain control of coincidence detection (Meek 1992b). Mormyrid and mammalian Purkinje cells are depicted in Figure 12.6, together with a representative Purkinje cell for most teleosts (fish).

Meek (1992a) pointed out that, in contrast to the basically similar intrinsic organization of the cerebellum of different tetrapods, the cerebellum of fish shows fundamental differences in this respect, the cerebellum of mormyrids being a case in point. Thus, mormyrids have a valvula (gigantocerebellum), no parasagittal zonal organization, projection neurons (eurydendroid cells) instead of deep cerebellar nuclei, a precerebellar nucleus lateralis valvulae (Fig. 12.7), olivocerebellar fibers that do not climb into the molecular layer (Fig. 12.6, right side), uni- and bilateral locations of granule cells, parallel fibers without a T-shaped bifurcation (Fig. 12.8) and

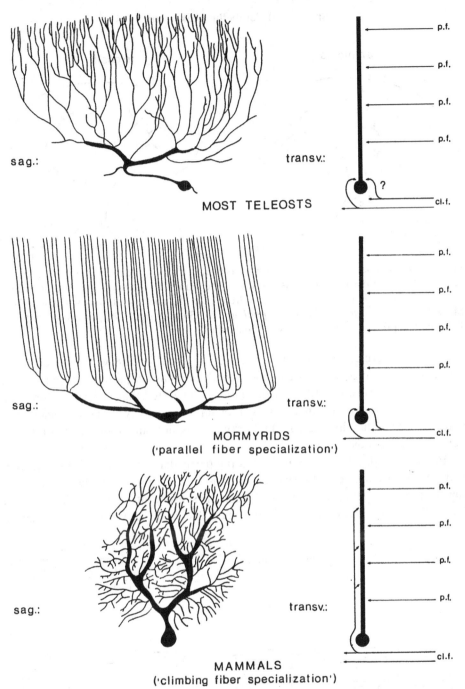

MOST TELEOSTS

MORMYRIDS
('parallel fiber specialization')

MAMMALS
('climbing fiber specialization')

Figure 12.6. Some characteristics of teleostean (including mormyrids) and mammalian Purkinje cells, showing their overall dendritic organization in the sagittal (sag) plane, and their connectivity pattern with parallel fibers (pf) and climbing fibers (cl.f.) in the transverse (transv) plane. In the sagittal views, the so-called "smooth" climbing fiber receptive surface has been drawn thick. The spiny dendritic compartment, making numerous spiny synaptic contacts with parallel fibers, has been drawn thinly, without the spines. (From Meek 1992a; *European Journal of Morphology*, Vol. 30, copyright 1992, Swets & Zeitlinger Publishers; reprinted by permission of the publisher.) (See also Meek and Nieuwenhuys 1991, Fig. 20.)

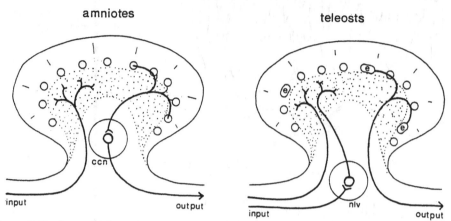

Figure 12.7. Summarizing scheme of some basic differences in the organization of extrinsic cerebellar connections in teleosts (fish) and amniote tetrapods (i.e., mammals, birds, reptiles). ccn, central cerebellar nucleus; e, eurydendroid cell; alv, nucleus lateralis valvulae. (From Meek 1992a; *European Journal of Morphology*, Vol. 30, copyright 1992, Swets & Zeitlinger Publishers; reprinted by permission of the publisher.)

with a coextensive distribution in the transverse plane (Fig. 12.8, valv.), and different Purkinje cell arrangements, including a dendritic palisade pattern (in the valvula [Fig. 12.6, morymids; Fig. 12.9]). Meek (1992a) suggested that these configurations reinforce the notion that a single main cerebellar function may exist (i.e., coincidence detection of parallel fiber activity by Purkinje cells, not only in mormyrids but also perhaps in tetrapods; Meek 1992b).

Earlier, mention had been made that the particular arrangement of the valvula had suggested that it could provide the capability of a precise evaluation of brief time differences that may be encountered in the sensory information reported from lateral line organs, and of the subtle differences in electric field strengths that may be

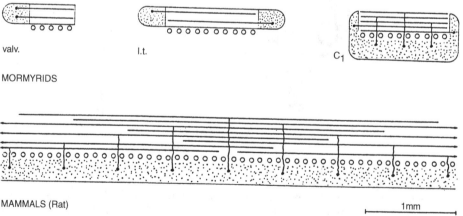

Figure 12.8. Transverse views of the granular cell–parallel fiber–Purkinje configurations encountered in the mormyrid valvula cerebelli (valv), lobus transitorius (l.t.), and lobe C_1 compared with the mammalian one. (From Meek 1992a; *European Journal of Morphology*, Vol. 30, copyright 1992, Swets & Zeitlinger Publishers; reprinted by permission of the publisher.)

INPUT   REGULARITY   GRADIENTS   NUMBERS
                                                (per cell)

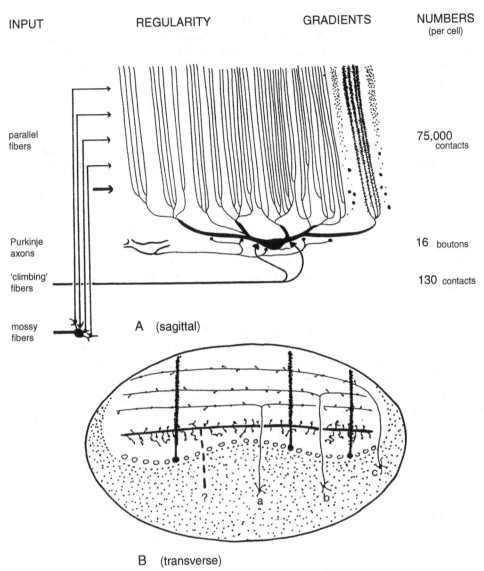

parallel
fibers

75,000
contacts

Purkinje
axons

16 boutons

'climbing'
fibers

130 contacts

mossy
fibers

A (sagittal)

B (transverse)

Figure 12.9. Summarizing scheme of the morphological and synaptic organization of Purkinje cells and their input in lobe C_1 (a part of the valvula). (A) Sagittal view showing the distribution of input, the regularity, the gradients in spine and parallel fiber density, and the numbers of synaptic contacts observed or estimated in lobe C_1. Medially lying granule cells give rise to symmetrical parallel fibers, but more laterally lying granule cells have asymmetrical or even unidirectional parallel fibers (not shown). (B) Transverse view showing the similarity in length of the parallel fibers contacting Purkinje cells in lobe C_1, but their variability in diameter (superficially: thin; deeply: thick) and site of origin: medially located granule cells give rise to symmetrical parallel fibers (a; i.e., a left and right branch of equal length), but more laterally located granule cells have asymmetrical (b) or even unidirectional (c) parallel fibers. Magnifications: A: × 150; B: × 75. (From Meek and Nieuwenhuys 1991; *J. Comparative Neurol.*, Vol. 306, copyright 1991, Wiley-Liss, Inc., a subsidiary of John Wiley & Sons, Inc.; reprinted by permission of the publisher.)

sensed by electroreceptors. A variant notion would be that the valvula of mormyrids may function as an adaptive signal processor (adaptive beamformer) for a signal-receiving array (compare Haykin 1994, p. 68, with Widrow and Stearns 1985, p. 368), specifically, the electroreceptor organs of mormyrids. However, as noted above, the close relationship that had been inferred earlier between the electroreceptors and the valvula has more recently become less well established.

12.2. The Mammalian Dorsal Cochlear Nuclear Complex and the Electro-Sensory (Electroreceptive) Lateral Line Lobe of Certain Fish

The mammalian cochlear nuclear complex spans the border between the pons and the medulla at the cerebellopontine angle, at which all primary auditory fibers (the central fibers from the auditory end organ) terminate (Webster 1992). Each primary auditory fiber bifurcates upon entering the cochlear complex. An ascending branch goes to the anterior ventral cochlear nucleus (AVCN). A descending branch goes first to the posterior ventral cochlear nucleus (PVCN) and then to the dorsal cochlear nucleus (DCN). It is the latter nucleus that is the subject of the present discussion.

That there are analogies between the DCN of the auditory system and the cerebellum has become evident (e.g., Mugnaini and Maler 1993). In the superficial layers of the DCN there is, in most mammalian species, a cerebellum-like microcircuit driven by a mossy fiber system presumably carrying polysensory information. The granule cells extend their axons as parallel fibers in the molecular layer where they innervate the other neurons in the superficial microcircuit, including the apical arbors (dendritic trees) of cartwheel cells and of the efferent neurons, the pyramidal (fusiform) cells. Associated with the granule cells are Golgi interneurons, which form an axonal plexus synapsing with granule cell dendrites at the periphery of glomerular synaptic fields, similar to those in the cerebellar granular layer. The flattened pyramidal (efferent) cells project to the contralateral central nucleus of the inferior colliculus.

The dorsal cochlear nucleus is, in most mammals, a layered structure perched on the dorsolateral aspect of the brain stem (Cant 1992). Lorente de Nó (1981) used the term, tuberculum acousticum, instead of dorsal cochlear nucleus, to indicate this anatomical relationship. In the human, the DCN is relatively large, but the lamination typical of other mammals (e.g., the three layers in Nissl-stained material from the cat [Cant 1992]) is not seen nor is it present in some other species of primates (Cant 1992; Moore and Osen 1979). Moore and Osen (1979) suggested that the entire dorsal cochlear nucleus of the human is equivalent to the pyramidal (efferent) and deep layers in other mammals. This suggestion is in accord with the observation that primates have very few, if any, granule cell areas because the molecular layer in other animals is made up largely of the parallel fibers that are the axons of the granule cells and their postsynaptic targets. Cant (1992) concluded that lack of knowledge of function of the DCN renders speculation about the significance of the differences between primates and other animals meaningless (cf. Moore and Osen 1979).

The mossy fibers probably do not originate from the spiral ganglion in the ear but may originate from higher auditory centers. In humans, unlike cat, the DCN is not stratified, the pyramidal cells (see below) have lost their orientation, and there is only a vestige of a molecular layer. The dorsal cochlear nucleus in humans cannot therefore be regarded as a structural analog of the cerebellar cortex (Brodal 1981, pp. 616–617).

Lorente de Nó (1981) pointed out that the total number of local fibers, association and centrifugal, entering the DCN is greater than the number of cochlear nerve afferents, and hence the cochlear nuclei cannot be regarded as an ensemble of simple relay stations. Indeed, this author concluded that the primary (dorsal and ventral) acoustic nuclei constitute a miniature brain that has a cerebellum of its own, the dorsal cochlear nucleus.

12.2.1. Features of Granule, Golgi, and Stellate Cells in Cochlear Nuclei

In the dorsal and ventral cochlear nuclei, collectively known as the cochlear nuclear complex, of cat, rat, and mouse, the small granule cells, evidently excitatory, participate in glomerular synaptic arrays similar to those of the cerebellar cortex (Mugnaini et al. 1980). The two cochlear nuclei, dorsal and ventral, differ in that the dorsal cochlear nucleus has a molecular layer, as does the cerebellum, but the ventral cochlear nucleus does not. Neurons, evidently inhibitory and resembling cerebellar Golgi cells, are also present. In raising the question of the possible functional significance of a circuit (i.e., of granule cells) in the acoustic system that resembles a portion of the cerebellar network, these authors reiterated the question of the origin of the mossy fibers that synapse onto granule cells (e.g., the olivocochlear bundle originating from the superior olivary complex).

Mugnaini, Warr, and Osen (1980) found that all, or at least the majority, of the granule cell axons project to the molecular layer of the DCN, forming parallel fibers similar to those of the cerebellar cortex. Further, the cochlear parallel fibers traverse the spiny apical dendrites of pyramidal cells (see below) and the stellate cells with smoother dendrites in the molecular layer (Fig. 12.10). (These authors point out that granule cells are known to be less frequent in the DCN in man, monkeys, and cetacea than in cat, rat, and mouse, whereas in the cerebellum, granule cells are present in great numbers in all mammals, including primates and cetacea.) In the rat, but not in the cat, dendrosomatic or dendrodendritic appositions between stellate cells are characterized by gap junctions (Mugnaini 1985; Wouterlood et al. 1984).

12.2.2. The Cartwheel Cell

Cartwheel cells do not appear to be present in humans (Adams 1986; Cant 1992). On the basis of Golgi preparations, electronmicroscopy, and transmitter immunocytochemistry (Fig. 12.11), possible analogies between spiny cartwheel and the aspiny stellate cells of the DCN, on the one hand, and the cerebellar Purkinje and stellate/basket cells, on the other hand, were suggested by Mugnaini (1985).

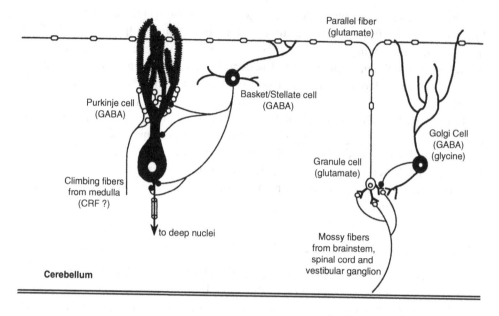

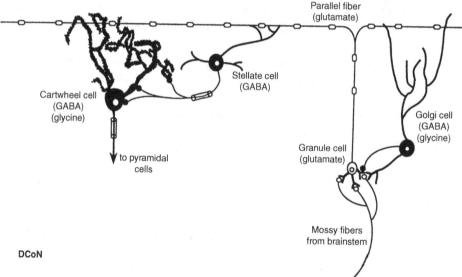

Figure 12.10. Diagram highlighting the differences between Purkinje cells of the cerebellum (*top*) and cartwheel neurons of the DCN (*bottom*). Details in text. (From Berrebi and Mugnaini 1993; reprinted from Merchán et al. (eds.): *The Mammalian Cochlear Nuclei: Organization and Function*, copyright 1993, Kluwer Academic/Plenum Publishers; reprinted by permission of publisher and author.)

Electronmicroscopy (Fine Structure) of the Cartwheel Cells. The electronmicroscopy of the cartwheel cell in the rat was studied by Wouterlood and Mugnaini (1984). Its cell body and dendritic shafts are covered by synaptic terminals, all of which contain pleomorphic vesicles and which may be of several types. The profuse dendritic spines characteristic of the secondary and tertiary dendrites of this cell type make synaptic

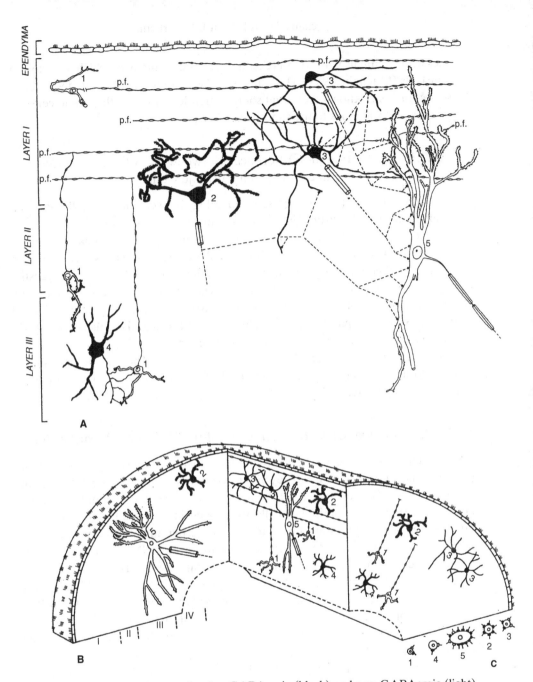

Figure 12.11. Schematic diagram showing GABAergic (black) and non-GABAergic (light) neurons in the superficial portion of the DCN. (A) Possible synaptic relations between the cells are indicated; (B) the orientation of parallel fibers (p.f.) along the DCN major axis and the anisotropy of the apical and basal dendritic arbors of pyramidal cells (5) are indicated by the block diagram. Dendrites of granule (1), Golgi (4), stellate (3), and cartwheel cells (2) (see below) are orientated in all directions. (C) The relative frequency of GAD-positive (black dots) and GAD-negative (open circles) boutons on the five categories of cells is indicated. Cartwheel cell bodies (2) are the only cell bodies contacted exclusively by GABAergic boutons. (From Mugnaini 1985; *J. Comparative Neurol.*, Vol. 235, copyright 1985, Wiley-Liss, Inc., a subsidiary of John Wiley & Sons, Inc.; reprinted by permission of the publisher.)

contact with terminals with round (excitatory) vesicles, many of which are axons of granule cells (Mugnaini 1985). The sources of the other terminals were described by these authors as unknown. Potential sources mentioned were other small cells and any source of projections to the superficial layers.

12.2.3. Similarities and Differences Between DCN Cartwheel Cells and Cerebellar Purkinje Cells

Berrebi and Mugnaini (1991) proposed a homology between the cerebellar Purkinje cell and the cartwheel neuron. The authors pointed out that both cell types synthesize GABA and the peptide, cerebellin (see below), among other cellular features in common. The DCN is involved in auditory signal processing, but it also receives fibers from the dorsal column nuclei, which relay somatosensory information, suggesting a polysensory integrative role for the DCN. The structure of the DCN has some resemblance to that of the cerebellum (Fig. 12.10), and there are granule cells with branched axons (i.e., parallel fibers), which thread through the apical dendrites of the inhibitory cartwheel cells (Berrebi and Mugnaini 1991). The cell bodies of the cartwheel cells lie in the pyramidal (fusiform) layer of cells. The multipolar or stellate cells are located in all three layers of the DCN. Granule cells in the DCN are found mainly in the pyramidal cell layer (Cant 1992).

12.2.4. Pyramidal Cells: Efferent Cells of the Dorsal Cochlear Nucleus

The efferent cells of the DCN, the pyramidal (fusiform) cells, are excitatory and project to the inferior colliculus. They may be considered a homologue of the cerebellar nuclear cells. The cell bodies of the cartwheel cells lie in the pyramidal (fusiform) layer. The stellate (or multipolar) cells are located in all three layers of the DCN. Granule cells in the DCN are found mainly in the pyramidal cell layer. There appear to be three types of inhibitory interneurons in the DCN: the stellate cells, the cartwheel cells (homologue of the cerebellar Purkinje cells), and the Golgi cells (Cant 1992). Granule cells throughout the cochlear nucleus (i.e., both dorsal and ventral parts) project to the molecular layer of the DCN (Mugnaini, Warr, and Osen 1980), where they form the parallel fibers that are in a position to terminate on the apical dendrites of the pyramidal cells and on the dendrites of the stellate and cartwheel cells (Cant 1992).

Mugnaini and Maler (1993) reiterated that the DCN granule cells are assumed to be excitatory and glutamatergic, whereas the Golgi, stellate, and cartwheel neurons are presumed to be inhibitory. As noted above, it had been proposed that the stellate cells are analogous to cerebellar stellate and basket neurons, and that the cartwheel neurons are analogous to Purkinje cells and modulate the activity of the efferent neurons, the pyramidal cells. It was suggested that, because the above-mentioned microcircuit of the mammalian cochlear nuclei does not have a counterpart in amphibians and reptiles, it may be considered a "newly rediscovered" neuronal machinery reproduced by the anlagen of the area octavolateralis in relation to mammalian hearing, paralleling the microcircuit in the flocculonodular cerebellar cortex, which receives primary input from the vestibular nerve.

12.2.5. Further Comparison of the Cerebellum and the Mammalian Dorsal Cochlear Nucleus

In a more recent formulation of similarities between the anatomy in the cerebellum and that of the nonhuman mammalian DCN of the auditory system (Dunn et al. 1996), several points were made. The DCN has a stratified organization and a cerebellar-like microcircuit in the superficial layers, the main neurons of which are the excitatory granule cells and the inhibitory cartwheel neurons, the homologues of cerebellar granule cells and Purkinje cells, respectively. The cerebellar-like system is driven by mossy fiber afferents evidently derived from multiple sources, suggesting that a variety of extrinsic neurons affect the processing of acoustic information within the DCN. Local circuit neurons include granule, unipolar brush, Golgi, stellate, and cartwheel cells. The axons of granule cells in the DCN are either branched or unbranched to become parallel fibers. The efferent neurons are the pyramidal (fusiform) cells, which project to the contralateral inferior colliculus. The detailed function of the DCN remains unclear. One suggested possibility is that it serves to coordinate information on auditory localization with the position of the pinnae (Dunn et al. 1996). (See also Mugnaini, Diño, and Jaarsma [1997] concerning the unipolar brush cells of the mammalian cerebellum and cochlear nucleus.)

12.2.6. Possible Role of DCN in "Cocktail Party" Effect

In view of the cerebellum-like structure of the DCN, and in view of the putative capacity of the cerebellum to act as an adaptive signal processor, the question may be raised of whether the DCN could also act as an adaptive signal processor or Kalman filter (Chapter 12) in which a "signal is to be separated from background noise." One example that could be cited is that of the common "cocktail party effect," in which one attends to a single voice selected from among several (compare Brodal 1998, p. 294). (In this connection, the ventral cochlear nucleus is believed to be related to, among other functions, localization of a sound [Brodal 1998, p. 292].)

12.3. Molecular Biology of Cerebellum and Cerebellum-Like Structures

12.3.1. Cerebellin and PEP-19 as Markers for DCN Cartwheel Cells and Cerebellar Purkinje Cells

Layers 1 and 2 of the DCN nuclei, as already mentioned, contain a system of mossy fibers that synapse onto granule cells and Golgi cells, thus resembling those in the cerebellar granular layer (Mugnaini and Morgan 1987). Axons of the DCN give rise to a system of parallel fibers in layer 1 (the molecular layer) that synapse onto the spiny cartwheel cells and the nearly aspiny stellate cells, and onto the apical spiny arborization of pyramidal cells, the output cells of the DCN. Thus, cartwheel and stellate cells have several similarities to cerebellar Purkinje cells and stellate cells, respectively. Further, Golgi, Purkinje, and stellate cells in the cerebellum, and Golgi, cartwheel, and stellate neurons in the DCN are GABAergic, and granule cells evidently use an excitatory amino acid neurotransmitter in both the cerebellum and DCN. In addition, the neuropeptides cerebellin and PEP-19 have been found to be markers both for Purkinje cells in the cerebellum and also the cartwheel cell, the homologue cell in the DCN, the primary targets of which are the DCN pyramidal cells (Berrebi and Mugnaini 1991; Mugnaini and Morgan 1987; Mugnaini et al. 1987). The pyramidal cells, in turn, can be viewed as the homologue of the cerebellar nuclear cells, as previously mentioned.

12.3.2. Granule Cell Mutation Weaver, Purkinje Cells, and Cartwheel Cells

Complementing the results summarized above, Berrebi, Morgan, and Mugnaini (1990) found that the cerebellar granule cell mutation, weaver, which primarily affects granule cells but spares most Purkinje cells in the lateral cerebellum, also spares cartwheel cells. These findings were considered to support the notion that the cerebellar germinative zone extends to the caudal portion of the rhombic lip, which gives rise to the dorsal cochlear nucleus.

Reviews of some aspects of the genetic basis for normal and abnormal development of the cerebellum and of its cell types (e.g., global and subcellular levels of compartmentalization, sagittal versus rostrocaudal compartmentalization) have appeared (Goldowitz and Hamre 1998; Oberdick, Baader, and Schilling 1998).

12.3.3. Molecular Similarities and Differences Between DCN Cartwheel Cells and Cerebellar Purkinje Cells

Berrebi and Mugnaini (1993) summarized moleculobiological similarities and differences between Purkinje cells in the cerebellum and cartwheel cells in the DCN; the cartwheel cells were presumed to represent the equivalent of Purkinje cells (Fig. 12.10). The two cell populations originate from neighboring regions of the neuroepithelium at the lip of the rhombencephalon, are generated during the same embryonic period, and share several ultrastructural and neurochemical phenotypes. Four independent mouse mutations – Lurcher (Lc), Purkinje Cell Degeneration (pcd), staggerer (sg), and nervous (nr) – cause similar defects in cerebellar Purkinje cells and DCN cartwheel neurons, strongly suggesting that the repertoire of genes expressed in these two cell types is very similar. The authors concluded that the neuronal cell populations of the cerebellar cortex and the superficial layers of the DCN form remarkably similar neuronal circuits.

Among the differences between the two types of cells, Berrebi and Mugnaini (1993) pointed out that cartwheel neurons, unlike Purkinje cells, do not receive a climbing fiber input onto their dendritic trunks, nor do they receive an inhibitory pinceau formation around their axon initial segments, as do Purkinje cells from basket cells. Further, the cartwheel neurons are not arranged in a single layer, their dendritic fields do not lie in a single plane, and their axons are relatively short, as are those of Purkinje cells. These features vary somewhat among different species.

Berrebi and Mugnaini (1993) reiterated that cartwheel neurons represent homologues of Purkinje cells in the cerebellar-like circuit of the DCN superficial layers (Fig. 12.10), and that cartwheel neurons are members of the Purkinje cell family that have become adapted to carry out cerebellar-like processing of auditory inputs, or perhaps play a role in the regulation of acoustic reflexes.

12.3.4. Recent Views Concerning the Dorsal Cochlear Nucleus

Nelken and Young (1996) summarized the DCN in cats and rodents as a layered structure divided into superficial and deep layers by the pyramidal (output) cell layer (Fig. 12.12). The pyramidal cells have two dendritic arborizations, extending into the superficial layer and into the deep layer, respectively. The pyramidal cell layer with the deep layer forms the auditory part of the DCN, in which the auditory input terminates. The superficial layer strongly resembles the cerebellum, in that there are terminals of cerebellar-like granule cells, the inputs to which are many and poorly understood (they appear to receive some somatosensory input, e.g., from the pinna, but little if any type I auditory nerve fiber input). As previously mentioned, the DCN cartwheel cells are closely related to the cerebellar Purkinje cells, both in terms of circuitry and in their biochemical and genetic properties. The organization of the superficial DCN can be viewed as two-dimensional, such that granule cell axons (parallel fibers) run perpendicular to the isofrequency sheets defined by auditory nerve fibers, with an auditory tonotopic map along one dimension and an unknown map carried by the granule cell parallel fibers along the other dimension. Most, if not all, the output axons of the DCN project to the inferior colliculus. It was pointed out that, in general, the comparative anatomy of the DCN is not well described, and extensive studies of DCN physiology have only been performed on the cat and, more recently, on the gerbil. As for function, Nelken and Young (1996) mentioned the possibility that the DCN participates in the startle reflex, in particular, the head-turning reflex. Detection of spectral notches conveying sound localization information could be a mechanism (Young, Nelken, and Conley 1995).

Noting that the granule cell-associated circuits of the superficial part of the DCN provide both excitatory and inhibitory (i.e., via stellate and cartwheel cells) pathways to the principal (i.e., pyramidal) cells from a variety of auditory and nonauditory inputs (specifically, somatosensory), Davis, Miller, and Young (1996) drew attention to the similar systems in the fish electrosensory and lateral line systems, which are used for gain control and to suppress self-generated stimuli arising from respiration and other movements. However, it remained unclear whether similar functions could be attributed to the DCN. It has been pointed out that there is also a need for a better understanding of the distribution of the inputs from descending pathways with respect to cell types. Almost all cells in the cochlear nucleus receive primary input from the cochlea (Cant 1992).

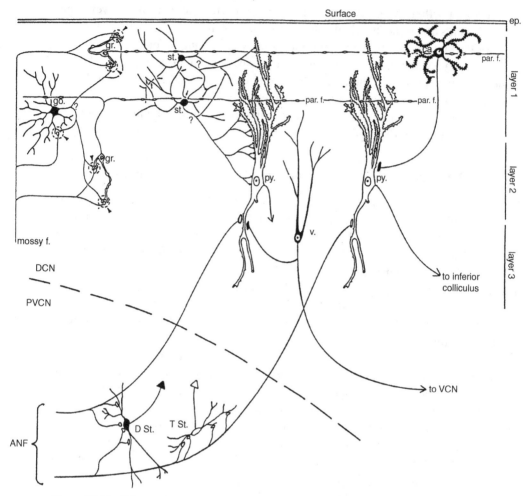

Figure 12.12. Schematic representation of the DCN. The layer of pyramidal cells (py) separates the superficial layer (layer 1) and the deep layer (layer 3). Layer 3 contains the basal dendrites of the pyramidal cells, vertical cells (v), and giant cells (not shown). Auditory nerve fibers (ANF) and projections from the VCN terminate in the deep layer. Type T stellate cells (T St.) from the PVCN presumably supply excitation to the DCN, whereas type D stellate cells (D St.) from the PVCN presumably supply inhibition to the DCN, Layer 1 contains parallel fibers (par f.), which are axons of granule cells. The cartwheel (ca.) and stellate (st.) cells are inhibitory interneurons of the superficial layer. The superficial stellate cells of the DCN are different from the stellate cells of the PCVN. The granule cell domains also contain a class of inhibitory neurons, the Golgi cells (go.). (From Nelken and Young 1996; reprinted from *Journal of Basic and Clinical Physiology and Pharmacology*, Vol. 7, copyright 1996, by permission of Freund Publishing House, Ltd.)

The recognition of the different neuronal populations in the cochlear nucleus has led to the view that the auditory system is made up of multiple neuronal pathways (e.g., Warr 1982). Presumably, the different pathways have different functions in auditory signal processing; in some cases, there is insight into what that role is (Cant 1992)

The inhibitory cartwheel cells of the DCN (the homologue of cerebellar Purkinje cells) are excited by parallel fibers from granule cells to yield both simple and complex spikes, the latter without a counterpart of climbing fibers, which are not present in the DCN (Davis and Young 1997). Somatosensory stimulation tended to induce (via granule cells) complex spike discharges, whereas stimulation of parallel fibers tended to induce only simple spikes. It was presumed that somatosensory stimulation to the granule cells produces greater calcium current (sufficient to activate complex spikes in the cartwheel cells) than stimulation of the parallel fibers.

12.4. The Mammalian Dorsal Cochlear Nucleus, the Electroreceptive Lateral Line Lobe of Fish, and the Cerebellum: A Comparison

Mugnaini and Maler (1993) compared the organization of the DCN with that of the ELL of gymnotiform fish. The structure of the ELL is itself interesting: there are not one but two systems of (excitatory) parallel fibers in a feedback arrangement that may serve to suppress irrelevant background activity, an arrangement that has been compared with the inhibition of thalamic relay cells by the reticular nucleus in Crick's (1984) searchlight hypothesis (Bastian 1993; Maler and Mugnaini 1993, 1994). Descending inputs to the ELL are said to be involved in gain control and in the spatial tuning of ELL E and I units (Nieuwenhuys, ten Donkelaar, and Nicholson 1998).

Young et al. (1992) pointed out that there are some aspects of the anatomy of the DCN that resemble those of the ELL, and that both resemble the anatomy of the cerebellum.

12.4.1. Sensory Prediction in Cerebellum-Like Structures in Fish

Against an underlying premise that sensory processing may be understood as the generation of predictions (expectations) that are removed from the actual sensory inflow, thus sharpening unusual or unexpected components of the latter, Bell et al. (1997; see also Sugawara et al. 1999) pointed out such a process in four distinct groups of fishes (*Mormyridae*; *Rajidae*; *Scorpaenidae*; and *Apteronotidae*) (see also Bell 1993). The responsible neuronal structure consists of a sheetlike array of principal (output) cells (which can be compared with Purkinje cells), from which apical dendrites extend out into a molecular layer where they are contacted by parallel fibers. The basilar regions of the arrays receive primary afferent inputs from electroreceptors, lateral line organs, or eighth nerve end-organs. The parallel fibers (originating from granule cells), which descend from higher levels of processing, convey a diversity of information including corollary discharge (efference copy) signals (for modifying sensory signals according to changes resulting from motor commands), and sensory information from other modalities (e.g., proprioception). Associations between the descending signals conveyed by the parallel fibers and particular patterns of sensory input to the basal layers lead (probably via diminished efficacy at the parallel fiber–principal cell synapses) to the generation of a negative image of expected sensory input within the principal cell array, which, when added to actual sensory input, results in the subtraction of expected from actual input. The unexpected or novel input thus stands out more clearly. The authors found that such a process is remarkably similar among the four groups of fishes, and suggested that it may generalize to cerebellum-like structures in other sensory systems and groups of species (e.g., the optic tectum in teleosts and the mammalian DCN). Analogous conclusions concerning elasmobranchs (cartilagenous fish, including rays and sharks, as opposed to teleosts or bony fish) were reached by Bodznick and Montgomery (1993). An alternative characterization of the process is that of an adaptive filter (Montgomery and Bodznick 1994).

12.4.2. Adaptive Gain Control

The converse effect, namely, maintaining a relatively constant level for a received electrosensory signal of varying intensity (i.e., adaptive gain control) has also been described (see, e.g., Maler and Mugnaini 1994), an effect that appears to entail GABAergic (inhibitory) feedback mechanisms.

In fish having electrosensory systems and an electric organ, the firing of the electric organ is accompanied by a corollary discharge that serves to modify the electrosensory system, a movement-induced reafferent input as in the lateral line system of fish and the echo-locating system of bats (Bell 1986; Bell and Szabo 1986).

12.4.3. Comment

Although there are several similarities of cell and fiber types, there appears to be one major difference between the arrangement of the valvula, the ELL, and the DCN, and the true cerebellum, namely, that the latter possesses the capability (via climbing fibers) of plasticity at the parallel fiber–Purkinje cell synapse. It is not evident that the other organs just mentioned have such a capability that is refined to the degree found in the true cerebellum. Thus, in the valvula of mormyrids, climbing fiber synapses are largely confined to the Purkinje cell body (Fig. 12.6), and the DCN is evidently devoid of climbing fibers (Davis and Young 1997).

However, in the absence of a mechanism for changing synaptic efficacy, the question can be raised as to whether a continuing capability of such synaptic plasticity is not needed in these organs and, for relatively fixed patterns of behavior, is even unnecessary. Were this the case, the synaptic efficacy could perhaps be fixed by means of some other mechanism (e.g., simply by repeated use), without the need for a formal inferior olive-climbing fiber mechanism. In any case, it would presently appear that only the true cerebellum can be considered fully adaptive (i.e., capable of adjusting its own parameters [synaptic weights] to a refined degree).

PART THREE

MODELS AND THEORIES

Nonadaptive Models, Forerunners of Adaptive Models, and Earlier Adaptive Control Models

In this chapter and in the following chapters, the terms "theory," "hypothesis," and "model" are used more or less interchangeably, although "theory" (or "hypothesis") could imply a mental construct, whereas "model" could refer to an actual implementation, in terms of a mathematical model, a device, or on a computer (thus, a computer model).

This group of chapters on models and theories (this chapter and Chapters 14, 15, and 16) presents a limited survey, in roughly chronological order, of cerebellar theories that have been advanced since the 1960s. A comprehensive detailed, comparative, critical evaluation is not attempted, rather, an overview of the principal trends in modeling the cerebellum is the objective. In several instances, critiques of particular theories by proponents of other theories have been included. Some of the theories summarized in this chapter are only of historical interest, but other older theories were forerunners of adaptive control models that are considered further in Chapters 14 through 16. Discussions of cerebellar theories (primarily in its motor aspects) can also be found in, for example, Llinás (1981b), Ito (1984), Miall et al. (1993), Houk, Buckingham, and Barto (1996), and Thach (1998a, 1998b, 1998c).

13.1. Types of Theories

On the one hand, theories of the cerebellum can perhaps be categorized by how the cerebellum is organized, and on the other hand, by how it functions. In this survey, emphasis is on the latter group.

Cerebellar theories have had their origins in many fields of interest, including, for example, anatomy, physiology, clinical neurology, and electrical or communications engineering. Such diversity probably arises in no small measure from the unique and relatively uniform anatomy of the organ.

In considering these various theories, it is well to keep in mind a distinction that has been emphasized by Kawato (1993), which can be rendered as follows: a problem is "well-posed" when its solution exists, is unique, and depends continuously on the initial data. An ill-posed problem fails to satisfy one or more of these criteria. Most motor-control (movement-control) problems are ill posed in the sense that their solutions (i.e., their trajectories, as in touching a finger tip to the nose) are not unique. Any computational theory or neural-network model of the cerebellum that is to have biological relevance should possess capability to resolve the ill-posed aspect of these problems.

To indicate the pace of development of models of the cerebellum, it is interesting to compare the minimal mention of models in the book on the cerebellum by Eccles, Ito, and Szentágothai (1967): "It is generally believed that in some way the cerebellum functions as a type of computer that is particularly concerned with the smooth and effective control of movement" (p. 300), which can be said to indicate design specifications for models, with the more extensive sections on modeling in the book by Ito (1984) on the cerebellum. In Ito's book, there are two chapters (Chapter 10, Neuronal Network Model, and Chapter 24, Control System Model of the Cerebellum) on this topic.

Historically, it may be noted that, after the appearance of the book by Eccles, Ito, and Szentágothai (1967), a tutorial paper by Szentágothai (1968), primarily on the detailed structure (anatomy) of the cerebellum, appeared in the *Proceedings of the Institute of Electrical Engineers*. Interestingly, the three authors whose theories are described immediately below (Marr, Albus, Fujita) cite the original book of Eccles, Ito, and Szentágothai (1967) rather than Szentágothai's tutorial paper.

Most papers on cerebellar theories and models have been multiauthored, but for convenience and brevity and only for convenience and brevity, the survey in this and subsequent chapters refers to the first or senior author or to the leader of a group, or to the author whose name is usually associated with a given theory or model.

13.2. Nonadaptive Theories and Models

13.2.1. Braitenberg's Timing-Organ Hypothesis

In this hypothesis, the cerebellar cortex is taken to be a clock in the millisecond range (Braitenberg, 1961, 1977; Braitenberg and Atwood 1958) or, perhaps more exactly, as a system of delay lines (in the form of the parallel fibers) to generate small but precise time intervals. Braitenberg was impressed by the anatomical fact that the parallel fibers and the dendritic trees of Purkinje cells are almost rigidly perpendicular to one another (Ramón y Cajal 1995) to form a lattice structure (i.e., axons of the parallel fibers and dendrites of the Purkinje cells in two planes perpendicular to one another), as described in Chapters 2 and 3. Braitenberg was also impressed by the minimal distortion of the molecular layer (and consequently of the lengthwise dimension of its parallel fibers; Fig. 13.1), which occurs as a result of folding or foliation, in contrast to the appreciably greater distortion of the granular layer (Braitenberg 1990).

Based on a conduction velocity of about 0.5 millimeter per millisecond per second along the very thin unmyelinated parallel fibers, the time of arrival of signals between neighboring Purkinje cell trees would be about a tenth of a millisecond,

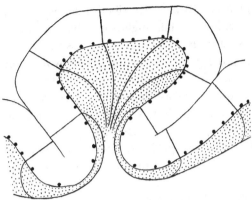

Figure 13.1. Diagram of a convolution of the mammalian cerebellum to show a constant thickness of the molecular layer (of parallel fibers and Purkinje cells) and a varying thickness of the granular layer, yet constant ratios between volume of molecular layer, number of Purkinje cells (black dots), and volume of granular layer. (From Braitenberg and Atwood, 1958; *J. Comparative Neurol.*, Vol. 109, 1958, copyright Wiley-Liss, Inc., a subsidiary of John Wiley & Sons, Inc.; reprinted by permission of the publisher.)

so a given parallel fiber would make contact with some 130 Purkinje cells in a time interval of the order of 20 milliseconds, for a 10-millimeters long parallel fiber. Correspondingly (Braitenberg 1967), a chain of parallel fibers reaching from one side of the human cerebellum to the other (about 100 millimeters) could be expected to give a total maximum delay of 200 milliseconds. Braitenberg (1987) indicated that time differences of such small orders of magnitude as just mentioned could be expected in the execution of complex movements such as playing a violin.

In Braitenberg's view, the notion of a timing organ that transforms spatial into temporal patterns and vice versa (a simple mathematical treatment appears in Braitenberg [1961]) applies to the entire range of vertebrates that have a cerebellum. Thus, he stated (1977, p. 78):

in its rudimentary form, in *Cyclostomes*, [see Chapter 2] the cerebellum is nothing more than a bridge of nerve tissue with parallel fibers and Purkinje cells between the right and left vestibular nuclei. In view of this connection to the obviously more static than dynamic function of equilibrium, can the idea of the cerebellum as a timing device still be upheld? I believe that one can show that in swimming aquatic animals (which prehistoric vertebrates that first developed a cerebellum certainly were) the problem of stabilization against rotation around a longitudinal axis could best be solved by a mechanism involving temporal coding.

Braitenberg (1961) drew attention to suggestive support for the timing-organ hypothesis from the experimental results of Calne (1959) in frogs that, in response to some sites of stimulation, a fixed delay between stimulus and response in Purkinje cells was found, whereas for other sites of stimulation, a range of delays was found.

More specific corroborative experimental evidence for Braitenberg's hypothesis was obtained by Freeman (1969, 1970) who found, in detailed studies of the frog cerebellum, that in response to different types of electrical and natural stimulation, Purkinje cells lying on the same beam of parallel fibers fired in sequence with a precise delay. Freeman (1969) also described a simple model for the precise sequential firing of Purkinje cells that might form the basis of a physiological timing mechanism as suggested by Braitenberg. In discussing Freeman's results, Bennett (1969) pointed out that there are several animals for which precise measurement of time intervals is necessary for processing of exteroceptive signals, including species that have electroreceptors for measuring small differences in electric field strength, such as electric fish, cetaceans (dolphins), and perhaps whales and, of course, bats in echolocation (see also Chapter 12, concerning the valvula).

Kornhuber (1971, 1974) also proposed the parallel fibers of the cerebellar cortex as a delay line for calculation of the burst duration for rapid preprogrammed movements.

The difficult problem in Braitenberg's theory of a maximum delay in one parallel fiber of not much more than 10 milliseconds in time resulted in a reformulation of the concept (Braitenberg 1983), which entailed chaining of elementary motor acts (controlled perhaps by the motor cortex), whereas the sequencing within the elementary episodes would be controlled by the cerebellum. In this connection, a given Purkinje cell in combination with the parallel fibers that synapse with it was envisaged as being able to perform velocity detection, by virtue of staggered firing of granule cells along a beam of parallel fibers (Braitenberg 1993). This capability would permit the cerebellum to respond to sequences of events, which, by their successive activation of Purkinje cells, would provide a series of inhibitory influences on the motor system via the inhibitory output of the Purkinje cells to the cerebellar nuclei (Braitenberg and Preissl 1992). Braitenberg (1993) considered this view of the cerebellum as an events-sequencer to be compatible with the cerebellar adjustable pattern generator of Houk (1987).

13.2.2. Braitenberg's Tidal Wave Hypothesis

In a formulation by Braitenberg, Heck, and Sultan (1997), the cerebellum is considered to be a large collection of individual lines (in the sense of Eccles' "beams"; Eccles, Ito, and Szentágothai 1967), which respond specifically to certain sequences in the input and result in sequences of signals in the output. The concept of the effect on Purkinje cells of sequences of stimuli in the mossy fiber input was tested experimentally in slices of rat and guinea pig cerebellum by sequential activation of a row of stimuli along a folium in such a way that the temporal differences between points of stimulation corresponded to the travel time along parallel fibers, resulting in a progressive buildup of a "tidal wave" of excitation and activation of Purkinje cells (Fig. 13.2). It was considered that, in the intact animal, the sequence of mossy fiber activation resulting in this effect on "beams" that are appropriately tuned are derived from the cerebral cortex in combination with information about ongoing movement reported from the spinal cord. The output from the cerebellar cortex is triggered by the tidal waves that travel through the excited beam. The beam passes to the cerebellar nuclei a sequence of signals produced by selected Purkinje cells at times specified by the moving wave of excitation. It was stressed that the beam is not limited to the length of parallel fiber branches; consequently, the sequence of output

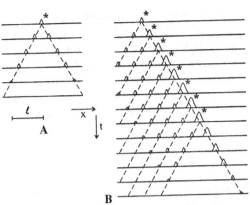

Figure 13.2. Schema of "tidal wave." (A) The effect of a short local stimulus (∗) to the cerebellum in time and space. The laterolateral direction of the cerebellum is plotted horizontally; time is plotted vertically downward, the horizontal lines representing a succession of points in time. The wave set up by the stimulus travels in both directions and dies out after it has traveled a length l, corresponding to one branch of the parallel fiber. (B) If a succession of stimuli (asterisks) imitating movement along the folium is presented, summation of activity in the parallel fiber system occurs. A wave of maximum amplitude builds up when the stimuli follow each other at the conduction velocity in the parallel fibers. Upon cessation of the stimuli, the tidal wave continues for the length l with diminishing amplitude and then dies out. (From Braitenberg, Heck, and Sultan 1997, in *Behavioral and Brain Sciences*, Vol. 20, 1997, copyright by Cambridge University Press (NY); reprinted by permission of the publisher.)

signals it emits may have a duration (e.g., up to 200 milliseconds) considerably exceeding the 10 milliseconds limit of a parallel fiber.

In their reformulation (which includes a synopsis of cerebellar anatomy), Braitenberg, Heck, and Sultan (1997) drew attention to certain contrasts between cerebellar cortex and cerebral cortex: (1) in humans, the anteroposterior length of the flattened cerebellar cortex is more than 2 meters, as compared with 0.3 meter for the flattened cerebral cortex; (2) the surface area of the cerebellar cortex is about that of one cerebral hemisphere; (3) the number of neurons is about the same in both; (4) in the cerebellar cortex itself, the only fibers running transversely (the parallel fibers) are excitatory, whereas axons running perpendicularly to them arise from inhibitory interneurons, suppressing activity on either side of an active beam of parallel fibers (an exception being the inhibitory Golgi neurons, whose axons do not exhibit a preferred direction); (5) in contrast to a relatively well-defined trend for cerebellar surface area for a number of species (including the macaque monkey), the surface area for the cerebellar cortex for humans is some 10 times higher in relation to body weight; (6) the thickness of the dendritic tree of a Purkinje cell along the folium is about one-tenth that of the approximately square enclosure encompassing its other dimensions (35 mu vs. 350 mu, approximately), and there is essentially no overlap of the dendritic trees of adjacent Purkinje dendritic trees (in contrast to a much higher overlap of pyramidal cell dendrites in the cerebral cortex, of the order of 1,000).

The paper by Braitenberg, Heck, and Sultan (1997) includes more than one quotable quote reflecting the view of a long-time worker in the cerebellum (Braitenberg):

In no other part of the nervous system does the shape of neuronal elements suggest their functional relations as clearly as in the cerebellar cortex (p. 234).

The whole arrangement seems to imply that for each dendritic tree there is a predetermined place along the length of the parallel fibers at which it is to receive its synaptic input. *The idea that what really matters is the time at which the synaptics become active is old but still enticing.* (p. 234). [Emphasis added].

which sees parallel fibers as generators of time delays between the activation of different muscles involved in one movement. And this was also the most vulnerable form of the timing hypothesis, since with the known length of parallel fibers of a few millimeters and the measured velocity of conduction of about 0.5 m/sec (Eccles, Ito, and Szentágothai 1967) the delays generated could hardly be more than 10 msec. This is not enough for the timing of movements which typically take about 200 or 300 msec for their completion.

Moreover, the vague hope that some internal circuitry could perhaps relay signals from one delay line to the next in order to generate the longer delays was thwarted by the finding (Eccles, Ito, and Szentágothai 1967) that, except for the granular cells/parallel fibers themselves, all interneurones in the cerebellar cortex are inhibitory. Today's estimates for 2l (i.e., the combined length of the two segments of a parallel fiber) vary between 4.7 and 6 mm (Brand, Dahl, and Mugnaini 1976; Harvey and Napper 1988; Mugnaini, 1983; Pichitpornchai, Rawson, and Rees, 1994) (p. 235a).

The authors (Braitenberg, Heck, and Sultan 1997) presumed that the functional unit is the beam of parallel fibers together with the associated postsynaptic synapses, the ensemble being excited by a sequence of events spelled out by the order of mossy fibers along its length.

The individual events are signals from the motor cortex interspersed with signals from the periphery. The output (to the cerebellar nuclei) is triggered by the resultant tidal wave, which travels through the excited beam (itself not limited to the length of the parallel fiber), the resultant being a series of signals produced by selected Purkinje cells at times specified by the moving wave of excitation. (The effect of the moving wave of excitation on the inhibitory neurons, i.e., stellate and basket cells was assumed to be one of inhibition of adjacent or off beam Purkinje cells.) In the cerebellar nuclei, the inhibitory Purkinje cell output is subtracted from the excitatory collaterals of mossy and climbing fibers, thus "sculpting" (Eccles 1973) the motor commands to the periphery, either via the motor cortex or the red nucleus.

Braitenberg, Heck, and Sultan (1997) pointed out that the experimental verification of tidal waves, using rat cerebellar slices, indicated that parallel fiber-to-Purkinje cell synapses were quite effective when the input is put to them in the right way, in comparison with synapses onto Purkinje cells from the ascending stems of granular cell axons (i.e., before bifurcation of the latter). It was also pointed out that the cerebellum is fed at least as much information from the surface of the body (somatosensory input) as from the deep (muscle, tendon, and joint) senses.

(The authors' target article [Braitenberg, Heck, and Sultan 1997] appears together with 26 open peer commentaries, which provide a rich diversity of ideas concerning the cerebellum and its function, ending with the authors' responses to the commentaries.)

That the cerebellum is a clock in the millisecond range can be considered a partial theory, limited by the fact that the maximum time delays (of about 10 milliseconds) appear to be too short (in comparison with movements of 200–300 duration), unless some additional time-delay mechanism becomes evident. It may be pointed out, however, that any theory that entails prediction (as does adaptive control) necessitates a capability of prediction (Chapter 17). But the "tidal-wave" hypothesis of sequences of events in and out of the cerebellar cortex appears to move the strict requirement on timing to structures outside the cerebellum, which raises its own set of problems about timing mechanisms such as the nature of the generators.

13.2.3. The Cerebellum as a Site of Learning Motor Skills

In a meeting report, Brindley (1964) suggested that the message sent down by the forebrain in initiating a voluntary movement is often insufficient as instructions for all the anterior horn cells that take part in the movement, even if elaborated as far as it can be according to fixed rules. It needs to be further elaborated by the cerebellum in a manner that the cerebellum learns with practice, and this further elaboration makes use of information from sense organs. It was concluded that the cerebellum is thus a principal agent in the learning of motor skills.

13.2.4. Eccles' Purkinje-Cell Readout Hypothesis

It had been observed (Eccles, Ito, and Szentágothai 1967; Eccles, Llinás, and Sasaki 1966) that the individual spikes of a complex spike of Purkinje cells in response to climbing fiber activity varied in number from 1 to 4, according to the level of inhibitory input from the basket and stellate cells (four spikes for minimal inhibition, one spike for maximal inhibition). Eccles suggested (Eccles, Ito, and Szentágothai 1967, p. 308) that the climbing fibers could effect a readout of the inhibitory level of the Purkinje cell (derived from its input from basket and stellate cells, and in turn from the mossy fiber system), because the climbing fiber excitatory input could overcome even the deepest inhibitory depression (see also Eccles, Llinás, and Sasaki 1966).

A difficulty with Eccles' "readout" theory was pointed out by Thach (1967, 1980) in that, in the lightly anesthetized cat, for all or at least half of all Purkinje cells, only one spike propagates down the Purkinje cell axon for each complex spike. Moreover, for the awake monkey, the number of secondary spikes (i.e., after the first) in the complex spike bears no correlation with the immediately prior simple spike frequency, which itself is a direct measure of the level of excitability of the cell. Further, the complex spike occurs during bursts and pauses in simple spike activity. Therefore, the "readout" theory seemed untenable. (Thach [1980] also reviewed other proposals for possible functions of the climbing fibers and provided a set of "Koch's postulates," with which subsequent proposals for climbing fibers, and therefore cerebellar function, could be evaluated.)

An alternative hypothesis to Eccles' somewhat coarse four-level scheme was offered in 1966 by R. Kado,* in which the function of the climbing fiber was to reset the excitability of the corresponding Purkinje cell to a "ground state" by depolarizing the entire dendritic tree of the Purkinje cell. Information about the inhibitory level of the Purkinje cell would then be contained in the (continuously variable) time interval between complex spike and the first following simple spike, rather than in the much more coarse one-to-four spike readout measure, thus providing information about the present state of the movement in question.

A related hypothesis was that of Bloedel and Roberts (1971), in which, as a result of the expected marked increase in conductance of Purkinje cell dendrites resulting from synaptic activity of the climbing fibers, the polarization produced by excitatory and inhibitory inputs arriving prior to the onset of the climbing fiber response would be "erased," which could prevent the output of a given Purkinje cell from reflecting transient instabilities arriving in the neuronal circuitry.

13.2.5. Eccles' Dynamic Loop Control Hypothesis

In this hypothesis (Eccles 1967, 1973; Eccles, Ito, and Szentágothai 1967; Eccles et al. 1972), it was postulated that the cerebellum effects the control of movement by the piecemeal integration of an immense number of subsets of information from receptor organs and from the command centers of the cerebral cortex, giving as an output a patterned mosaic of independent units of integration. The hypothesis further postulated that the ultimate synthesis is effected in the maintained posture and in the evolving movement. The postulated dynamic loop is from the command centers of the cerebrum via the pontine and olivary nuclei to the cerebellum with return circuits to the cerebrum via the cerebellar nuclei and the ventrolateral thalamus. This process is viewed as a dynamic one, in which it is continuously subject to revision by the feedback of information to the cerebellum, as reflected, for example, in an increase and a decrease, respectively, of simple spike firing rates of Purkinje cells nearby one another.

13.2.6. Allen and Tsukahara's Cerebral Cortex–Cerebellum Cooperative Hypothesis

Allen and Tsukahara (1974) envisaged a two-stage planning–execution cooperative endeavor between the cerebral cortex and the cerebellum for carrying out

---

* Kado's concept was presented during discussions at a Neurosciences Research Program work session on the cerebellum held near Portland, Oregon, May 3–5, 1966, but the concept does not appear in the summary proceedings of that meeting (*Neurosciences Research Symposium Summaries*, Vol. 2 [1967], pp. 515–616). A projected volume in which this idea was to appear in a chapter on the cerebellum, although cited more than once by workers on the cerebellum, was not actually published for various reasons. The projected chapter was to have been: Harman, L.D., Kado, R.T., and Lewis, E.R. (1971): "Cerebellar modeling problems." In L.D. Harmon (Ed.); *To Understand Brains*, New York: Prentice Hall. Kado, R.T., personal communication, 1996.

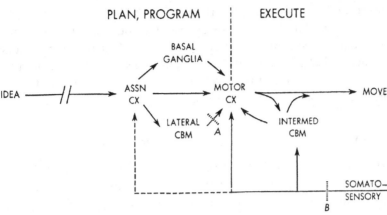

Figure 13.3. Allen and Tsukahara's schema showing proposed roles of several brain structures in movements. Thin dashed lines represent a pathway of unknown importance. Heavy dashed lines at *A* and *B* represent cooling of the cerebellum and sectioning of the dorsal roots or dorsal columns, respectively. It was proposed that the basal ganglia and cerebellar hemispheres are involved with association cortex in programming of volitional movements. At the time that the motor command descends to motor neurons, engaging the movement, the pars intermedia of the cerebellum updates the intended movement, based on the motor command and somatosensory description of limb position and velocity on which the movement is to be superimposed. Follow-up correction can be performed by motor cortex when cerebellar hemisphere and pars intermedia do not effectively perform their functions. (From Allen and Tsukahara 1974; *Physiological Reviews*, Vol. 54, 1974, copyright American Physiological Society; reprinted by permission of the publisher.)

movements, as depicted in Figure 13.3. The schema incorporates the idea that the association areas participate in the translation of the idea to move into a patterned activation of certain motor cortical columns and their elemental movements. The association areas that project to the cerebellar hemispheres are among those in the premotor chain. Because the cerebellar hemispheres appear to perform their function without the aid of direct peripheral inputs, it seems that the hemispheres are more suited for participation in planning the movement than in actual execution and updating of the movement, which was proposed to be a function of the intermediate zone. (The fact that the cerebellar hemispheres may receive somatosensory information from association areas does not imply that the lateral cerebellum is primarily a processor for sensory information relayed by the association areas.) Once the movement has been planned within the association cortex, with the help of the cerebellar hemisphere and basal ganglia, the motor cortex issues the command for movement. At this point, the intermediate cerebellum updates the movement based on the sensory report of the limb position and velocity on which the intended movement is to be superimposed. This is a kind of short-term planning as opposed to the longer-range planning of the association cortex and lateral cerebellum (Fig. 13.3).

Upon cooling of the dentate (Fig. 13.3, line **A**) of a monkey conditioned to perform movements between two target zones: (1) the movement becomes slower; (2) external cues (e.g., auditory, visual) are used to locate the target zones; and (3) errors appear in rate and range in attempting the movement. Each of these alterations in the movement was considered to be consistent with the notion that the movement is primarily preprogrammed. However, after sectioning the dorsal columns or dorsal roots (Fig. 13.3, heavy dashed line B), the movements are still performed markedly well, indicating preprogramming at the level of the association areas and the cerebellar hemispheres (Allen and Tsukahara 1974).

13.2.7. Calvert and Meno's Spatiotemporal Filter Model

Calvert and Meno (1972) modeled the cerebellar cortex as an anisotropic (different in different directions) spatial filter with particular temporal properties, suggesting that one function of the cerebellum may be to enhance the detail in spatiotemporal patterns. In particular, the model suggests that the cerebellar cortex may act as a filter that can emphasize the high-frequency content of the input patterns, both in space and time.

13.2.8. Hassul and Daniels' Lead-Lag Compensator Model

Focussing on the mossy fiber input, the model of Hassul and Daniels (1977) described the cerebellar cortex qualitatively as a higher-order lead-lag compensator, which, if the strengths of the coupling coefficients between its neural elements were varied, could match its dynamics to that required by any particular control system involving the cerebellum. The model, which includes granule, Golgi, basket, stellate, and Purkinje cells, predicted that if Purkinje cell collaterals have a weak effect on the basket and stellate cells, the cerebellar cortex would act as a lead compensator, whereas if there is a strong effect, it would act as a lag compensator.

13.2.9. Pellionisz' Tensor Theory

Against a background of prior work directed at computer simulations and neuronal net modeling of the cerebellum and its components (Pellionisz 1970; Pellionisz and Szentágothai 1973, 1974), Pellionisz drew attention, in a series of papers (e.g., Pellionisz and Llinás 1979, 1980, 1982, 1984), to the problem for the cerebral cortex of planning the execution of movements in one space or system of coordinates, and executing them in another. Thus, the planning space could be ordinary extrinsic three-dimensional space, whereas the space for execution could be that of the limbs-on-limbs-on-trunk, a multidimensional space or hyperspace (more than three dimensions), a quite different frame of reference. For the solution of this problem, Pellionisz proposed the cerebellum as a tensor (tensorial) transformer.

In tensor theory, the coordinate axes, unlike the conventional mutually perpendicular three-dimensional xyz axes, are not necessarily mutually perpendicular. This is the case, for example, in a corner of a parallelogram. Tensor analysis arises, for example, in deformations of a medium that has different properties (e.g., compressibility, heat transfer) in one direction from another (i.e., it is anisotropic), in contrast to one that has the same properties in all directions (i.e., that is isotropic). (The general question of movement in space, frames of reference, and coordinate systems was considered by Soechting and Flanders [1992]; see also Andersen et al. [1993], and Stein [1992], concerning representations of space and their transformations [or transformations of sensory vectors] by distributed neural networks.)

A specific example entailing such transformations is that of the VOR, in which the coordinate systems for the tensions exerted by the extraocular muscles are different from those for the semicircular canals, along roll, pitch, and yaw axes. In tensor terminology (Pellionisz and Graf 1987; Pellionisz and Llinás 1980; Pellionisz, Peterson, and Tomko 1990), the cerebellum would function by transforming the *covariant* (sensory frame of reference) components of the intended movements into their *contravariant* (motor-executive frame of reference) components. Computer simulation of use of covariant components of an intended movement, that is, without proper transformation, was reported to result in the equivalent of ataxia. Further, by adding time as another dimension, the possibility of predictive cerebellar action arises (Pellionisz and Llinás 1982). It should be noted that the prediction was based on higher derivatives of a Taylor expansion (representation), rather than on (adaptive) linear prediction (see Arbib and Amari, 1985, and Chapter 16 concerning the use of Kalman–Bucy [Kalman and Bucy 1961] filtering for purposes of prediction).

According to Arbib and Amari (1985), however, the depiction by Pellionisz and Llinás (1980) of the transformation of motor planning into motor execution in terms of tensor theory was miscast, because the latter authors had not demonstrated that the cerebellum implements a metric tensor (i.e., accomplishes a transformation of coordinates according to tensor theory). In the face of results from neural network modeling of the VOR, Robinson (1992a, 1992b) raised questions about the utility for understanding of brain function at a detailed level of such specific mathematical formulations as tensor theory.

13.2.10. Boylls' Synergistic Parameterization Theory

In Boylls' (1975a, 1975b; see also Llinás 1981b) mathematical theory of synergic parameterization, motor synergies (i.e., proper reciprocal balance of agonist and antagonist muscle groups) are considered, as well as the methods by which such "synergic parameterizations" can be computed. There are four main postulates of the theory, which principally introduced a new view of the role of cerebellar climbing fibers and does not entail synaptic plasticity: (1) Synergic parameters are modulated by cerebellar outflow, to control overall muscular intensity and the distribution of activity among the various muscles within a muscle group; (2) Synergic structure and activation intensity are encoded in cerebellar outflow; (3) Time courses of cerebellar physiological activity and their association with synergic parameterization entail at least two different time constants (short, of 20 milliseconds or less; long, 5–30 seconds). The short time constant regulates real-time fluctuation (e.g., during locomotion), whereas the long time constant governs alterations in background activity upon which the short-time variations are superimposed (e.g., modulation of the vestibular nuclei during afternystagmus); (4) Short and long time-course cerebellar processes are identified with mossy and climbing fiber afferent systems, respectively.

In brief, the mossy fiber pathways are taken to be a force-producing agency, whereas the olivocerebellar (climbing fiber) system is taken to be a directionality-postural skewing mechanism. Such an arrangement is presumed to exist in Voogd-type compartments (Fig. 5.9) so the background or baseline activity (under the influence of the climbing fibers) could be different in adjacent compartments (by recurrent lateral inhibition). At the same time, mossy fiber activity would produce immediate "memory-less" changes of activity in the two adjacent compartments without spatial patterning. The redistribution of activity among a specific class of muscles that would be affected by such a mechanism when applied to the spino-olivocerebellar system and the anterior cerebellum would constitute one means whereby intrinsic spinal locomotor circuits could bias cerebellar outflow to accord with muscle activation in different gaits (Boylls 1975a).

In a companion report (Boylls 1975b), the author discussed application of the model to locomotor behavior in the cat and to the VOR, stressing that movement is centrally programmed, not in terms of individual muscle contractions but rather in accordance with linkages (ensembles) of many muscles.

13.2.11. Mano's Climbing Fiber Synchronizing Pulse Hypothesis

Based on known anatomical facts and on their own observations of discharge characteristics of the complex spike of cerebellar Purkinje cells in behaving monkeys, Mano, Kanazawa, and Yamamoto (1986, 1989) formulated their hypothesis as follows (Fig. 13.4). First, several (numbering N_i) inferior olivary neurons form a synaptic cluster by virtue of their electronic coupling via gap junctions (Llinás, Baker, and Sotelo 1974; Sotelo, Llinás, and Baker 1974). Second, an axon from one inferior olivary neuron branches into more than 10 (N_j) climbing fibers, and each climbing fiber makes a one-to-one synaptic contact with a Purkinje cell, for a total of

$$N = (N_i) \times (N_j).$$

Purkinje cells. These N Purkinje cells, firing complex spikes synchronously, are conjectured to converge on a cerebellar nuclear neuron to form a functional unit in controlling movement, as suggested, for example, for the "cerebellar efferent modules" postulated by Voogd and Bigaré (1980; Fig. 5.9).

The hypothesis then presumes that, when a prompt motor command (i.e., response) is required, for example, to an external stimulus, the synchronously firing complex spikes (CS, Fig. 13.4) simultaneously accelerate the simple spike patterns in the individual Purkinje cells for a rapid onset of movement. When precise timing is not crucial (as in self-paced movement), the complex spikes are not activated.

13.3. Other Nonadaptive Theories

13.3.1. Bloedel's Dynamic Selection Hypothesis

This hypothesis (Bloedel 1992; Bloedel and Kelly, 1992) is based on the recognized sagittal organization of the cerebellum, in particular, of the climbing fiber system

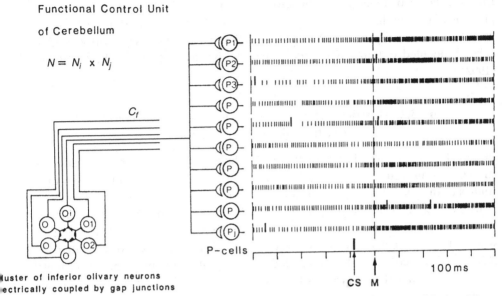

Figure 13.4. Mano's synchronizing pulse hypothesis. Explanation in text. (From Mano, Kanazawa, and Yamamoto 1989; In Strata (ed.) *The Olivocerebellar System in Motor Control*, copyright 1989, Springer-Verlag, Heidelberg; reprinted by permission of the publisher.)

(Voogd and Bigaré 1980; see Fig. 5.9), and also of the cerebellar nuclei. The hypothesis was posed in opposition to the hypothesis of the establishment of engrams in the cerebellar cortex for motor learning (see also Bloedel and Bracha 1995) as the prime function of the climbing fibers. It was proposed instead that the climbing fibers have their prime role in relation to real-time operations by the cerebellum during execution of movements. This view was considered to be supported by a demonstration of a specific short-term (some 200 milliseconds) action rather than any long-term effect such as LTD of climbing fibers on simple spike responses. In brief, only a short-lasting enhancement of the Purkinje cell's simple spike response (i.e., a gain change) to the mossy fiber–granule cell–parallel fiber input was envisaged, rather than a prolonged alteration in Purkinje cell responsiveness resulting from pairing climbing fiber and parallel fiber inputs.

Thus, according to the "dynamic selection hypothesis," the distribution of climbing fiber inputs activated by specific patterns of convergence in the inferior olive determines those populations of sagittally aligned Purkinje cells that will be most highly modulated by mossy fibers activated under the same behavioral conditions. The mossy fibers are viewed as conveying critically important quantitative information regarding ongoing changes in the periphery or in activity in the descending pathways.

More generally (Bloedel 1992), the cerebellum is viewed as a "mediator" that serves to integrate properties of external target space with other movement-related information so optimum execution coordination of movement occurs.

The hypothesis was considered to build on the tensor hypothesis of the cerebellum elaborated by Pellionsz (see above), and was viewed as being consistent with

Llinás' concept of inherent rhythmicity in the olivocerebellar system and the expression of this rhythmicity in the activation of sagittal strips of Purkinje cells, which would serve to modify the correlation among climbing fiber inputs to nearby Purkinje cells. A detailed critique of Bloedel's hypothesis was given by Gilbert and Yeo (1992).

13.3.2. Bloedel's Theory of Cerebellum and Derivation of Strategies of Movement

In a slightly later formulation of the cerebellum in relation to the derivation of strategies of movement, Bloedel, Bracha, and Milak (1993) concluded, from their studies of the role of cerebellar nuclei in the learning and performance of forelimb movements in the cat, that the principal role of the cerebellum in motor learning is not as the storage site for the engrams, but rather as a structure critical for deriving the strategy required to perform the movement successfully. Thus, the involvement of the cerebellum was considered to be related to coordinating the performance of novel movements rather than serving as the site of the actual plastic changes underlying the acquisition of the behavior.

13.3.3. Houk's Model of Adjustable Pattern Generators (APGs)

Houk (1987), having become convinced from experimental studies that the movement signals apparent in the magnocellular part of the red nucleus probably represent the output of pattern generators in the brain rather than the effect of continuous feedback from the periphery, implicated the cerebellum as a site for the pattern generators. ("Adjustable pattern generator" (APG) means the ability of a pattern generator to generate an elemental burst command with an adjustable intensity and duration.) A basic schema of the model is shown in Figure 13.5, in which the feedback paths to the cerebellum are mossy fibers. These motor patterns are assumed to be under the control of the Purkinje cells, which are also taken to be the site of learning of the motor patterns. Triggering of the patterns, from the motor cortex, could occur anywhere along the olivo-cerebello-rubral pathway, and feedback from proprioceptors provides corrective information and turns off the pattern generators (see also Schöner and Kelso 1988). A neural network of the model was later implemented (Berthier et al. 1992; Houk et al. 1990). A more recent description of these ideas and the inclusion of the basal ganglia, cerebral cortex, and cerebellum in a concept of distributed modular architectures in relation to movement is presented in Houk, Keifer, and Barto (1993) and in Houk and Wise (1995).

The motor command output of the red nucleus itself was concluded to be in a muscle-based coordinate system (perhaps after conversion by a distributed representation of target position known to be present in the posterior parietal cortex, and by the cerebellum [Miller and Houk 1995]) in a whole-limb coordinated manner for reaching movements (Sinkjær et al. 1995).

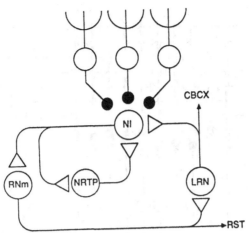

Figure 13.5. Model of an adjustable cerebellar pattern generator. Bursts of RNm (magnocellular red nucleus) are postulated to be produced by regenerative excitatory connections from NI (nucleus interpositus) to NRTP (nucleus reticularis tegmenti pontis) to NI and from NI to RNm to LRN (lateral reticular nucleus) to NI. Inhibitory input to NI from several Purkinje cells (three are shown) in the cerebellar cortex is postulated to control the frequency and duration of bursts of patterened output, which is sent to the spinal cord as a motor command via the RST (rubrospinal tract). CBCX, cerebellar cortex. (From Houk 1987; in Glickstein, Yeo, and Stein (eds.) *Cerebellum and Neuronal Plasticity*, copyright 1987, Kluwer Academic/Plenum Publishers; reprinted by permission of publisher and author.)

In the adjustable pattern generator model, the programs for generating the motor commands are learned by adjusting the synaptic weights of parallel fiber to Purkinje cell synapses, using training signals transmitted by climbing fibers. The model also included positive feedback loops interconnecting the deep cerebellar nuclei with the brain stem and motor cortex (Peterson and Houk 1991).

13.3.4. Houk's Adjustable Pattern Generators Model for Two Joints

In a later paper (Berthier et al. 1992), the earlier single adjustable pattern generator (APG) model (Houk et al. 1990) was expanded to an array of APGs for control of movement of a simple two-degree of freedom simulated limb (i.e., two joints). Rubrocerebellar and corticocerebellar information-processing modules function as APGs, the motor programs being stored in the cerebellar cortex in the weights of parallel fiber synapses onto Purkinje cells. Training signals derived from sensory information are conveyed by climbing fibers to direct the adaptation of parallel fiber synapses and, after learning, selection of the motor patterns initiated by a trigger mechanism is controlled by basket cells. Links with other models were pointed out, including Kawato's feedback error learning model (Kawato, Furukawa, and Suzuki 1987).

Somewhat later, Barto, Buckingham, and Houk (1996) proposed a predictive switching model, a simplified version of the APG model, to control movement in the presence of significant feedback delays, but without using a forward model of the motor plant. The model incorporates Purkinje cell bistability and a synaptic

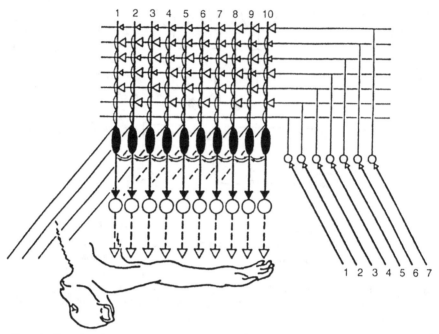

Cerebellar circuitry is a candidate because of:

- *Climbing fibers* — one source, one-to-one contact on Purkinje cells, powerful synapse, low firing
- *Mossy fibers* — many sources and types of information, high frequency firing
- *Granule cells* — multiplex mossy fibre input, $>10^9$ in number
- *Parallel fibers* — spread the context over several motor 'mode' zones, link the response elements across several mode zones

Experimental support

- Ablation of cerebellar cortex impairs/prevents movement adaptation and learning
- Neural recording during movement shows CS (climbing fiber response) firing at low rate, unrelated to movement, while SS (parallel fiber response) fires at high rate, related to movement.
- Neural recording during learning shows CS related to performance error and learning, and SS changing as a function of CS occurrence.
- Paired electrical stimulation of climbing + mossy fibers shows that CS occurrence causes changes in SS response to parallel fiber input (long-term depression).

Figure 13.6. Schema of cerebellar circuitry (top), and logic behind implication of cerebellar circuitry in motor control and points of experimental support (bottom). Top: Model of granule cell–parallel fiber control of muscular coordination which has the following features: (a) within each nucleus, there is a use-specific (modal) representation of somatic musculature; (b) the orientation of the myotome is in the coronal plane; (c) the orientation of the parallel fibers is also in the coronal plane; (d) the output of the parallel fiber beam of Purkinje cells falls on "eligibility trace" that constitutes a short-time memory trace. The learning rule includes both long-term depression (LTD) and long-term potentiation (LTP), in a formulation similar to that of Albus (1971). The authors related their model to adaptive control methods of the direct predictive adaptive controller type.

For exploratory purposes, Barto et al. (1999) developed a simplified version of the APG for adaptive predictive control based on delayed feedback information. The model consisted of a single module comprising a single unit representing a Purkinje cell with multistable properties that consisted of a collection of nonlinear switching elements termed dendritic zones that represented segments of a Purkinje cell dendritic tree. The model was explored in conjunction with a simulated single degree-of-freedom limb.

13.3.5. Thach's Neural Network Mechanism for Multiple Synergistic Muscles and Joints

Thach and colleagues (Thach 1998a; Thach, Goodkin, and Keating 1992; Thach, Kane, et al. 1992) came to the conclusion that the cerebellum is arranged to function over multiple synergistic muscles and joints (Fig. 13.6, top), as opposed to single joints. In advancing this concept, clinical data and more recent anatomical information and experimental support were taken into account (Fig. 13.6, bottom), for example, that the length of parallel fibers was greater than previously assumed (i.e., for chicken, of just under 10 millimeters instead of 2 millimeters as had been reported earlier for the cat; Palkovits, Magyar, and Szentágothai 1972; see also Chapter 3). Also taken into account in formulating the concept was the apparent representation of the myotomes (groups of muscles) perpendicular to the long axis of the cerebellum (i.e., roughly parallel to the trajectory of the parallel fibers).

An additional part of the formulation of these authors was the representation of body maps in each of the three deep cerebellar nuclei, each coding a different type and context of movement, and an adaptive role of the cerebellar cortex for combining simpler elements of movements into more complex synergies. Thus, the medial or fastigial nucleus controls muscles only in the modes of sitting, standing, and walking, the intermediate or interposed nucleus controls stretch and other somatosensory reflexes, and the lateral or dentate nucleus helps initiate (via thalamus and motor cortex) those movements that are triggered by mental or arbitrary sensory cues, and are therefore called volitional (Thach, Kane, et al. 1992).

Figure 13.6. (*contd.*)
the nuclear representation of the myotome; (e) different uses of the muscles in a limb may be coded by different subsets of parallel fibers and their differential effects on the Purkinje cells (coordination of synergist muscles); and (f) parallel fiber beams that span the nuclei in their Purkinje cell projection may influence two or more nuclei simultaneously (coordination of modes of movement). (From Thach, Goodkin, and Keating 1992, in *Annual Review of Neuroscience*, Vol. 15, copyright 1992, Annual Reviews; and from Thach 1998a, in *Novartis Symposium 218*, copyright 1998, John Wiley & Sons Limited; reproduced by permission of publishers and author.)

According to Thach (1998b), a critical function of the cerebellum is to help to combine the actions of muscles so they all work together toward a common goal, without the necessity of having to think about them. Thus, coordination of the many body parts to achieve smooth movements is generally agreed to be the specific role of cerebellar control. Hence, the role of the cerebellum as learning the coordination of movement (i.e., the coordination of movement involving several joints), employing mechanisms that are consistent with the Marr–Albus theory of motor learning, was stressed (Thach 1998b)

Accordingly, patients with lateral cerebellar lesions (i.e., lesions of the cerebellar hemispheres) show impairment of compound movements (i.e., across several joints), with relative or absolute sparing of simple movements made at a single joint by loaded agonist muscles only. (In contrast, inactivation of the motor cortex impairs both compound and simple movements.) It was concluded that parallel fibers implement both the coordination of complex movements and the learning of new movements. The basic Marr–Albus theory of motor learning was thus extended to reflect the point that the size of the response combinations (i.e., the repertoire) would be proportionate to the length of parallel fibers. The essential change (i.e., learning) was concluded to be a change in parallel fiber–Purkinje cell synaptic efficacy.

Thach (1998a) pointed out that, without the cerebellum, single-jointed movements (i.e., the load conditions are simple and the movement is made by the action of one or a few muscles only) are accurate, but multi-jointed movements lack coordination. Thus, when reaching out to grasp and pluck an apple, the first muscle to contract is the tibialis anterior in the lower leg, which compensates the moving arm's inertial torque on trunk and legs, preventing falling over backward. In contrast, when patients with a cerebellar injury reach to grasp an object, the tibialis anterior muscle no longer leads the response. (Diener et al. 1989).

Evidence was also cited suggesting a dissociation between the control of simple movements and compound movements: unit recordings in and inactivation of the deep cerebellar nuclei suggested control of compound but not simple movements, and consequently the Marr–Albus model was extended to propose that the parallel fiber contacts on the beam of many somatomotor-coded Purkinje cells could be the mechanism combining downstream motor nuclei elements and, ultimately, muscles (Thach, Goodkin, and Keating 1992; Thach, Kane, et al. 1992).

An anatomic model to account for a cerebellar role in coordinate compound movement and in motor learning was created (Thach, Goodkin, and Keating 1992; Thach, Kane, et al. 1992). In the model, different modes of control are mapped discretely within each of the deep nuclei, as follows: The fastigius controls equilibrium, stance, and gait under vestibular, somesthetic and visual control. The interpositus controls agonist-antagonists muscle couplings in various somatosensory reflexes. The dentate controls synergists in movements directed into extrapersonal space, under control from frontal, premotor, prefrontal, and parietal cortex. Each nucleus appears to contain a complete body map. Body parts within each body map, as well as adjacent body maps, are coupled by the parallel fiber beam, which contains many Purkinje cells, thereby combining muscles. Complementarity may be due to the many different body part configurations all being stored at the level of the parallel fiber–Purkinje cell synapse.

The authors further pointed out that damage of the cerebellum prevents control of interaction torques during reaching (Bastian et al. 1996). Thus, multijointed movement was deemed more complex than a summed combination of single-jointed movements because interaction torques (inertial, centripetal, Coriolis) are generated by one linkage moving on another. Further, fast compound reaching movements increase the magnitude of the interaction torques, and normally require prediction and compensation. Mathematical studies of patients and normal control subjects performing two-jointed reaching movements showed that patients had curved trajectories that overshot the target because of abnormal net torques, due to the patients' inability to control interaction torques. Patients attempted to eliminate the need to control interaction torques by reducing velocity and by decomposing the reach into movements made at each joint in sequence. As reach velocity increased, the errors increased, consistent with an inability to control interaction torques. Errors were made in the initial direction of movement, consistent with an inability to predict and compensate interaction torques.

The data were interpreted as being consistent with views that the cerebellum both helps to initiate movement and sends predictive signals to prevent errors that otherwise would occur because of uncontrolled interaction torques (Thach 1998a). It was speculated that the cerebellum uses motor commands and somatosensory feedback during early phases of the movement to trigger ad hoc learned patterns of muscle activity so selected, scaled, and timed to compensate the interaction torques that develop during later phases of the movement. The learned predictive compensation requires somatosensory feedback and is apparently removed by damage to the cerebellar cortex, from which it is inferred that the learned program is stored within the cerebellar cortex.

Such mechanisms of the cerebellum, it was suggested, might theoretically also underlie "cognitive" contributions of the lateral cerebellum, thus allowing multiple parallel background mental operations (analogous to multiple automatic muscle actions) concurrently with conscious foreground mental operations (Thach 1998a).

13.3.6. Thach's Concept of Context Linkage

Thach (1996a, 1996b, 1996c), in a review of the role of the cerebellum in motor learning and cognition, and following in the tradition of Brindley (1964), Marr (1969), and Albus (1971) (see below), posited that initially, movements are generated consciously. However, with repetition, the cerebellum establishes within itself a linkage (established by input from the inferior olive), with the context in which the movement is made, to the lower-level movement generators. When the linkage is complete, the occurrence of the context (i.e., a certain input to the cerebellum) will trigger (via the cerebellum) the appropriate motor response, now being automatic, rapid, and stereotyped. This concept was considered to be equally applicable to executing movements and thought. The premotor area of the cerebral cortex (for movement) and the "prefrontal areas" (for thought) would still plan without the help of the cerebellum, but not so smoothly, efficiently, and effectively (Thach 1996a, 1996b, 1996c).

13.3.7. Llinás's Theory of Inherent Rhythmicity and Electrotonic Spread in the Inferior Olivary Nucleus

In attempting to answer the question of the role of the cerebellum in motor coordination, Llinás and his colleagues (Welsh et al. 1995) attributed special importance to the organization of the olivocerebellar system. These authors used a technique of multiple Purkinje cell recording (Sasaki, Bower, and Llinás 1989). Having found that there are domains or regions of Purkinje cell activity that are highly rhythmic and time-locked to movement (skilled tongue movements in rats) and thus synchronous, the authors concluded that the inferior olive organizes movement both in time (by entraining motor-neuronal firing through rhythmic activation of the cerebellum) and in space (by synchronous activation of cell ensembles, owing to electrotonic coupling among cells in the inferior olive). Thus, specific motor patterns can be reflected both in the size of an ensemble of Purkinje cells firing in unison and in the rate of firing of the individual Purkinje cells in an ensemble. In connection with the former, a fixed conduction time from inferior olive to the occurrence of the Purkinje cell complex spike was reported (i.e., the conduction time was independent of the length of climbing fiber; Sugihara, Lang, and Llinás 1993).

In the theory, Welsh et al. (1995) postulated that the axons of synchronously firing Purkinje cells converge on specific motor zones within the cerebellar nuclei. In turn, dynamic repatterning or sculpting of olivocerebellar synchrony, postulated to occur under the control of the cerebellar nuclei, may allow different combinations of muscles to be used for movements intended to have varying spatial organizations.

In a summary of the theory (Welsh and Llinás 1997), oscillatory activity of olivary neurons is postulated to provide a pacemaking signal and to restrict the control process to particular moments in time, while the process of electrotonic coupling and uncoupling of assemblies of olivary neurons is proposed to underlie the spatial distribution of synergistic muscle activations.

In recordings from awake behaving monkeys, however, Keating and Thach (1995) found that discharges from olivary neurons, as reflected in complex spikes from Purkinje cells in monkeys performing noncyclic wrist movements, were random rather than rhythmic and synchronized. An absence of clocklike timing in awake behaving animals was also reported for cerebellar nuclear cells (Keating and Thach 1996).

13.3.8. Silkis' Three-Layer Olivocerebellar Neural Network with Modifiable Connections

Silkis (2000) proposed a model of a three-layer olivocerebellar neural network with modifiable excitatory and inhibitory connections, the same Hebbian modification rules (Chapter 14) being assumed for Purkinje cells, granule (input) cells, and deep cerebellar nuclei (output) cells. (The modification rules for Golgi cells were assumed to be different.) Modification of excitatory transmission between parallel fibers and Purkinje cells, mossy fibers and granule cells, and mossy fibers and deep cerebellar nuclei cells, respectively, was considered to depend on inhibition from stellate/basket cells, Golgi cells, and Purkinje cells, respectively. The nature of modifications of the different synapses in the three layers of the network was assumed to be determined by olivary cell activity. Thus, in the absence (or, alternatively, presence) of a signal from the inferior olive, the long-term potentiation (or, alternatively, depression) of the efficacy of a synapse between input mossy fiber and output cell could be induced.

13.3.9. Commentary

Among the theories mentioned to this point, it is perhaps not surprising that there is little overlap because the theories are very diverse. Thus, for example, emphasis is laid on tapped delay lines and their modifications (Braitenberg), Purkinje cell complex spike readout as a measure of inhibition (Eccles), the special coordination between the association areas of the cerebral cortex and the lateral cerebellum, (Allen and Tsukahara, Thach), ongoing control by the climbing fibers of Purkinje cell simple spike rate (Mano, Bloedel, Llinás), transformations of various kinds by the cerebellar cortex (Calvert and Meno, Hassul and Daniels, Pellionisz), reverberating circuits (Eccles, Houk), and multimuscle/multijoint synergy (Boylls, Thach). In short, there is little in the way of themes common to all these theories of the cerebellum. In contrast, the next group of theories have in common the feature of storage at the parallel fiber–Purkinje cell synapses, under the conjoint control of the climbing and mossy fibers.

13.4. Cerebellar Learning Theories – Forerunners of Adaptive Control Theories

A recurring theme in several theories is that of the learning of the elements of motor acts by the cerebellum, the learning taking place at the interface between parallel fibers and Purkinje cell dendritic tree. The idea of the cerebellum as a site of learning of motor skills was mentioned in an early meeting report by Brindley (1964), as indicated previously.

13.4.1. Grossberg's Parallel Fiber–Climbing Fiber Correlation Model for Cerebellar Learning

Emphasizing the basic orthogonality (perpendicularity) of parallel fibers and climbing fibers (i.e., of Purkinje cell dendritic trees), Grossberg (1969) proposed that a correlation between the two types of fibers results in a two-dimensional correlational matrix, according to which the growth of new Purkinje cell dendritic spines is determined, thus implementing motor learning of spatiotemporal patterns. (Compare

Seijnowski's [1977] theory of motor learning [see below] by storage of covariance of parallel and climbing fibers.)

The publication of the book on the cerebellum by Eccles, Ito, and Szentágothai (1967), if not the paper in an engineering journal by Szentágothai (1968) on the cerebellum, may have inspired or at least spurred the publication of two major theories of this type, namely, the ones of Marr (1969) and of Albus (1971).

13.4.2. Marr's Instruction Learning Theory

One of the first of this group of theories was that of Marr (1969), which he considered applicable both to learning by the cerebellum of motor skills as well as learning to maintain posture and balance. Some revisions appeared subsequently (Blomfield and Marr 1970), in light of the then recent developments concerning the cerebellum.

The key to the theory was the close relationship between Purkinje cells and cells of the inferior olive via their climbing fibers terminating on the Purkinje cells. In the learning phase, it was presumed that movement is organized by the cerebral cortex, and either directly or via a corollary (parallel) discharge of the cerebral movement commands to peripheral muscles, the appropriate olivary cells (in which single elemental movements are individually represented) fire in a particular sequence. The consequent activation of the Purkinje cells, via their corresponding climbing fibers, causes the Purkinje cells to learn the corresponding elemental movement from the parallel fibers, which report the same movement as was reported over the climbing fibers, but instead over the mossy fiber system.

The mossy fiber–granule cell–Purkinje cell arrangement, it was suggested, could operate as a pattern-recognition device, so a given Purkinje cell, by virtue of different patterns of alterations of its mossy fiber synapses, could store different contexts (in effect, different combinations of parallel fiber activity). Golgi cells were viewed as a kind of automatic level control (i.e., on excitability) for granule cells, with stellate cells and basket cells acting in the same capacity for Purkinje cells. After learning, particular contexts (carried by the parallel fiber input) were themselves adequate to fire the Purkinje cell, the output of which would then induce the next elemental movement, and so on.

The learning itself, at the synapses from parallel fibers to Purkinje cell dendrites, was considered to be *facilitated* (in the sense of a Hebbsian [Hebb 1949] modifiable synapse) by the conjunction (essentially simultaneous firing, i.e., within some 50–100 milliseconds) of climbing fiber activity and presynaptic activity at the parallel fiber–Purkinje dendritic tree synapses. No other cerebellar synapses were required to be modifiable, although they were considered to contribute to the learning process.

In brief, in Marr's theory, Purkinje cells learn to execute elements of movements on the basis of their parallel fiber inputs, under the direction of, or upon instruction from, the cells of the inferior olive and their associated climbing fibers. The inferior olivary cells themselves were presumed to receive instructions for elemental movements from the cerebral cortex, in the learning process. The initiation of a sequence of learned elemental movements in Marr's (1969) original formulation was evidently presumed to result from an initialization at the periphery (effected by the cerebral cortex), which would then be reported to the cerebellum via the mossy fibers, thus initiating a chain of elemental movements. An essential point, however, was that of modifiability of synapses of the parallel fibers onto the Purkinje cells.

Marr considered that the main test of the theory would be whether the synapses from parallel fibers to Purkinje cells are facilitated by the conjunction of presynaptic and climbing fiber (or postsynaptic) activity. Marr also discussed the possibility that the cerebellum could be the site of storage of conditioned reflexes.

Soon after his theory of the cerebellum appeared, Marr (1970) also published a theory for the cerebral neocortex; however, it is perhaps Marr's theory of the cerebellum that will be his most enduring legacy (see Llinás 1981b).

13.4.3. Albus' Pattern-Recognition Data-Processing Theory

Albus' theory was perhaps the first neural network model of the cerebellum (Chapter 14). The theory, which was developed independently of Marr's theory but agrees with it on a number of points, according to Albus (1971), was viewed by him as modifying and extending Marr's theory. Albus indicated that his theory was modeled after a classical Perceptron (Chapter 14) pattern-classification device (Rosenblatt 1961), in which the mossy fiber–granule cell–Golgi cell input network performs a divergence or fan-out operation (Fig. 13.7) that enhances the pattern-discrimination capacity and learning speed of the Purkinje cells. Modifiability of parallel fiber synapses was postulated for stellate and basket cells, as well as for Purkinje cells, including the inhibitory and excitatory synapses onto the latter. An essential difference from Marr's theory was that pattern storage is accomplished primarily by *weakening* synaptic weights rather than by strengthening them. Albus also included a role for the cerebellar nuclei.

As explained by Albus, the prototype of a pattern-recognition device in the form of a Perceptron (which was originally conceived as a model for the eye) consists of cells having adjustable-strength synaptic inputs of excitatory and inhibitory influences that are summed and compared with a threshold (Fig. 13.7). If the threshold is exceeded, the cell fires; if not, the cell does not fire. Patterns to be classified or recognized are presented to the input layer of sensory cells (i.e., the first of three layers of cells). The sensory cells are connected to associative cells, which perform transformations (e.g., perhaps random, perhaps feature detecting) on the sensory pattern. Outputs of the associative cells then act upon response cells through weights of various strengths. It is the firing, or failure to fire, of the response cell that results in a classification or recognition on the set of input patterns presented to the sensory layer (e.g., retina). The Perceptron exhibits an ability to learn, under instruction (i.e., by being presented with the desired classification), in response to which it adjusts its own weights according to a set of rules. This latter process basically consists of a negative feedback (not shown in Fig. 13.7) to the weights so as to effectively diminish the proportion of incorrect classifications.

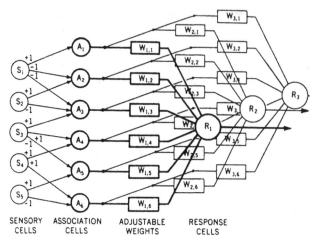

Figure 13.7. Classical Perceptron. Each sensory cell receives a stimulus of either +1 or 0 (e.g., light or dark). This excitation is passed on to the association cells with either a + 1 or −1 multiplying factor. If the input to an association cell exceeds 0, the cell fires and outputs a 1; if not, it outputs 0. This association layer output is passed on to response cells through weights $W_{i,j}$, which can take any value, positive or negative. Each response cell sums its total input and, if it exceeds a threshold, the response cell R_j fires, outputting a 1; if not, it outputs 0. Sensory input patterns are in class 1 for response cell R_j if they cause the response cell to fire, in class 0 if they do not. By suitable adjustment of the weights $W_{i,j}$, various classifications can be made on a set of input patterns. (From Albus 1971; in *Mathematical Biosciences*, Vol. 10, copyright 1971, Elsevier Science; reprinted by permission of the publisher.)

In comparison with the Perceptron, the parallel fibers are viewed, in Albus' theory, as containing information coded in an ideal manner to serve as the input to the Perceptron association (intermediate) cells, and the Purkinje cells are considered to serve a function similar to the Perceptron response (output) cells (Fig. 13.7). In comparison with the fan-out (divergence) of the Perceptron association cells and the fan-in (convergence) of the Perceptron response cells, Albus drew attention to the large fan-out of each granule cell and the enormous fan-in of each Purkinje cell. Thus, the closely stacked single-plane Purkinje dendritic tree makes possible the maximum fan-out for each parallel fiber. At the same time, the flat Purkinje dendritic tree with its input parallel fibers pierces it at right angles, thus maximizing the fan-in for each Purkinje cell. These layouts were considered optimal for the cerebellum's task of recognizing patterns of information from proprioceptive receptors and of generating the appropriate motor command signals.

In relation to synapse modifiability, Albus viewed the inactivation pause in Purkinje simple spikes following climbing fiber activation as a classical unconditioned response (UR), the unconditioned stimulus (US) being the activation of the climbing fiber. The conditioned stimulus (CS) was taken to be the ongoing mossy fiber activity at the time of the climbing fiber activation. If so, then the effect of learning should be that the particular mossy fiber pattern (CS) should elicit a pause (CR) in Purkinje cell activity similar to the inactivation response (UR) previously elicited by the climbing fiber activation. Such a pause would require that the relevant parallel fiber synapses be weakened, rather than strengthened.

In Albus' formulation, it was postulated that parallel fibers activating the Purkinje cells toward the end of the inactivation pause in Purkinje cell simple spikes, which follow climbing fiber activation, generate an error signal that weakens any parallel fiber synapses that tend to cause the Purkinje cell to fire during the inactivation response. The more strongly the excitation of that parallel fiber–Purkinje synapse, the greater the weakening. After learning is complete, the Purkinje cell pauses when the appropriate constellation of parallel fiber activation occurs, even in the absence of climbing fiber activation. The parallel with the Perceptron is that, if the response cell fires or tends to fire when it should not fire, then all synapses from active parallel fibers would be weakened, whereas if the response cell does not fire improperly, no adjustments are made.

It was assumed that inhibitory synapses (from basket and stellate cells) are also subject to the same weakening, because otherwise, firings of Purkinje cells would cease entirely. Thus, parallel fiber synapses on Purkinje cells, basket cells, and at least some stellate cells are weakened by incorrectly firing during climbing fiber activity. (However, other stellate cells, presumed to be subject to climbing fiber influence, were viewed as exhibiting a strengthening, rather than a weakening, of their parallel fiber synapses.) Purkinje cell collaterals were viewed as maintaining the average Purkinje cell activity at a relatively constant level over the entire cortex, as well as engendering of lateral inhibition (i.e., across different folia). To the recurrent Purkinje collaterals (and perhaps also to climbing fiber activity) was also attributed a bistable effect in the firing rate of Purkinje cells (i.e., either spontaneously active or completely silent).

Because, according to Albus' theory, learning is associated with a *decrease* in Purkinje cell inhibitory output, the net effectiveness of the (excitatory) input from mossy fiber collaterals to the cerebellar nuclei is increased, so less and less (excitatory) input to the nuclear cells from collaterals of the climbing fibers is necessary to produce the same amount of nuclear cell response.

Albus (1975a, 1975b; see also Miller, Glanz, and Kraft 1987) described a robotics application of his theory of the cerebellum in the form of an adaptive system (Chapter 14) in which control functions for many degrees of freedom operating simultaneously could be computed by referring to a table (the latter analogous to the stored modifications of parallel fiber–Purkinje cell synaptic weights) rather than by mathematical solutions of equations.

13.4.4. Eccles' Instruction-Selection Theory

Eccles (1977a) indicated that his instruction-selection theory could be considered a detailed neurophysiological formulation of conjunction-potentiation theory of Marr (1969) and the related theory of Albus (1971). In Eccles' theory, the precisely targeted climbing fibers (i.e., synapsing onto a very few Purkinje cells) effect a synaptic strengthening of a small volume of parallel fibers from among a much larger region of termination of parallel, and thus of mossy fibers, so the synaptic effectiveness of the latter would be selected in accordance with the climbing fiber territory traversed, provided the activation of the parallel and climbing fibers approximate one another quite closely in time. In this way, an originally diffuse cloud of mossy fiber input would become greatly sharpened.

13.4.5. Synaptic Mechanisms

Neither Marr nor Albus indicated specific mechanisms whereby parallel fiber–Purkinje dendrite synapses could be strengthened (Marr) or weakened (Albus). Such mechanisms were developed later by other workers (Chapter 7).

In a commentary on the Marr–Albus–Fujita models (see below), Ito (1982b) stressed the need for models of the cerebellum to include coordination and prediction, as well as the preprogramming of complex voluntary movements and their execution.

13.4.6. Gilbert's Distributed Memory Theory

Gilbert's (1974) theory has some features in common with Marr's (1969) theory of the cerebellum as a memory device, except for having a much larger memory capacity. Thus, for a single memory, all the (parallel fiber–Purkinje cell) synapses are viewed as being modified, not just a small group out of the total number of synapses of an ensemble of Purkinje cells. Thus, every synapse is envisaged as holding information relating to every memory stored in the neuronal network. Further, it is assumed that a Purkinje cell could learn to respond to a particular input from the parallel fibers (i.e., a certain pattern of frequencies of firing in these fibers) with any arbitrary output (frequency of firing). Any change in the Purkinje cell output causes a change of input to the muscle on which that cell acts, resulting in turn, via muscle receptors, in a change in the parallel fiber input to the same Purkinje cell. It is assumed that, in this way, an entire motor sequence would follow automatically. The Purkinje cell outputs would be determined by the cerebral cortex and conveyed to the former via the climbing fibers. Storage in the cerebellum is assumed to occur at synapses between parallel fibers (and basket cell axons) and Purkinje cells. Changes in climbing fiber rate during motor learning in a subsequent experimental series (Gilbert and Thach 1977) were considered to be consistent with the theory.

13.4.7. Seijnowski's Theory of Motor Learning by Storage of Covariance of Parallel and Climbing Fibers

Seijnowski (1977) treated motor learning in the cerebellum as a problem of storage of covariance, such that the change in synaptic strength between a parallel fiber and a Purkinje cell would be proportional to the covariance between discharges in the parallel fiber and the climbing fiber. It was predicted that both facilitation and inhibition should occur (under different conditions) at the same synapse, thus obviating the problem of saturation if only a unidirectional change were postulated (i.e., either LTD or LTP). The synapses maintain a constant average strength when

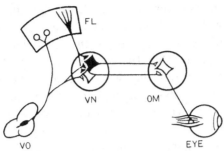

Figure 13.8. Sidepath connections through the cerebellum of the rabbit. VO, vestibular organ; FL, flocculus; VN, vestibular nucleus; OM, motorneurons innervating eye muscles. See also Figure 8.1, of which this is a simplified version. (From Ito 1984; *The Cerebellum and Neural Control*, copyright 1984; Lippincott Williams and Wilkins; reprinted by permission of publisher and author.)

the climbing fiber and the parallel fiber are uncorrelated; when they are correlated, the synaptic strength could be flexibly adjusted anywhere within its dynamic range. (Compare Grossberg's [1969] parallel fiber–climbing fiber correlation model above.)

13.5. Early Adaptive Control Models

13.5.1. Ito's Computer/Control Model: An Internal Neocerebellar Model

Ito (1970) drew attention to the participation of the cerebellum in the formation of skilled movements (see also Chapter 7). Thus, in voluntary unskilled movements, the initial order arising from association cortex is transferred to the motor cortex and then through the pyramidal tract down to the spinal motor centers; the final outcome being verified via sensory pathways by the association cortex. However, with practice, the movements become refined and become voluntary skilled movements, the sensory feedback loop from the periphery being replaced by an *internal model in the neocerebellum* that is a faithful miniature of the combination of the spinal motor system, the external world, and the sensory pathways.

In light of control theory, according to Ito (1970), this arrangement may be understood as a type of model reference adaptive control system. Cerebellar syndromes such as dysmetria and intention tremor could then be understood in terms of impairment or loss of the internal model in the neocerebellum, just as in the stage before learning.

Ito (1970, 1972, 1976b) also suggested that the flocculus and the fastigial nucleus act as an adaptive control system with a variable gain element to regulate brain stem neuronal activity producing the VOR.

In pointing out the relevance of control theory to cerebellar function, Ito (1970, 1972, 1979) drew attention to two reflex arcs: the VOR, as mentioned above, and the vestibulospinal reflex. The VOR (Fig. 13.8) entails a three-neuron chain that includes primary vestibular afferents, vestibuloocular relay neurons (with a side chain through the flocculus of the cerebellum), and oculomotor neurons. The vestibulospinal reflex also operates as a three-neuron chain: primary vestibular afferents, vestibulospinal relay neurons, and spinal neurons. As a specific example, the vestibulocollic (neck) reflex arc (for holding the head stable) acts through neck and trunk muscles to reposition the head; this output is sensed by the vestibular organ, thus closing the loop, in control theory terminology. There is no cerebellar side loop in this instance. In the case of the VOR, however, the loop is not closed, because movement of the eye is not detected by the vestibular organ, but rather by the retina, and is reported to the cerebellar side chain via the inferior olive (Maekawa and Simpson 1973). The vestibulo-ocular arc, therefore, functions in an open loop manner (i.e., as a feedforward control system), the cerebellum having the effect of closing the loop by adjusting the gain in the open loop. This constitutes Ito's "flocculus hypothesis of the VOR control" (Ito 1970, 1984).

Ito (1984, p. 328) gave several additional examples of such a modifiable sidepath model, as well as some examples in which the cerebellum is included not as a side path, but within a loop itself, and also a hypothetical lateral interaction type in which there are facilitatory or inhibitory influences from one control system to another. In general, Ito suggested that the critical requirement for involvement of the cerebellum in a control system should be lack of an effective feedback loop, but not necessarily lack of a feedback loop altogether.

An open-loop control system, Ito (1984) indicated, is simpler to design and construct than a closed loop one, because a feedback path is not required. An open-loop system, however, can be more subject to external disturbances and to changes in parameters of the control system. These drawbacks of an open-loop control system could be removed by a computer. Ito pointed out that the cerebellum could have this role in motor control and, further, it could be the site of the learning process then recently postulated by Marr (1969). Ito then expanded his control system model of the cerebellum to include, in general terms, adaptive (i.e., self-modification or optimization of parameters) and predictive (anticipatory) control, as well as some aspects of motor learning (Ito 1984).

In more recent formulations (Ito 1990, 1993d) that incorporate more formally the phenomenon of LTD in Purkinje cells as the basis of long-term storage (Ito, Sakurai, and Tongroach 1982), Ito (1984) advanced the concept of a cerebellar microcomplex, consisting of a cortical microzone (Oscarsson 1979) and a small group of cells in a cerebellar or vestibular nucleus, the ensemble of which acts as an adaptive controller. The error signals for modification of the Purkinje cells (in relation to parallel fiber synapses) were considered to arrive via the climbing fibers. Such adaptive-control microcomplexes, it was postulated, are inserted in reflex arcs, command systems of voluntary motor control, and probably even in cortical systems performing certain mental activities (Ito 1990).

The corticonuclear microcomplexes were postulated to function as follows: (1) Purkinje cells have an inhibitory action on cerebellar nuclear cells, whereas both mossy and climbing fibers give off excitatory collaterals to nuclear cells. (2) Climbing fibers convey encoded error signals. (3) These act to induce LTD in those parallel fiber–Purkinje cell synapses that were coactivated with the climbing fiber input.

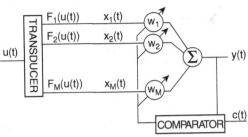

Figure 13.9. Fujita's diagram of an adaptive filter. In the counterpart cerebellar model, u(t) is a mossy fiber signal; $F_1 \ldots F_M$ represent the output, at various delays (phases), of the mossy fiber–Golgi cell–granule cell phasing system; $w_1 \ldots w_M$ are the weights of the parallel fiber–Purkinje cell synapses; y(t) is the output of the Purkinje cells; c(t) the training signal from the climbing fibers, which is compared with the output y(t) in an iterative manner to readjust the weights to minimize the error (in a "mean square" sense) between y(t) and c(t). (From Fujita 1982a; *Biological Cybernetics*, Vol. 45, copyright 1982, Springer-Verlag, Heidelberg; reprinted by permission of publisher and author.)

As theoretical models for this concept, Ito (1990) cited Albus' (1971) Perceptron model and Fujita's (1982a) adaptive filter model (see below). In actuality, Ito (1993c, 1993d) suggested, ordinary voluntary movement is learned during repeated practice in a feedback mode, but after learning is completed, it is executed in a feedforward mode.

13.5.2. Fujita's Adaptive Filter Model

Fujita (1982a), who characterized the models of Marr and of Albus as spatial pattern-classifier models with learning capacities, based his own model on the theory of adaptive filters (Widrow et al. 1975; Widrow et al. 1967; see also Widrow and Stearns 1985). Fujita considered his model, in which "adaptive" means "self-modifying," to be a reformulation of the models of Marr and Albus in such a way as to be more relevant to the operation of the cerebellum. Fujita's diagram of an adaptive (linear) filter is reproduced in Figure 13.9. The Golgi cells (themselves functioning as a phase-lag element), which together with the granule cells make up the transducer or phasing system (left side of Fig. 13.9), receive input from both climbing fibers and mossy fibers. The error-correcting feedback loop in Figure 13.9 is such that a positive correlation between a given phase of the signal, x_j, with the error signal itself results in a diminution of the corresponding weight, whereas a negative correlation results in an increase.

According to the learning principle of Fujita's schema, the synaptic weight of a given parallel fiber onto a given Purkinje dendrite decreases when the activity of its climbing fiber is smaller than the spontaneous discharge rate of that climbing fiber and, conversely, increases when the activity of the climbing fiber is less than the resting rate. The weight change is proportional to the product of the impulse rate of the parallel fiber and the deviation of the climbing fiber rate from its resting rate.

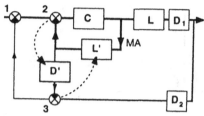

Figure 13.10. Schematic diagram of the Smith Predictor. The Smith Predictor consists of the boxes labeled L' and D', and lies within a negative feedback loop in which errors (sensed by Comparator 1) are converted by a controller (C) to torques that are sent to the limb (L). The feedback loop contains delays on the forward (D_1) and backward (D_2) paths. The dynamic (time-varying) model of the limb (L') lies on a fast internal feedback loop that receives a moving average of the torques sent to the muscles (MA). The output of the dynamic model is sent to Comparator 2, and also through the model delay ($D' = D_1 + D_2$) before comparison (by Comparator 3) with the delayed feedback. The dashed lines indicate training signals for modifying the two models to make the Predictor adaptive or time varying. (From Miall and Wolpert, 1995, in Ferrell and Proske, eds., *Neural Control of Movement*, copyright 1995, Kluwer Academic/Plenum Publishers; reprinted by permission of publisher and author.)

As Marr and Albus assumed in their models, Fujita assumed that a coincidence of parallel fiber activity and climbing fiber activity onto Purkinje cells resulted in an alteration in the efficacy of the parallel fiber–Purkinje cell synapses.

For the filtering function, a Golgi cell was considered to act as a (relative) phase-lag element, so various lead-lag versions of the incoming mossy fiber signals were available to the parallel fibers from mossy fiber–granule cell–Golgi cell input network (Fig. 13.9). The parallel fiber signals are gathered together through the adjustable weights of their synapses onto the Purkinje cells, to form the output signals of the Purkinje cells.

In a companion paper, Fujita (1982b) applied his adaptive linear filter model to the VOR (Chapter 8), obtaining good agreement with experimental data on alterations of the reflex by prisms.

13.5.3. The Cerebellum as a Smith Predictor

Starting with existing forward predictive models that were proposed by others for the motor apparatus (limb and muscle) and that provide a rapid prediction of the sensory consequences of each movement, Miall et al. (1993) and Miall and Wolpert (1995) proposed adding a second model for the time delays (of 150–200 millisec-onds) in the control loop due to receptor and effector delays, axonal conductances, and cognitive processing delays (Fig. 13.10). This model delays a copy of the rapid prediction so it can be compared in temporal register with actual sensory feedback (e.g., visual) that results from the movement, with the delay that the feedback in-curs. The result of this comparison serves to correct for errors in performance and to be a training signal to learn the first model. The authors suggest that such a Smith Predictor, comprised of adaptive neural networks, is present in the lateral cerebellum, predicting movement outcome in visual, egocentric, or peripersonal coordinates, and another is in the intermediate cerebellum, where the predictions are in motor coordinates. The second model (the delay model) is a type of Smith Predictor, a form of controller originally devised for engineering systems subject to long feedback delay, and which have internal representations of the object being controlled. By using error signals from the comparators, the Smith Predictor can be made adaptive.

In summary, first, the Smith Predictor provides a rapid prediction of the outcome of a motor command, and second, it provides a delayed copy of the prediction that will match in time the actual feedback arising from the movement. By combining these two functions, which should be easier to generate than inverse dynamic models, fast and stable control can be achieved even in the presence of long loop delays. Thus, as long as the predictive model and the delay models are accurate, the transport delays are effectively moved outside the feedback control loop because the actual and predicted feedback cancel one another. The authors further suggest that the comparison between expected (i.e., reafference) and actual sensory signals, from which a teaching signal is provided for the cerebellum, is carried out by the inferior olive (Miall et al. 1993; Miall and Wolpert 1995).

13.5.4. Models of the Saccadic System

Schweighofer, Arbib, and Dominey (1996a, 1996b) described an adaptive control model of the cerebellum for control of saccadic gain that includes adaptation to repeated presentations of two-step visual targets (Goldberg et al. 1993). (The latter authors found that, after lesions of the fastigial and interpositus nuclei, monkeys had lost and never regained saccadic adaptation to such stimuli.) In the model, the inferior olive is an error detector and includes a "window of eligibility" to ensure that error signals that elicit a corrective movement are used to adjust the original movement, not the second movement. In comparison with the feedback error learning scheme of Kawato and Gomi (1992a, 1992b, 1993), the authors indicated that in their own model, the cerebellum is only part of the inverse model of the plant (limb system), there being other noncerebellar, nonadaptive pathways that provide an approximate inverse model of the plant.

In view of clinical and experimental evidence that damage to the cerebellar vermis results in permanent loss of saccadic accuracy, Dean (1995) simulated this finding in a model in which the vermis adjusts the gain of the saccadic internal feedback loop in response to information about the amplitude of the intended saccade. The conclusion was reached that appropriate timing of burst onset and duration in the fastigial nuclei (which receive the output from the vermis) is essential for producing accurate saccades.

13.6. The Cerebellum as a Sensory Processor

Fahle and Braitenberg (1985), in raising the issue of whether the task of the cerebellum is to adapt motor coordination to the passive mechanical propagation of some disturbance through the body and therefore function as a detector of movements, pointed out that such a view would place the cerebellum more on the sensory side.

13.6.1. Paulin's Hypothesis of the Cerebellum as a Kalman–Bucy Filter

Paulin (1989) expressed the view that the cerebellum is basically a sensory-processing organ, the correct operation of which is essential for motor control. In his view, the cerebellum is an analog of a Kalman–Bucy filter (see below), and by analogy, the cerebellar patient is forced to break normally extended smooth movements with many degrees of freedom into small, manageable pieces. It was also suggested that adaptive arrays may provide possible realistic models for cerebellar structure and function, especially in view of the parallel organization of the cerebellum (Paulin 1989).

13.6.2. Bower's Hypothesis of the Cerebellum as a Sensory-Data Processing Aid

Bower (1997) suggested that the cerebellum is involved in coordinating the sensory data on which the motor system depends. The conclusion was based on the different types of influences the ascending segment and the two parallel fiber segments of the granule cell axon, in conjunction with the background synaptic input of stellate cell synapses, may have in controlling the physiological responsive state of the Purkinje cell dendrite to the synaptic input from the ascending segment of the granule cell axon. In this view, the cerebellum has no direct responsibility for any behavior, including motor coordination. Rather, it facilitates the computational efficiency of a large number of other neural systems by supervising the acquisition of the data on which these other systems depend. Thus, slowed execution of motor tasks by cerebellar patients is considered to result from the longer computing time necessary to process poorly controlled sensory data.

Miall (1997; see also Miall, Malkmus, and Robertson 1996) advanced the related view that the cerebellar cortex does not generate motor sequences, but does generate sensory predictions about the sensory consequences of motor acts.

It may be mentioned that, in the role of the posterior parietal cortex (PPC) in the transformation of visual coordinates into motor coordinates and the issuing of motor commands, the question also arises as to whether the role is better characterized as "sensory" or "motor" (Eskandar and Assad 1999).

13.6.3. Results from Imaging Studies

From their positron emission tomography (PET) cerebral blood flow (CBF) studies, Jueptner and Weiller (1998) suggested that the neocerebellum (i.e., the hemispheres of the posterior lobe) is more engaged when lines were retraced as compared with new line generation, and that the neocerebellum is involved in monitoring and optimizing movements using sensory (proprioceptive) feedback. Comparison of active and passive movements suggested that 80–90% of the neocerebellar signal could be attributed to sensory information processing. The authors concluded that the neo-cerebellum may be concerned with monitoring the outcome (the afferent sensory component) and optimizing movements using sensory (feedback) information.

From a functional magnetic resonance imaging (fMRI) study of normal subjects, Parsons et al. (1997) concluded that the lateral cerebellum and dentate nucleus is primarily concerned with sensory rather than motor processing (see also Paulin 1993). Thus, activation of the dentate occurred during sensory stimulation when there were no accompanying overt finger movements or discrimination, but substantial finger movements (when not associated with tactile discrimination) did not result in significant activation. However, dentate activation was greatly enhanced when a sensory discrimination was required, with or without overt finger movements. The strongest activation occurred when sensory discrimination was combined with finger movements.

13.6.4. The Importance of Proprioceptive Sense

From study of patients with loss of proprioceptive sense because of severe sensory neuropathy, Ghez et al. (1990) concluded that proprioceptive input (sensory receptors of muscles and joints, especially the spindles and tendon organs) is necessary both to program movement trajectory accurately and to specify the muscle activation pattern necessary for the subsequent maintenance of posture. As a result of the loss of proprioceptive input, the deafferented patients were unable to compensate for the complex inertial properties of their limbs, although performance improved appreciably by vision of the limb at rest prior to movement or during a prior movement. In contrast to the relatively good accuracy of direction, distance, and acceleration in movements by normal subjects (which movements the authors assume to be pre-programmed; compare McIntyre and Bizzi 1993), the patients made large errors in direction and distance, indicating that, in contrast to conclusions from studies of single-joint movement, proprioceptive information from the limb is critical for the programming of multijoint movement. The authors proposed that proprioceptive input (from the sensory receptors in muscles and joints, especially the spindles and tendon organs) is used by the central nervous system to update an internal representation, or model, of the mechanical properties of the limb.

For an extensive case history of loss of proprioceptive sense resulting from severe sensory neuropathy, see Cole (1991).

13.7. The Cerebellum as a General Preparatory Organ

Courchesne and Allen (1997) reiterated their hypothesis that the fundamental purpose of the cerebellum is to predict internal conditions needed for a particular mental or motor operation and to set those conditions in preparation for the operation at hand (Akshoomoff and Courchesne 1992). Such a cerebellar preparatory function is neither a sensory nor a motor activity, but rather a general one, preparing the relevant neural system (sensory, motor, memory, attention, language, etc.) that may be needed in upcoming moments. Cerebellar preparatory actions thus facilitate and improve sensory processing, as well as mental and motor performance, in response to subsequent sensory events.

13.8. Some Reviews and Critiques of Models and Theories of Cerebellum

Houk, Buckingham, and Barto (1996) reviewed several models of the cerebellum and motor learning, including the parallel fiber–Purkinje cell modifiable synapse model of Marr (1969) and Albus (1971); the APG model (Berthier, Singh, and Barto 1993); the control theory models of Paulin (1989), Miall et al. (1993), and Kawato and Gomi (1992a); the multijoint coordination model of Thach, Goodkin, and Keating (1992), as well as several conditioned reflex models, and models for saccadic and smooth eye movements. Four prerequisites for models of motor learning were then enumerated: (1) identification of what is being learned in an information processing sense; (2) a rule for modifying synaptic efficacy (i.e., a "learning rule"); (3) a means of directing of training signals to the appropriate sites and appropriate times in the training process so that the learning is adaptive; and (4) the training information that is provided to the model must be defined and realistic. The authors then considered the various theories in relation to these criteria, tending to favor the APG model.

(The authors' article [Houk, Buckingham, and Barto 1996] and seven other target articles are followed by 42 commentaries and in turn by the responses of the authors of the target articles.)

13.8.1. The Modifiable Parallel Fiber–Purkinje Cell Synapse Theories

Several apparent difficulties with the Brindley (1964)–Marr (1969)–Albus (1971) concept of cerebellar motor learning were raised by Llinás, Lang, and Welsh (1997), for example, (1) LTD evidently does not require climbing fibers; (2) the unidirectionality of LTD, which would soon suppress all parallel fiber synapses unless a complementary mechanism such as LTP is also present; and (3) data from certain knockout mice indicating that neither motor learning nor classical conditioning requires cerebellar LTD. An alternative function for LTD was proposed, namely, that of a neuroprotective function for Purkinje cells against any Ca-mediated excitotoxicity, arising both from parallel fiber and from climbing fiber activity. In closing, the authors reiterated their own view of the olivocerebellar system as being directly involved in the ongoing modulation of movements, acting to time appropriately the activation of different muscle groups in complex movement sequences.

Llinás, Lang, and Welsh (1997) also raised concerns of whether LTD can underlie the unique types of learning that are commonly studied in this regard, namely, classical conditioning of eyeblink reflexes and gain modification of the VOR, because the stimulus conditions under which they occur are very highly specific.

However, Thach (1996a) expressed the view that much evidence favors the Marr–Albus theory for trial and error modification of certain kinds of behavior that is within the province of cerebellar control.

13.8.2. Artificial Neural Network Models

According to Kawato (1996b), several artificial neural-network learning algorithms, such as the recurrent back-propagation or forward-inverse modeling approach that have been used for trajectory learning, cannot be easily mapped onto the cerebellar circuitry in a biologically plausible way.

In Kawato's view, one of the most important predictions of the cerebellar feedback–error learning model – that is, that the inverse dynamics model of a controlled object resides in the cerebellar cortex – requires that some mossy fiber inputs represent the desired trajectory information.

Kawato (1996b) also concluded that the sensory-motor transformation occurs at the parallel fiber–Purkinje cell synapse, or speaking in more computational terms, the cerebellar cortex is the major site of inverse-dynamics transformation. For cognition (Chapter 9), Kawato proposed bidirectional architecture (i.e., using both the forward and inverse models in a reciprocal fashion; Chapter 16).

13.8.3. Adjustable Pattern-Generator Models

Kawato (1996b) observed that the APG model does not provide any concrete computational mechanism for learning invariant features of multijoint arm movements, such as roughly straight paths of the hand in Cartesian space and bell-shaped velocity profiles, in a recurrent network when only the target error information is provided.

In setting forth their own view that the cerebellum makes sensory predictions (or "state estimates") that are based on outgoing motor commands and sensory feedback, Miall, Malkmus, and Robertson (1996) differed with Houk, Buckingham, and Barto (1996) on the latter group's view of the cerebellum as an APG, pointing out the lack of support from comparative anatomy (as had Paulin [1993]) and the difficulty of controlling positive feedback loops (in the brain stem), an essential part of the APG hypothesis.

From the perspective of Kalman filtering (Kalman 1960), Paulin (1996) also took issue with the APG theory of Houk, Buckingham, and Barto (1996) and the notion that elemental movement commands are generated by positive feedback in distributed neural loops regulated by Purkinje cells, the cerebellum itself regulating premotor networks.

13.8.4. The Hierarchy of the Cerebellum in Motor Processing

Paulin (1996) took issue with Thach's (1996b) conclusion of the ordering of the hierarchy within which the cerebellum is placed (i.e., whether it is upstream or downstream from other structures involved in motor processing), which in Paulin's view results in the conclusion that the cerebellum initiates movements (see also Paulin 1993).

FOURTEEN

Neural Networks and Adaptive Control: Neural Network Models

In the survey of models in Chapter 13, several different types of cerebellar models, including some adaptive control and some neural network models, were treated more or less equally. In this chapter, by contrast, emphasis is placed on general features of (the closely interrelated) adaptive control and neural network models, especially concerning the question of plasticity (memory; i.e., changeability of weights), as a model for changes of efficacy of mossy fiber–Purkinje cell dendrite synapses under the influence of the climbing fibers. This chapter paves the way for Chapter 15, in which the features of adaptive controllers (as well as, in principle, neural network models) are illustrated with the aid of a specific implementation. Thus, a look is taken inside the "black box" or schematic diagram. In turn, more advanced and recent adaptive control and neural network models are considered in Chapter 16.

A brief word should be mentioned about terminology and synonyms, a topic that will also arise later. Neural nets, nerve nets, or (artificial) neural networks, are also known as connectionist models (theories) of computation (Rumelhart 1990). Adaptive controllers are also known as adaptive filters, adaptive signal processors, state estimators, and Kalman filters or Kalman–Bucy filters. These terms are used more or less interchangeably in this text. (The term, *adaptive controller*, has a slightly different meaning from that of adaptive signal processor; the latter implies that there is no specifically controlled object; see also Chapter 16.)

Haykin (1996, p. 17) characterizes an (artificial) neural network as consisting of a large number of interconnected nonlinear processing units called *neurons*, the development of which from the beginning has been motivated by the way the human brain performs its operations, hence the name.

Surveys of the history of and tutorials on the topic of neural networks can be found, for example, in Sutton and Barto (1981), Cowan and Sharp (1988a, 1988b), Lockery (1992), Vemuri (1992), Fetz (1993), Gupta and Rao (1994), Arbib (1998), Rolls and Treves (1998), and Haykin (1995, 1996). For the field of adaptive control, standard references include Widrow and Stearns (1985), Haykin (1996), and Ioannou and Sun Jing (1996). A comparative survey of the two fields, with particular emphasis on historical aspects, is given by Widrow and Lehr (1990).

14.1. Neural Networks

14.1.1. History

The field of neural networks is often considered to have begun with the publication of Rosenblatt's (1958, 1961) description of his Perceptron. As mentioned in Chapter 13, the Perceptron, in its most specific form, was a visual pattern-recognition device. However, Rosenblatt himself originally intended the term *perceptron* (not capitalized) as a generic name for a variety of theoretical nerve nets (i.e., to refer to a set of signal-generating units, or "neurons") connected together to form a network. Rosenblatt considered the neuron model to be a direct descent of that proposed by McCulloch and Pitts (1943), in which the fundamental thesis, as summarized by Rosenblatt, was that all psychological phenomena can be analyzed and understood in terms of activity in a network of two-state (i.e., all or none, or one bit) logical devices. Indeed, Arbib and Amari (1985) pointed out that Pitts and McCulloch (1947) modeled the superior colliculus as a distributed controller of eye movements, in which spatial distribution of activity, rather than localized decision making based on a lumped variable, provided the appropriate transformation from retinal activity to muscle contraction.

Werbos (1975) completed a doctoral dissertation at Harvard University entitled, "Beyond Regression: New Tools for Prediction and Analysis in the Behavioral Sciences" (see also Werbos 1990). Werbos' dissertation, although unnoticed for a time, was the forerunner of a blossoming of activity in the neural networks field. Werbos' starting point had been to attempt to improve on the work of Box and Jenkins (1970) concerning the method of prediction known as autoregressive moving average (ARMA) analysis. The essential contribution of Werbos (1975) was to implement two separate methods, using dynamic (time-varying) feedback to accelerate the estimation of the coefficients in an ARMA process. A brief digression is made concerning the ARMA approach.

In ordinary autoregressive analysis or linear prediction (see e.g., Barlow 1985; Haykin 1996; Makhoul 1975), a time series or signal (e.g., a voltage–time graph) is "regressed on itself," by which a model of the time series is made. In the equivalent terms of linear prediction, the immediate past sample points of the signal (i.e., the most recent set of values resulting from periodic sampling) are used iteratively to predict the value at the next sample points. The term *linear* implies that the predicted output is a *sum* of weighted portions (weighted, of course, implies multiplication) of the most recent sample values. The ensemble of weights or coefficients to be applied to the sequence of the immediately previous sample points must be computed, for which methods exist (e.g., the so-called least-mean-square [LMS] technique; see e.g., Makhoul 1975). The error signal, itself a time series, is just the time sequence of the difference between the predicted values and the actual values.

In ARMA analysis (Haykin 1996), the error signal itself (i.e., the prediction error) is also expressed as a linear combination of its own past. Correspondingly, the weights for the error-signal sample points must also be computed, so the ARMA procedure is clearly a more complex computational procedure than is the autoregressive method.

In both autoregressive (AR) analysis and in ARMA analysis, the original signal is assumed to be unchanging in its statistical characteristics (e.g., its power spectrum). However, in Kalman filtering (or Kalman–Bucy filtering, in the analog case; see, e.g., Barlow 1985; Haykin 1996), the original signal can be changing or nonstationary. The output error signal is fed back iteratively in such a way as to adjust the weights to maintain a minimum output error, even though the input itself is nonstationary or changing with time. It is this essential principle of self-adjustment that lies at the basis of both adaptive control and neural network methods and makes them powerful (e.g., for prediction of stationary and nonstationary signals), and at the same time, makes them relevant to the problem of modeling the cerebellum.

14.1.2. Kalman (Kalman–Bucy) Filtering

A Kalman filter is an example of the implementation of an adaptive system, either in the original time-sampled form (Kalman 1960) or its continuous form (Kalman and Bucy 1961).

The basic principle of operation of the Kalman–Bucy filter is to extrapolate (predict) a given curve consisting of the set of most recent sampled values by applying recurrently a correction based on the difference between the most recent value and the prediction for that value, based on a (small) set of the most recent values. The Kalman–Bucy filter can be considered to be an extension to nonstationary time series (i.e., signals) of the Wiener filter to predict the trajectory of aircraft for anti-aircraft fire control (Wiener 1950). Because its transfer function may vary continuously, the Kalman filter is often called an adaptive filter (Haykin 1996).

Arbib and Amari (1985) suggested possible neural analogues of the Kalman–Bucy filter for realistic motor control problems, particularly in relation to a look-ahead module (predictor). These authors indicated that use of the Taylor series (i.e., expression of the next point in time as a function of the present point, its first derivative, and its second derivative) were not satisfactory because of inherent drawbacks. These include that it uses differentiation, a highly noisy operation, and presumes noise-free data. For one sample-point look-ahead, the first of these problems (but not the second) can be diminished by periodic sampling and taking successive differences, together with successive differences of the successive differences. The results are equivalent to the first and second derivatives, respectively. The Kalman–Bucy filter, however, permits multiple-point look-ahead, the accuracy of the prediction being inversely related to the prediction interval.

Paulin (1989, 1993, 1997) suggested that the cerebellum is a neural analogue of a Kalman filter, as previously mentioned.

Also, as previously mentioned in Chapter 9, Droulez and Cornilleau-Pérèz (1993, p. 491) have drawn attention to the relevance of Kalman filtering to the problem of multisensory fusion in the moving organism.

14.1.3. Learning by Back-Propagation

Werbos' approach was later rediscovered, or discovered independently, by Rumelhart, Hinton, and Williams (1986a, 1986b). In the learning procedure that these authors described, which was termed "back-propagation," the weights of the second layer (the internal or "hidden" layer of units between the input and output layers in a three-layer neural net) are repeatedly adjusted to minimize the error in the output vector or outputs. (It may be noted in passing that, generally speaking, a neural network can comprise more than, but not less than, three layers.) The learning procedure that these authors described differed from previous, simpler methods such as the perceptron-convergence procedure (in which the connections to the intermediate layer are fixed by hand) in its ability to create new features (Widrow and Stearns 1985; see Widrow and Lehr [1990] and Haykin [1994, p. 41] for additional points of history of the back-propagation algorithm). Albus' approach, described in Chapter 13, could be considered an example of the perceptron-convergence procedure.

The arrangement and the procedure is schematized in Figure 14.1. The three layers of units are depicted in C. Of these, the input units form the bottom layer, the hidden units form the middle layer, and the output units form the top layer. For the hidden (middle) layer, only one weight (w_{ij}) is shown. In A in Figure 14.1, the inputs and outputs of a single intermediate cell are depicted; the shape of the curve through which outputs are passed, a sigmoid, is shown in B. The sigmoid curve has the effect of making the output much less sensitive to extreme fluctuations than to fluctuations near the middle section of the curve. Alternative curves (also known as squashing functions, activation functions, transfer characteristics, or threshold functions) through which the outputs could be passed are shown in Figure 14.2, along with the sigmoid curve; they include a threshold or step function, and a diagonal line for linear modeling (output proportional to input). (See also below.) The sigmoid curve of neural net theory can be compared with sigmoid transfer curves for neurons shown in Figure 14.3. (It may be noted, in passing, that the sigmoid transfer curve has the effect of converting a Gaussian or normal amplitude distribution function to a rectangular (equally probable) amplitude distribution function [cf. Barlow 1993, p. 348 ff].)

The term *back-propagation* arises from the method of (automatically) setting the weights of the hidden layer of units. In brief, in a three-layered system consisting of input, hidden, and output layers (Fig. 14.1), for example, the total error between each of the set of actual outputs (i.e., of the output vector) and the desired output vector (e.g., the input vector itself, or a teaching vector) is fed back (i.e., back-propagated) iteratively to the individual weights of the hidden or middle layer, in such a way as to decrease progressively the total error. Initially, the weights are randomized. This procedure is known as the gradient-descent method of minimizing the error; it is equivalent to a least-squares or LMS approach. In the case of multiple hidden layers,

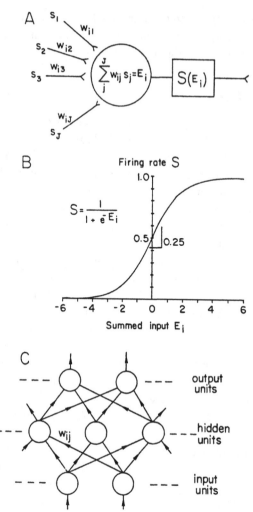

Figure 14.1. Properties of the units and network used for simulating the vestibulo-oculomotor system. A, Sample intermediate cell, with weighted inputs and summed and shaped (S(E$_j$)) output. B, Sigmoidal transfer characteristic for summed output to firing rate. A zero input result in a spontaneous rate of 0.5. C, General network architecture. Ordinarily, each unit projects to all units in the subsequent layer (note that direction of flow is from bottom to top). (From Anastasio and Robinson 1989b; *Biological Cybernetics*, Vol. 61, copyright 1989, Springer-Verlag; reproduced by permission of publisher and author.)

the weights for the ones nearest the outputs are processed first, followed by those for the successively earlier hidden layers. (Fig. 14.1 is considered further below.)

In effect, back-propagation networks have internal (hidden) units that are free to take on response properties to best accomplish a given computational task (Zipser and Andersen 1988).

In recurrent or feedback networks (which have their equivalent in more complex arrangements of feedforward networks), multiple hidden layers can propagate backward as well as forward, with weights for both directions in some instances. An example of a single-layer feedback neural network is shown in Figure 14.4. (It should

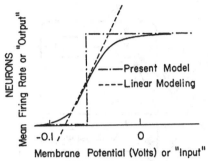

Figure 14.2. Sigmoid transfer function (solid line) together with linear (dashed line) and stepfunction or threshold (dotted-dashed line) transfer functions. Note that, in the linear case, the mean firing rate does not take on negative values. (From Hopfield, 1982; in *Proceedings of the National Academy of Sciences*, Vol. 79; reprinted by permission of the author.)

be noted that the feedback path is separate from the back-propagation, [which can also be viewed as feedback] for weight adjustment for time-varying inputs].) (A recurrent or feedback network can be viewed as the counterpart of a recursive adaptive filter, that is, one having an infinite impulse response [IIR] – see below and Chapter 15.)

A development in neural networks by Williams and Zipser (1989) made it possible to run continuously (i.e., for time-varying inputs) recurrent (i.e., using feedback)

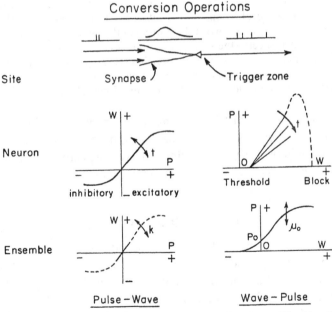

Figure 14.3. The operations of conversion (top) between the wave W and pulse P modes of activity for the single neuron and for the ensemble. At the single unit level, P to W is time varying and nonlinear, and W to P is time varying (t) but linear between threshold and cathodal block. At the macroscopic level, W to P is static and nonlinear, whereas P to W is constrained to a small-signal linear range. (The slope dW/dP changes with learning; the slope dP/dW changes with arousal.) (From Freeman 1983; in Basar et al. (eds.), *Synergetics of the Brain*, copyright 1983 Springer-Verlag, Heidelberg; reprinted by permission of publisher and author.)

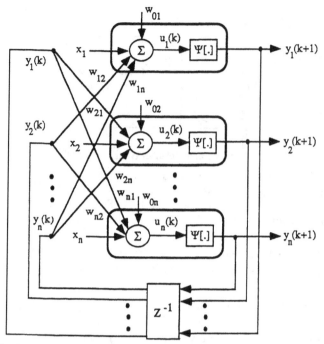

Figure 14.4. Single layer feedback neural network. The inputs are $x_1, x_2, \ldots x_n$; the weights are $w_{12}, w_{21}, \ldots, w_{n2}$, etc.; the bias inputs are $w_{01}, w_{02}, \ldots w_{0n}$; the transfer characteristic curve (Fig. 14.2) is indicated by the $\psi[.]$'s; and the outputs are $y_1(k+1), y_2(k+1)\ldots y_n(k+1)$. Note that the feedback (recurrent) input, shown at the bottom of the figure, is delayed one unit of time (indicated by z^{-1}) with respect to the $x_1, x_2, \ldots x_n$ inputs. (This feedback path is independent of the feedback path employed to determine the weights.) (From Gupta and Rao 1994; reprinted from *Neuro-Control Systems: Theory and Applications*, copyright 1994, IEEE; reprinted by permission of the Institute of Electrical and Electronics Engineers.)

networks. For such continuously operating neural networks, Williams and Zipser used the term *back-propagation through time*, as opposed to back-propagation. Such dynamic recurrent networks incorporating time-varying activity may include lateral as well as feedback connections within the same layer (Fetz 1993).

14.2. Adaptive Control

Numerous treatises concerning adaptive control and adaptive signal processing (i.e., in which there is not a specific controlled object) are available (e.g., Haykin 1996). Shynk (1995) presented a more mathematical treatment of adaptive filtering, and a comparison of the LMS algorithm and Rosenblatt's (Perceptron) algorithm. An overview of adaptive control can be found in Åström (1995), and a précis of adaptive signal processing can be found in Haykin (1995). Narendra (1995) gave a discussion of neural networks in adaptive control.

Sanner and Slotine (1995) pointed out that the rapid development and formalization of adaptive signal processing algorithms loosely inspired by biological models can be potentially useful in flexible new learning control algorithms for nonlinear

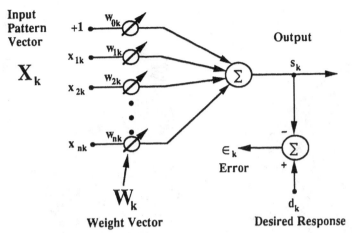

Figure 14.5. Adaptive linear combiner. (The method of computing the weight vector from the error signal is not shown.) (From Widrow and Lehr, 1990; reprinted from *Proc. IEEE*, Vol. 78, copyright 1990, IEEE, by permission of the IEEE.)

dynamic systems (e.g., robot manipulators) based on "neural" nets, provided, however, stability is ensured and performance is quantified.

14.2.1. Operation of Adaptive Controllers

A schema of one of the simplest adaptive controllers, an adaptive linear combiner, is shown in Figure 14.5. The unit receives multiple simultaneous inputs that are individually weighted and then summed (thus the characterization, linear); the latter are then compared with the desired response (method not shown in Fig. 14.5), from which comparison the weights are automatically and iteratively adapted so as to minimize the error, ϵ_k, using a least-mean-square (LMS) criterion (Widrow and Hoff 1960). Thus, the sum of the squares of the errors for each input is minimized. (The process of error minimization is described and illustrated in Chapter 15.)

The LMS algorithm or Widrow–Hoff rule (Widrow and Hoff 1960) was described at about the same time as the Perceptron (Rosenblatt 1958, 1961), and independently of the latter. Actually, the idea of a nonlinear adaptive filter (and predictor), using a minimum mean-square error criterion, was conceived by Gabor (1954) and successfully implemented several years later (Gabor, Wilby, and Woodcock 1961). With the addition of a threshold device, yielding a $+/-1$ output in parallel with the analogue output, the adaptive linear combiner becomes an adaptive linear element (Fig. 14.6).

The error signal is computed by obtaining the difference between the desired response or signal (also known as the training signal) and the output signal; from this difference, the weights are computed. Figure 14.6 shows the same linear combiner, but with three alternatives for computing the error: linear, sigmoid, and sigmum (threshold). The minimum square error (MSE) surfaces for each case are also shown; these indicate the manner in which the error approaches a minimum (i.e., the lowest

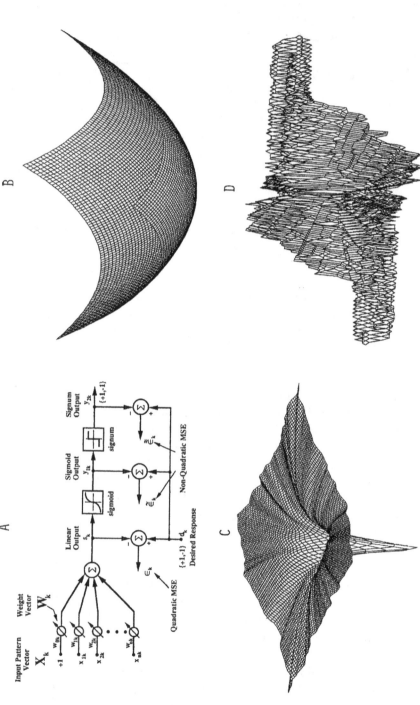

Figure 14.6. A, Adaptive linear combiner with linear, sigmoid, and sigmum (threshold or binary) output. B, C, D, Corresponding MSE surfaces for each of the three transfer functions. (Same functions as in Fig. 14.2.) Note that, in the linear case, the rate of error correction (i.e., adaptation) is maximum for the largest error; in the sigmoid case, the rate of correction is the faster the smaller the residual error. The surface for the sigmum (threshold or hard-limiting case), in which only the sign (+ or −) of the error is used, is very irregular, in effect reflecting the one-bit quantization of the error. Note that with the sigmum output, this schema is the same as that of the neural net schema in Figure 14.1A. (From Widrow and Lehr 1990; reprinted from *Proc. IEEE*, Vol. 78, copyright 1990, IEEE, by permission of the IEEE.)

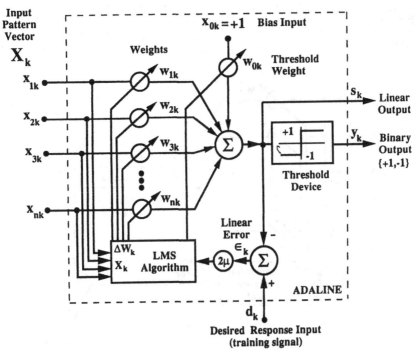

Figure 14.7. Adaptive linear element with inclusion of the return loop for automatically adjusting the weights by the LMS algorithm. In this instance, provision for a bias (offset) input is included (top). (From Widrow and Lehr 1990; reprinted from *Proc. IEEE*, Vol. 78, copyright 1990, IEEE, by permission of the IEEE.)

point on the respective surfaces). For the linear output, the surface is quadratic or paraboloid – the larger the error, the faster the error decreases. In the sigmoid case, the smaller the error, the more rapidly the error decreases. (Only the linear output is used for the illustrations in Chapter 15 [e.g., Fig. 15.2]). In the sigmum (sign only or binary) case, the error surface is very irregular; in a mathematical sense, the error function is not differentiable.

A redrawing of the adaptive linear combiner of Figure 14.5 to include the LMS algorithm, by means of which the weights are determined from the inputs and the error signal, is shown in Figure 14.7. Note that both linear and binary outputs are shown.

If the error signal is evaluated as the difference between the training signal and the binary output, rather than the linear output, the configuration shown in Figure 14.8 results; with the substitution of the Rosenblatt Perceptron Rule or Perceptron convergence procedure (as previously described) for the LMS algorithm, this configuration becomes equivalent to the Perceptron (Widrow and Lehr 1990). However, if the sigmoid function (Fig. 14.6) is used, the approach becomes mathematically equivalent to back-propagation (Widrow and Lehr 1990).

The adaptive linear combiner, when fitted with a sigmoid output characteristic, becomes equivalent to the back-propagation method or algorithm. The sigmoid

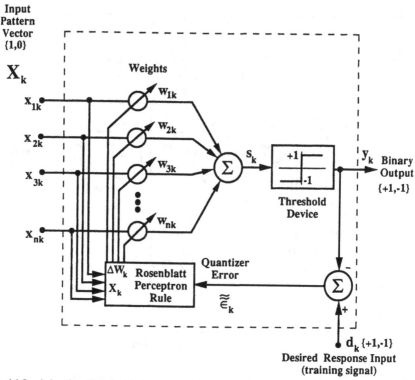

Figure 14.8. Adaptive threshold element of the Perceptron. Note that in the adaptive linear element (Fig. 14.6), the return loop for adjusting the weights (the linear error) is taken before the threshold device, whereas in the Perceptron, it is taken (as the quantizer error) after the threshold device. The Perceptron rule or convergence procedure does not change the weights if the output decision, the y_k,'s are correct (i.e., if the quantizer error is zero.). However, if there is an error, then the weight vector (the ensemble of weights) is combined either positively or negatively with the input signal (vector) to diminish the (quantizer) error. (From Widrow and Lehr, 1990; reprinted from *Proc. IEEE*, Vol. 78, copyright 1990, IEEE, by permission of the IEEE.)

shape provides saturation for decision making (i.e., the size of the error is limited in both directions), yet its mathematically differentiable input–output characteristic facilitates adaptivity. Widrow and Lehr (1990) gave a comparison of analogue versus digital implementation of the linear combiner with a sigmoid output characteristic. As mentioned previously, the sigmoid function has the effect of converting a Gaussian amplitude distribution to a rectangular (equally probable) amplitude distribution.

To reiterate, in the linear combiner as shown in Figure 14.5, there are multiple inputs, for the ensemble of which a weight vector (i.e., a set of weights) is computed. After scaling according to the weights, the inputs are then summed. From comparison with the desired response or training signal, the error signal is generated, with which the error is still further minimized.

Such multiple inputs can also be derived from the same source but at a series of different times (i.e., the input to the linear combiner becomes a time series),

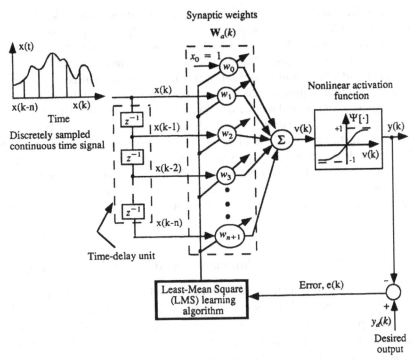

Figure 14.9. A time-delay (dynamic) neural network. The weights $W_a(k)$ are automatically adjusted according to the LMS learning algorithm. (A bias input $[x_0]$ and weight $[w_0]$ are included in the event that the desired output signal has an offset.) (From Gupta and Rao 1994; reprinted from *Neuro-Control Systems: Theory and Applications*, copyright 1994, by permission of the IEEE.)

as shown in Figure 14.9. This configuration makes possible the capability of linear prediction, which is considered and illustrated in Chapter 15. In particular, means for implementing the LMS algorithm are considered.

14.2.2. Finite Impulse Response vs. Infinite Impulse Response Adaptive Filters

In the design and implementation of adaptive controllers, a distinction is to be made between those controllers having a finite impulse response (FIR) and those having an infinite impulse response (IIR). Haykin (1996) compared FIR filters and IIR filters as follows:

> The choice of a finite-duration impulse response (FIR) vs. an infinite-duration impulse response (IIR) for the filter is dictated by practical considerations. An FIR filter is inherently stable, because its structure involves the use of forward paths only. In other words, the only mechanism for input-output interaction in the filter is via forward paths from the filter input to its output. Indeed, it is this form of signal transmission through the filter that limits its impulse response to a finite duration.

In contrast, an IIR filter involves both feedforward and feedback. The presence of feedback means that portions of the filter output and possibly other internal variables in the filter are fed back to the input. Consequently, unless an IIR filter is properly designed, feedback in the filter can indeed make it unstable, with the result that the filter oscillates; this kind of operation is clearly unacceptable when the requirement is that of filtering for which stability is a "must." By itself, the stability problem in IIR filters is manageable in both theoretical and practical terms. However, when the filter is required to be adaptive, which brings with it stability problems of its own, the inclusion of adaptivity combined with feedback that is inherent present in an IIR makes a problem that much more difficult to handle. It is for this reason that in the majority of applications requiring the use of adaptivity, the use of an FIR filter is preferred to an IIR filter even though the latter is less demanding in computational requirements. (pp. 195–196)

14.2.3. Neural Networks and Adaptive Controllers – A Brief Comparison

From the preceding, it is evident that with respect to the essential points, there are similarities and parallels between the approach of neural networks and the approach of adaptive controllers (adaptive filters). The essential similarities are that both compute the weights automatically by minimizing error by the LMS method. The "classical" adaptive controller usually employs a linear output characteristic whereas the neural network back-propagation method usually employs a sigmoid output characteristic (Figs. 14.2 and 14.6, top). Configurations of neural networks characteristically employ more (linear) mixing at all levels (input, intermediate [hidden] and output), the weights being imposed just before the hidden level (Fig. 14.1C). The similarities and differences between the topics of neural networks and adaptive control (adaptive signal processing), which as previously mentioned were originally developed independently, are well summarized by Widrow and Lehr (1990).

Additional aspects of adaptive control are discussed in Chapters 15 and 16.

14.3. Neural Network Models of the Cerebellum

The Albus model described in Chapter 13 is a forerunner of neural network models of the cerebellar system (or of certain of its components, e.g., the cerebellar nuclei, the inferior olive). Additional neural network models are now considered.

Treating the question of parallel fiber–Purkinje cell synapses in the context of conditioned reflex theory, Melkonian, Mkrtchian, and Fanardjian (1982), in their neuronal network model, placed the site of alteration of synaptic strength (i.e., the site of cerebellar memory), on the presynaptic side of the parallel fiber–Purkinje cell dendritic tree.

Dunin-Barokowski and Larionova (1985a, 1985b) considered several arrangements of the mossy fiber–granule cell interface as a neural net in relation to questions of coding, and the neural net of granule cells (numbering 20,000 in their particular example) and Purkinje cells in relation to the information-storing capacity of single parallel fiber–Purkinje cell synapses.

14.3.1. Neural Network Models and the Vestibulo-Oculomotor System

Anastasio and Robinson (1989a, 1989b; see also Arnold and Robinson 1991, 1992) used the back-propagation algorithm to program distributed neural network models of the vestibulo-oculomotor system. The networks were trained to combine vestibular, pursuit, and saccadic eye velocity command signals. Figure 14.1, previously discussed in part, shows the general properties of this system. After training, the model neurons in the neural networks were found to have diverse combinations of vestibulo-oculomotor signals that were qualitatively similar to those reported for actual vestibular nucleus neurons in the monkey (i.e., the behavior of the neurons correlated neither with the semicircular canals nor with the eye muscles). This similarity was considered to implicate a learning mechanism as an organizing influence on the vestibulo-oculomotor system. These authors contrasted their approach with the more commonly employed, lumped black box approach, which although modeling the overall behavior of the vestibulo-oculomotor system, indicates little about how real eye-movement signals would be propagated and processed by real neural networks.

In a related effort, Anastasio (1992) was able to simulate vestibular compensation, after unilateral loss of the organ, by means of a three-layered neural network employing back-propagation (weight adjustment) and connections (which were considered to be recurrent) among hidden-layer units for the two sides.

In a subsequent paper, which included a short tutorial on neural nets, and in a paired commentary paper, Robinson (1992a, 1992b; see also Arnold and Robinson 1997) argued that, in view of the apparent success of the approach of neural nets, and using the oculomotor system (mentioned above) as an example, the attempt of trying to explain how any biological neural network works on a cell-by-cell (i.e., reductionist) basis is futile, so one may have to be content with attempting to understand the brain at higher levels of organization. In a word, it could be said that the main work in neural nets is done not at the input and output levels (layers), but by the hidden units of the intermediate layers, and although the self-organization that characterizes the neural net accomplishes the desired task (e.g., of modeling the oculomotor system), the details of this distributed, internal organization may be impenetrable and incomprehensible and even meaningless from the outside, and in the biological case, even with microelectrodes. As an example, Robinson (1992a, 1992b) considered that mathematical descriptions of what a system is trying to do (e.g., a metric tensor representation [transformation] in the cerebellum [Pellionisz and Llinás 1980]), are likely to be truly impossible, and that neural networks subserving sensorimotor transformations appear to be shaped by error-driven learning rather than by mathematical constructs such as tensor theory, at least cocerning the vertical vestibulo-ocular reflex (VOR) (Anastasio and Robinson 1990).

Robinson (1992a, 1992b) was equally unenthusiastic, as indicated above, about black box modeling in general, which in his view seldom makes testable predictions and has largely proven to be a blind alley. On a similar note, Fetz (1993) pointed out the basic limitation of conventional physiological (and anatomical) data in that they provide a very selective sample of a complex system. Fetz called for a combination of unit recording techniques and neural modeling.

Using the VOR as a model, Lisberger and Seijnowski (1992) demonstrated that changes in the transient component of a neuron's responses can be transformed into changes in the steady-state output of a neural network by the use of recurrent (feedback) connections. The model was made more general by Qian (1995), by including two additional time constant variables and two synaptic weight variables.

As mentioned in Chapter 8, Arnold and Robinson (1997) described a neural network model that learned to simulate the integration necessary for conversion of eye-velocity commands (e.g., from the semicircular canals) to eye-position commands for the motor neurons of the extraocular muscles process. The model could also change its gain (by minimization of retinal slip) and, at the same time, compensate for orbital mechanics. The model included an equal number (14) of excitatory and inhibitory neurons. The integration employs positive feedback through lateral inhibition conveyed by an inhibitory commissure.

In the static neural net model of the VOR described by Coenen, Seijnowski, and Lisberger (1992), biologically plausible local learning rules that included both vestibular nuclei and the cerebellum were explored.

14.3.2. Rubrocerebellar and Corticocerebellar Neural Network Models

Berthier et al. (1992) described a neural network model of the cerebellum, starting from the concept of rubrocerebellar and corticocerebellar information-processing modules, arranged in parasagittal arrays in the cerebellar cortex, which function as adjustable pattern generators (APGs; see Chapter 13) capable of storage, recall, and execution of motor programs. The model consists of three parts: a neural network that generates control signals, a muscle model that controls joint angle, and a single-plane arm (Fig. 14.10). A learning rule, based on long-term depression (LTD; Chapter 7) adjusts the subsets of APGs that are selected, as well as characteristics of their activity, to achieve desired movements. Each APG consists of a positive feedback loop and a set of Purkinje cells (PCs), constituting a cerebrocerebellar recurrent network. Upon being triggered (by sufficiently strong activation), the neurons in these loops fire repetitively in a self-sustained manner. An APG's motor command is generated through the action of its PCs, which inhibit and modulate the buildup of activity in the feedback loop. The activity of loop cells is conveyed to spinal motor areas by rubrospinal fibers. PCs receive information that specifies and constrains the desired movements via parallel fibers.

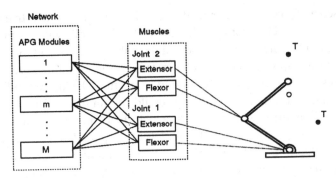

Figure 14.10. Neural network model for control of joint angles by APG. A collection of APGs (network) controls a simulated two-degree-of-freedom kinematic planar arm with antagonistic muscles at each joint. The task is to move the arm in the plane from a central starting location to one of eight symmetrically placed targets. Activation of an APG causes a movement of the arm that is specific to that APG and the magnitude of an APG's activity determines the velocity of that movement. The simultaneous activation of selected APGs determines the arm trajectory as a superposition of these movements. (From Berthier et al. 1992; in Moody, Hanson, and Lippmann (eds.), *Advances in Neural Information Processing 4*, copyright 1992, Academic Press/Morgan Kaufmann; reprinted by permission of the publisher.)

Testing the predictions based on an adaptive cerebellar model in the form of a dynamic (time-varying) neural network represented by a set of differential equations, Olivier, Coenen, and Seijnowski (1995; Coenen 1999) employed computer simulations of the model to show how the cerebellum could construct predictive modifications of the VOR to compensate for retinal slips occurring up to hundreds of milliseconds later.

Lukashin et al. (1995) proposed a recurrent neural network of interconnected, randomly spiking neurons to simulate the spiking activity of motor cortical cells recorded in behaving monkeys during two tasks. The first was a mental rotation task that required a movement at an angle from the stimulus direction. The second task entailed a memory scanning task, which required the selection of a direction of movement that depended on the serial position of stimuli in a sequence. The simulation was found to be possible by virtue of a large repertoire of neural activity stored in the connectivity matrix (i.e., the ensemble of weights), which, once initiated by specific external inputs, evolves in a sequential manner.

14.3.3. A Neural Network Model for Arm Movement

Keeping in mind that inertial, gravitational, and interaction forces must be taken into account when necessary in limb movements, and that the limb feedback in slow movements begins, with increasing speed, to arrive too late for online control, Contreras-Vidal, Grossberg, and Bullock (1997) proposed a neural network model of opponent (agonist–antagonist) cerebellar learning for arm movement. The model assumes a central pattern generator in the cerebral cortex and in the basal ganglia, a neuromuscular force controller in the spinal cord, and an adaptive cerebellum. For the latter, both LTD (from parallel fiber–Purkinje cell synapses in response to conjunctive stimulation of parallel fibers and climbing fibers), and long-term potentiation (LTP) (in response to parallel fiber signals alone, enabling previously weakened synapses to recover) are incorporated in the model. Clinical findings of delay in onset, ataxia, and terminal oscillations could be simulated. The model was considered to be compatible with models in which the command for movement originates outside the cerebellum (e.g., the models of Ito [1984] and of Thach, Goodkin, and Keating [1992]), in contrast to models that postulate the cerebellum as an adjustable pattern generator responsible for primary trajectory generation (e.g., Houk et al. 1990).

14.3.4. Olivo-Cerebellar-Nuclear Complex Models

Spatiotemporal patterns of activity in the sagittal olivo-cerebellar-nuclear complex were explored by Contreras-Vidal, Bloedel, and Stelmach (1995), with the aid of a neural net model that included nonlinear ordinary differential equations to model membrane potentials. In the network model, Purkinje cell dendritic trees were characterized as a single summing node at the soma, and short-term enhancement (rather than depression, as in LTD) of Purkinje cells was accounted for. The results were considered to be consistent with the Dynamic Selection Hypothesis of Bloedel and his group (Bloedel and Kelly 1992; see Chapter 13), concerning the importance of climbing fiber function in real-time cerebellar operations.

Fetz and Shupe (1990) successfully trained neural network models that incorporated time-varying activity and that allowed unrestricted connectivity by backpropagation to generate discharge patterns that had been previously seen in cells of behaving monkeys. The latter patterns, which were used as training signals for the networks, included phasic-tonic, tonic, decrementing, etc. The function of specific hidden units in the network were tested by making selective "lesions" of particular units, or by stimulating the latter and determining the resultant behavior of the remaining network.

Simulation of response properties of a subset of posterior parietal neurons in vision was reported by Zipser and Andersen (1988), employing a back-propagation programmed neural network.

14.3.5. Neural Network Generation of Timed Responses

In what they considered to be an elaboration of the model by Marr (1969) and by Albus (1971), Buonomano and Mauk (1994) described a neural network model of the cerebellum that can generate timed responses in the range of milliseconds to seconds without conduction delays (e.g., in the parallel fibers). In the neural network, the subset of granule cells that is active is time varying owing to a granule cell–Golgi cell–granule cell negative feedback. The duration of the interval following a stimulus is selectively altered by changing the strength of granule cell–Purkinje cell connections for those granule cells that are active during the target time window. Memory of the reinforcement at that interval is subsequently expressed as a change in Purkinje cell activity that is appropriately timed with respect to stimulus onset.

14.3.6. Neural Network Models of the Cerebellar Cortex

In the three-layered (i.e., glomeruli, granule cells, and Purkinje cells, respectively) neural network model of the cerebellar cortex proposed by Chapeau-Blondeau and Chauvet (1991), a schema was introduced that makes explicit use of a side feedback loop (granule cells to Golgi cells to granule cells), as well as propagation delays (primarily along the granule cell dendrites) of neural signals. The schema permits the ability, in response to mossy fiber input patterns, of storing temporal sequences of motor and associated sensory patterns in the Golgi cell–granule cell system, upon which sequences a perceptron-like association is then performed by the Purkinje cell layer according to Hebbian rules (rather than by gradient-descent minimization, i.e., by mean square error). The model was based on the hypothesis that a movement or trajectory in real space is coded and memorized by the cerebellar cortex as a trajectory in the (multidimensional) state space of a neural network. The climbing fibers are inactive in the retrieval phase, during which a temporal sequence is generated on the Purkinje cell axons (i.e., coding for the sequential commands necessary to perform or control the desired movement in the specified sensory context). All the different types of excitatory and inhibitory synapses of the cerebellar cortex are included in the network. Also included in the model is synaptic plasticity of the parallel fiber–Purkinje cell synapses under the control of the climbing fibers, which during the learning phase are viewed as conveying an error signal (as opposed to a teacher or desired signal), the method of generation of which was not specified. The resulting neural network was capable of learning and retrieving temporal sequences of patterns.

Finally, Lansner and Ekeberg (1994) reviewed several neuronal network models of motor generation and control in invertebrates and vertebrates, with particular emphasis on swimming by the primitive vertebrate, the lamprey (see Chapter 2). Neuronal network models of the motor cortex, cerebellum, and oculomotor system in various higher vertebrates were also reviewed.

14.3.7. Neural Network Model of the Dorsal Spinocerebellar Tract

On the basis of an earlier finding that a prominent feature of dorsal spinocerebellar tract (DSCT) responses (conveying muscle and cutaneous inputs from the hindlimbs) was that the timing pattern of their poststimulus activity was largely independent of the stimulus, Osborn and Poppele (1992) proposed that the response timing was established by neural circuitry rather than by afferent firing patterns. In this connection,

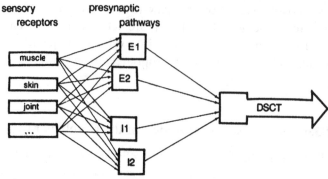

Figure 14.11. Functional neural net model of dorsal spinocerebellar tract DSCT circuitry. Sensory receptor afferents diverge onto four types of presynaptic pathways: two types of excitatory (E1 and E2) and two types of inhibitory (I1 and I2) pathways responsible for early- and late-peaking responses. DSCT cells receive convergent input from each type of pathway. (From Osborn and Poppele 1992; in *Journal of Neurophysiology*, Vol. 68, 1992, copyright American Physiological Society; reprinted by permission of the publisher.)

the authors proposed a parallel distributed network model of the DSCT (Fig. 14.11). A consequence of the distributed organization is that the signals transmitted to the cerebellum by single DSCT cells do not simply represent inputs from specific receptors. Rather, the information is transmitted in ensemble form, so a key element in the signaling was considered likely to reside in the temporal patterns of activity of DSCT neurons.

FIFTEEN

Specific Features of Adaptive Controllers and Adaptive Signal Processors

This chapter is devoted to a relatively technical discussion of adaptive control and adaptive signal processors (ASPs; as mentioned previously, the two terms are used more or less interchangeably), as a preliminary to the continuation of the consideration of adaptive control models of the cerebellum in Chapter 16 and to Chapter 17.

The discussion in Chapters 13 and 14 suggests that two of the leading and more promising approaches to modeling the cerebellum have been the closely interrelated approaches of neural networks, on the one hand, and adaptive controllers, on the other hand. These two approaches share the feature of self-adjustments of weights to adapt themselves automatically to a given training signal or to a desired output, or to a succession of desired outputs.

In this chapter, a closer look is taken at the process of adaptive control in the form of a specific ASP of the author's own design and construction, which functions on-line and in real time. (As previously indicated, the term *adaptive controller* is used in reference to a system that adaptively controls a specific object [e.g., a biological or robotic limb], and *adaptive signal processor* is used to indicate basically the same process, but without controlling a specific object.) This exercise begins with a simple task and progresses to a series of more complex tasks. Sample results (i.e., waveforms) are given from which a better impression of the operation of these devices can be obtained than from descriptions and block diagrams alone. These illustrative examples also serve to illustrate the adaptive features of neural networks since the operation of the latter is quite similar in principle to adaptive signal processors. The significance of the features that emerge from this survey in relation to modeling the cerebellum are considered in Chapter 17, after some additional, recently described adaptive controllers are considered in Chapter 16.

It should be emphasized that the topic at hand is that of modeling the function cerebellum, in the present case, by principles of adaptive control, or in the terminology of this chapter, ASP. To the extent that this premise is correct, the inner details of the models are clearly different from those of the biological systems of the cerebellum

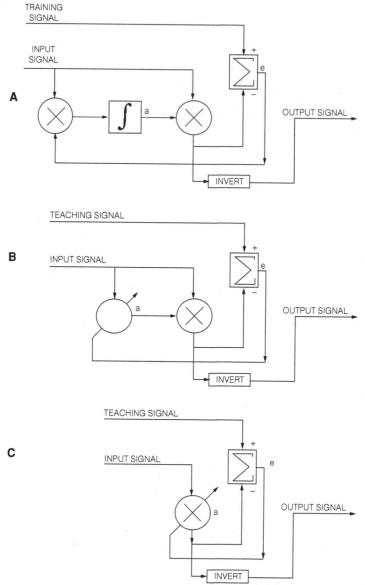

Figure 15.1. A. schema for carrying out the repeated adaptation shown in Figure 15.2, trace 2. An error signal, *e*, (Fig. 15.2, trace 3) is generated as the difference between the training signal (teaching signal) and the input signal (differencer, upper right), after the latter is passed through a multiplier (lower right) for scaling. The error signal is fed back in such a way as to minimize the difference between the training signal and the output signal as follows. The training signal and the input signal are in phase so that, if their amplitudes at the differencer are equal, the error signal is zero. If not, the error signal will have either the same phase as, or be inverted in phase with respect to, the training and input signals. Multiplication of the error signal by the input signal (multiplier at the lower left) will yield a signal (Fig. 15.3, trace 2) having positive values if the amplitude of the training signal is greater than the input signal, and negative values if the training signal is less than the input signal. The product signal is then passed through an operational-amplifier integrator (integral sign), the output (Fig. 15.3, trace 3.) of which is fed to the second multiplier,

itself. In short, there are, of course, no Purkinje cells in an adaptive control device, nor are there any electronic multipliers in the cerebellum. However, that there are principles of operation common to both is the presumption behind this chapter.

15.1. Adaptive Signal Processors

15.1.1. Automatic Amplitude Matching (Scaling)

To illustrate the basic principle of adaptive control, the simple operation of automatically adjusting a fixed-amplitude input sine wave to yield a variable-amplitude output sine wave to match the amplitude of a training sine wave is considered.

A schema of a device to accomplish this objective is shown in Figure 15.1A, and sample waveforms are shown in Figure 15.2 and 15.3. The training sine wave is depicted in the top trace of Figure 15.2, and the output sine wave is shown in the second trace. (The fixed-amplitude input sine wave, which is not shown, is of the same frequency as that of the training sine wave.) The third trace in Figure 15.2 shows the error signal, e, or difference between trace 1 and trace 2. The error signal is used to drive the scale factor, a (Fig. 15.1A), for the input signal in such a way as to decrease the error signal exponentially to zero (Fig 15.2, bottom trace) repetitively. The direction of change (increase or decrease) of the scale factor is established by comparing the polarity of the individual waves of the error signal with the polarity of the individual waves of the input signal by means of the multiplier on lower left in Figure 15.1A. Thus, if the two waveforms are in phase, a fluctuating positive voltage will appear at the output of the multiplier, and if the two are out of phase, a fluctuating negative voltage will appear (Fig. 15.3, trace 2). Integration, or fine-grained summation (box with integral sign, Fig. 15.1A) of this fluctuating voltage, yields the scale factor (Fig. 15.3, trace 3) for scaling the input signal (multiplier on the lower right in Fig. 15.1A). Note that the waveform for the scale factor is just the envelope of the output signal (Fig. 15.3, trace 4).

Within limits, this schema can be viewed as a model for the vestibulo-ocular reflex (VOR), as described in Chapter 17.

15.1.2. Parameters of an Adaptive Signal Processor

It is relevant to examine the effect of changes in certain design parameters of an adaptive controller.

Figure 15.1 (*contd.*).
the second input for which is the input signal. The latter is thus scaled up or down to minimize the amplitude of the error signal, e, from the differencer. Inversion of the scaled input signal yields the output signal (Fig 15.2, trace 2). B and C show successively more compact forms of A: in B, the first multiplier has been combined with the integrator; and in C, the two multipliers and the integrator have been combined. The latter form is used in Figures 15.11, 15.12 and 15.15. (From Barlow 1993; in Barlow, *The Electroencephalogram: Its Patterns and Origins*; copyright 1993, The MIT Press; reprinted by permission.)

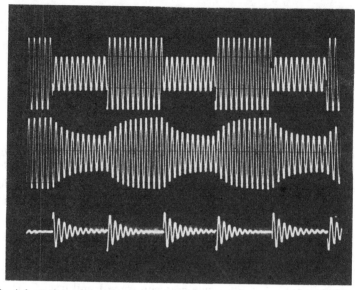

Figure 15.2. Adaptation of amplitude of output signal (trace 2) to a training signal that alternates abruptly in amplitude (trace 1); the error signal (trace 3) is the difference between traces 1 and 2. (Note that the adaptation curve [i.e., the envelope of trace 2] is a succession of exponentials, corresponding to the linear error case (Fig. 14.6A, B); for the cases of sigmoid error and sigmum error (Fig. 14.6C, D), different forms of the adaptation curve would result, a difference that may be of importance in relation to the possible function of the inferior olive as a differencer [Chapter 17].)

Amplitude of Input and Training Signals. The effect of a congruent decrease in amplitude of both the input and training signals by a factor of 2.5 is shown in Figure 15.4. It is evident that adaptation takes appreciably longer for the smaller amplitude signals, as is to be expected since the rate of adaptation is inversely proportional to the product of the amplitudes of the two signals. (The rate of adaptation varies linearly if only one of the two signals is varied.) This dependence of adaptation time on signal amplitude would imply the necessity of a narrow dynamic range (range of operating amplitudes; e.g., feedback stabilization) for optimum performance of an adaptive system.

Integrator Time Constant. The effect of a change of the time constant of the integrator components (resistor and capacitor) is illustrated in Figure 15.5. The adaptation rate (traces 3 and 4) is faster for the shorter time constant (by a factor of approximately 10:1), but the corresponding traces in *B* are appreciably more irregular than the corresponding ones in *A*, reflecting greater fluctuations in the multiplying coefficient (scale factor, weighting factor) for the shorter time constant.

True Multiplication vs. Approximations. In Figure 15.1A, the operations of multiplication of input signal and error signal (multiplier on the left), and scaling the input signal (multiplier on the right), are indicated as being carried out on true arithmetic

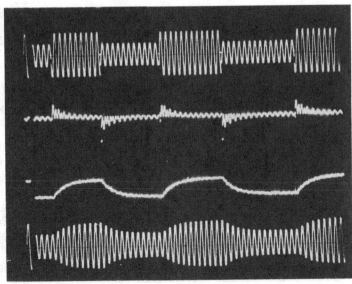

Figure 15.3. Adaptation of the amplitude of a sine wave (trace 4) to a sine wave of abruptly changing amplitude (trace 1). Trace 2 shows the error signal multiplied by the constant-amplitude input sine wave (not shown); trace 3 shows the integrated output of the latter (i.e., the scaling factor, a). The fixed-amplitude input sine wave is multiplied by the coefficient to yield the output (trace 4), which adapts exponentially to each of the stepwise changes in the training signal. Note, especially, the relatively slow time course of the coefficient (trace 3) in comparison with the much faster time course of the individual oscillations of the training signal (trace 1). Such a difference in frequency range also characterizes the signals in the climbing fibers and the mossy fibers, respectively (Chapter 17).

multipliers, which corresponds to operating on the linear output of Figure 14.6A, with its associated quadratic (paraboloid) mean square error (MSE) surface, depicted in Figure 14.6B. It should be noted that use of the sigmoid (signal compression) output results in a different MSE surface (i.e., Fig. 14.6C), and that use of the signum (sign only) output results in yet another MSE surface (Fig. 14.6D). Thus, for the linear output, the greater the error, the greater the rate of decrease of error (i.e., of the "strength of the restoring force"), whereas for the sigmoid output, the greater the error, the lesser the rate of decrease of error (i.e., of the "strength of the restoring force"). It may be mentioned that the sigmum (sign only) can be implemented by using the principle of synchronous detection (synchronous rectification), which implementation yielded rather satisfactory results in the author's experience, despite the rather complex MSE surface shown in Figure 14.6D.

15.1.3. Other Aspects of an Adaptive Signal Processor

Effect of Zeroing the Integrator. This effect is illustrated in Figure 15.6, from which it is apparent that the scaling factor (coefficient, a) is zeroed, the output signal becomes zero, and the error signal becomes the same as the input signal (except for polarity). In principle, Purkinje cell impairment could have an analogous effect.

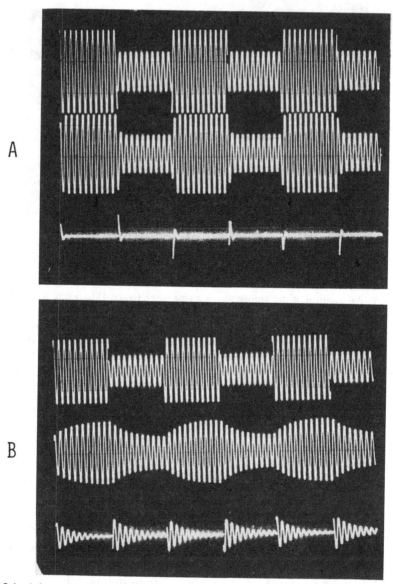

Figure 15.4. Adaptation of output signal (trace 2) to an alternating-amplitude training signal (trace 1) before (*A*) and after (*B*) a decrease in the amplitude of the training signal and of the input signal by a factor of approximately 2.5. The oscilloscope sensitivity was increased, by a factor of 2.5 in *B*. Note the appreciably longer adaptation time at the lower amplitude.

Effect of Fixed (Frozen) Coefficient. Illustrated in Figure 15.7, this effect could result from an interruption of the input to the integrator, or of either input (or both) to the first multiplier (Fig. 15.2A, lower left).

In principle, Purkinje cell climbing fiber impairment could have an analogous effect.

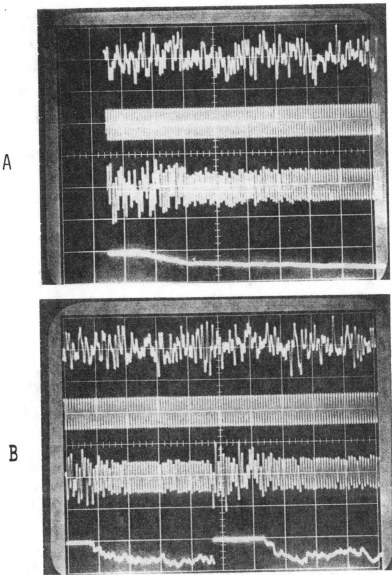

Figure 15.5.   Effect on the adaptation process (removal of random noise from a random noise–sine wave mixture) of integrator time constant change from 10 sec (A) to 1 sec (B). Trace 1: random noise. Trace 2: sine wave. Trace 3: mixture of noise and sine wave (sum of traces 1 and 2). Trace 4: multiplying coefficient. Note that the latter is much more irregular for the shorter integrator time constant. (In both A and B, the coefficient increments negatively after having been set to zero. For these results, the training signal is the sine wave (trace 2), and the input signal is the mixture of sine wave and noise. Note that the noise component of the mixture is progressively eliminated – a process termed *adaptive interference canceling*.)

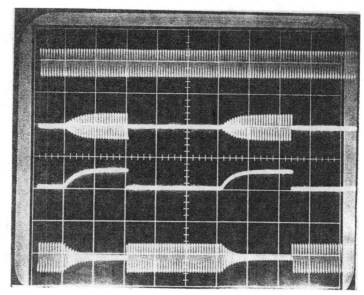

Figure 15.6. Effect on output (trace 2) of intermittent zeroing of the multiplying coefficient (trace 3). Trace 1: training and also input signal. Trace 4: error signal. Note that traces 2 and 4 summate to yield the same as trace 1.

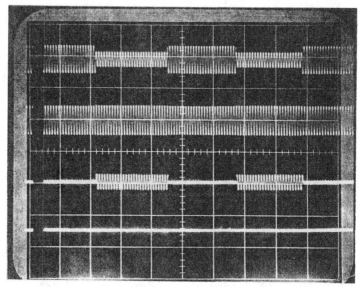

Figure 15.7. Effect of "freezing" the weight (multiplying coefficient, a) at a nonzero level (trace 4). Trace 1: training signal; trace 2: output signal; trace 3: error signal. (The coefficient was "frozen" in the higher-amplitude phase of the training signal.) Under these conditions, the error signal is generated, but it is ineffective because the connection to the input to the integrator (Fig. 15.1A) is open; hence, the output remains constant in amplitude, showing no adaptation (compare Fig. 7.3).

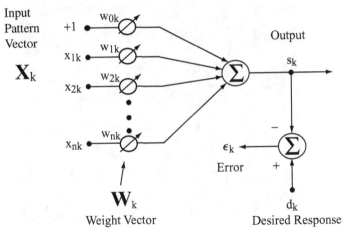

Figure 15.8. Schema of a three-input adaptive linear combiner (same as Fig. 14.5). The weights, the ensemble of which is termed the *weight vector*, are determined as indicated in Figure 15.1, each independently, from the common error signal. (From Widrow and Lehr, 1990; *Proc. IEEE*, Vol. 78, copyright 1990, IEEE, by permission of the IEEE.).

15.2. The Linear Combiner

The previous review of some features of a single-channel ASP will now be followed by a consideration of a multichannel one, termed an *adaptive linear combiner* (Widrow and Lehr 1990). A basic schema for a three-input adaptive combiner, or more exactly, an adaptive linear combiner, already briefly considered in Chapter 14, is shown in Figure 15.8. The operation of such a unit in which sine waves of three different frequencies were combined to match a prescribed combination of the same signals in the form of a training signal is shown in Figure 15.9. In principle, the resulting values of the respective three weights could be stored and reloaded at some later time, to obtain the same output pattern, given the original three input waveforms, but without the need of the training-signal combination of the three. (Note that in Figure 15.9, a single weight-determining mechanism could have served for the three sine waves since their amplitudes were the same.)

15.3. Linear Prediction – Adaptation to a Time Series

15.3.1. Finite Impulse Response Predictors

As indicated in Chapter 14, an adaptive combiner, rather than used to process several independent signals (Fig. 15.8), can be used to process several delayed versions of the same signal (Fig. 14.9). In the latter case, the set of delayed versions are obtained from a tapped delay line, as indicated in the left middle of Figure 14.9 (boxes) labeled z^{-1}. Examples of an ensemble of successively delayed versions of the same signal are illustrated in Figure 15.10 for a sine wave and for a random noise signal. Thus, the tapped delay line provides an ensemble of the immediate past sample values of the input signal as it moves stepwise through the tapped delay line.

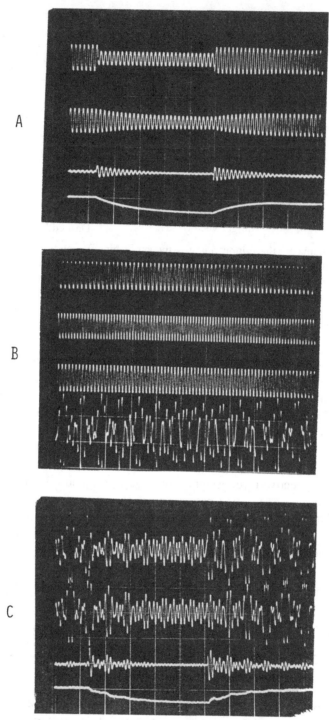

Figure 15.9. Sample results from a three-input linear combiner. *A.* Adaptation of output (trace 2) to a 50% decrease of amplitude of a single, 12.5 Hz, sine wave training signal (trace 1), the input signal remaining constant in amplitude (not shown); trace 3: error signal (difference

Carrying out the process that is performed with a linear combiner on the ensemble of delayed signals, y_{k-1}, y_{k-2}, y_{k-n}, permits prediction, as follows from the relation,

$$y_k - (+a_1 y_{k-1} + a_2 y_{k-2} \cdots + a_{ny k-n}) = e. \tag{1}$$

The equation states that the next (sample) value, y_k, of a time series (voltage-time graph) can be predicted (estimated) as a linear (thus, the + signs) combination of a small series of its immediate past sample values, multiplied by the respective weights (predictor coefficients), $a_1, a_2, \ldots a_n$. The error of the prediction is e (i.e., the difference between the first term on the left and the sum of the remaining terms on the left). The sequence of values (i.e., time series) of the error constitutes the error signal. If the prediction is perfect, as is possible for a sine wave (see below), the error signal will be zero after the predictor coefficients have become adapted.

A block diagram of an ASP configured as a linear predictor is shown in Figure 15.11. When such an ASP is arranged as a linear predictor, the input signal is also used as the training signal (top left).

The error signal (there is only one, not eight) in Figure 15.11 is fed back and multiplied by the respective versions of the delayed signal from the appropriate tap of the delay line, for modifying the respective weights (i.e., the as). In turn, the delayed signal from the respective tap of the delay line is multiplied by its corresponding weight so computed, and the resultant products are summated to yield the (negative) of the predicted next sample point. Thus, the schema in Figure 15.11 represents a straightforward implementation of the predictor equation (1). In brief, the processor "attempts" to predict the next value of the signal on the basis of a small fixed number of its immediate past sample values. (Note, in Figure 15.11, that if the "desired [or training] signal" were taken after the first delay step of the tapped delay line rather than before it, no prediction would be entailed. Indeed, only the first coefficient would be necessary and the device would reduce to that depicted in Figure 15.1A.)

The linear predictor of Figure 15.11 is of the finite impulse response (FIR; sometimes termed finite-duration impulse response) type, for which the error signal is fed back to adjust the weights, from which in turn the next sample point is predicted on the basis of the immediate past sample points, the latter being obtained from the tapped delay line. FIR arises because input information traverses the unit only once, from left to right through the tapped delay line (top part of Fig. 15.11).

Figure 15.9 (contd.).
between traces 1 and 2); trace 4: weight (coefficient), which parallels the envelope of trace 3. B. Individual sine waves of 10, 15, and 15.5 Hz (traces 1–3), and their sum (trace 4). C. Adaptation of output (trace 2) to a 50% decrease of amplitude of the sum of 3 sine waves as the training signal (trace 1); the input signal (B, trace 4) remained constant in amplitude; trace 3: error signal; trace 4: weight. Note that with each of the two changes in the amplitude of the training signal (trace 4), the error signal (trace 3) exhibits a sudden increase followed by an exponential decrease. In C, each of the 3 sine waves was weighted independently (only one weight is shown as trace 4) and adapts independently of the others. Correspondingly, the percentage changes of their amplitudes could have been made independent of one another.

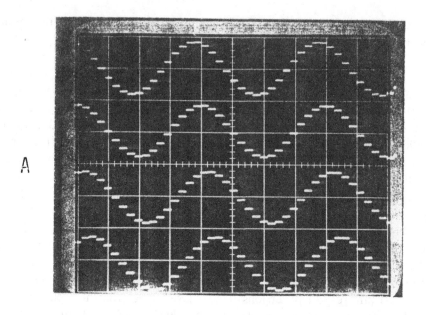

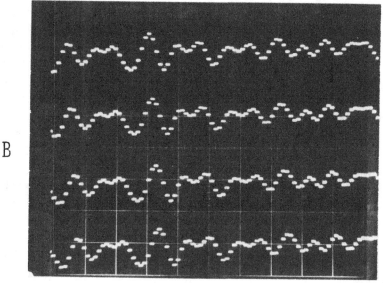

Figure 15.10. Output of four successive taps of a tapped delay line for A: 5 Hz sine wave; B: random noise (10 Hz narrow-band); note the slower oscilloscope sweep speed in B. The output signals from the successive taps are progressively shifted to the right (i.e., later in time).

If there are separate input and training signals (as in Fig. 15.1A), ASP can be used; such a unit (which is of the FIR type) is depicted in Figure 15.12.

Figure 15.13A shows the actual behavior of the eight weights or coefficients from the ASP operated in the linear predictor (FIR type) model (Fig. 15.11) for a sine wave abruptly alternating in frequency between 17 and 27 Hertz. The input and

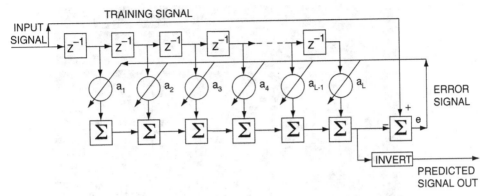

Figure 15.11. Schema of linear predictor (ASP) having a FIR. The chain of boxes at top labeled z^{-1} constitute a tapped delay line. Each of the weights or predictor coefficients ($a_1 \ldots a_L$) is computed independently and continuously, according to the principle depicted in Figure 15.1. Note that, for a predictor, the training signal is the same as the input signal, but the first weight is ordinarily computed on the input signal after it has been delayed by one step (top left). It is relative to the output from the first tap of the delay line that the prediction is carried out and is compared with the actual (desired or training) signal. (Modified from Barlow 1993; in Barlow, *The Electroencephalogram: Its Patterns and Origins*, copyright 1993, The MIT Press; reprinted by permission.)

output signals for the predictor are shown on a compressed time scale in Figure 15.13B. The same coefficients are shown in multiplexed form (i.e., in sequence) in Figure 15.14.

There is a rather striking behavior of the weights of the ASP as illustrated by the following example, which cannot very well be conveyed in illustrations. Let the series of weights (in the present case, eight) be displayed on an oscilloscope screen; the first one will always be the largest. Then, after the eight coefficients have been manually zeroed simultaneously, let adaptation take place to an input sine wave of a particular frequency. The weights will exhibit some pattern (e.g., upper trace of Fig. 15.14). Then, if the sine wave is changed to another frequency (say 1.2 times higher), the pattern of weights on the oscilloscope screen will undergo a change (e.g., Fig. 15.14, lower trace). If now the sine wave frequency is restored to the original, there is a

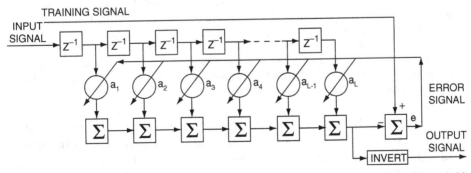

Figure 15.12. Schema of ASP with independent input and teaching signals (at the upper left). (Compare with the linear predictor of Figure 15.11, for which the two signals are the same.)

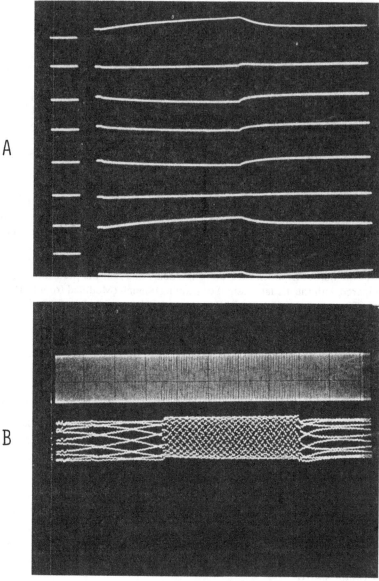

Figure 15.13.   Display of ASP weights *A*. Response of the eight weights (predictor coefficients) of the ASP (one-step prediction) to a sine wave input alternating between 17 and 27 Hz at a rate of 0.3 Hz (trace duration: 10 seconds). The short traces at the left indicate the baselines for the respective weights. Note the largely independent behavior of the weights during adaptation. *B*. Input signal (top trace) and predicted signal (bottom trace). (The moiré pattern evident in the latter results from the periodic sampling.)

further adaptation, but not as pronounced as the previous one. And so on, for a series of sine waves of different frequencies, so that after several such changes, the amount of adaptation necessary appears to diminish progressively. It is as though the ASP had "learned" to generalize from multiple prior trials of adaptation to minimize the

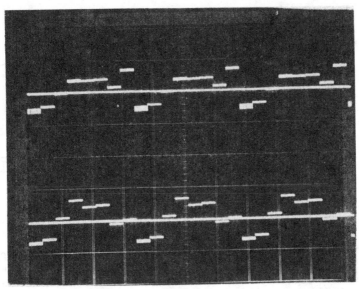

Figure 15.14. Sequential (multiplexed) display of weights (same as those in Fig. 15.13) displayed in relation to the baseline (unbroken horizontal traces) after adaptation had occurred, for two frequencies: 25 Hz (top trace) and 35 Hz (bottom trace). For each of the two frequencies, three sequences of the eight weights are shown. Note that the ensemble of predictor coefficients for the two frequencies are quite different.

extent of succeeding changes. (This behavior is doubtless related to the fact that, for a sine wave, there is redundancy among the eight weights.) It may be noted in passing that the weight-determining units (middle portion of Fig. 15.1A) are the counterparts of the hidden layer of a three-layer neural net, for which not dissimilar behavior has been described (Chapter 14).

15.3.2. Infinite Impulse Response Predictors

In the infinite impulse response (IIR; also termed infinite duration impulse response) type of ASP (Fig. 15.15), the predicted signal itself is used to improve the prediction (Haykin 1996; White 1975; Widrow and Stearns 1985). The predicted signal is fed back through a second tapped delay line (lower part of Fig. 15.15), its own set of weights are computed, and it makes its own contribution to the next sample point. (The details of the implementation of the FIR and the IIR ASPs are described in Appendix A.) The term *infinite duration impulse response* arises because the predicted signal is recirculated back through the unit (bottom tapped delay line in Fig. 15.11), and hence in principle could make itself felt for an extended time.

There are important differences between adaptive signal processors of the FIR type and the IIR type.

IIR units characterize an unknown system (or carry out prediction) more accurately than do FIR units. However, IIR units can be unstable (develop disabling sustained oscillations) because of the positive feedback in the "b" chain, unless careful

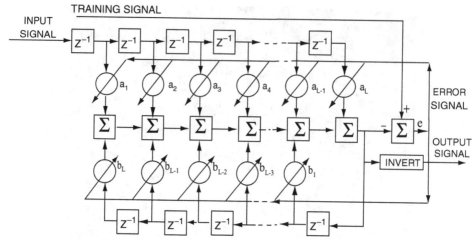

Figure 15.15. Schema of an ASP having an IIR, with weights in the feed-forward (upper) chain (as), and also in the feedback or recursive (lower) chain (bs). Note that the predicted signal itself is fed back through the lower chain to improve the prediction of itself (compare with Fig. 15.12). (Modified from Barlow 1993; in Barlow, *The Electroencephalogram: Its Patterns and Origins*, copyright 1993, The MIT Press; reprinted by permission.)

attention is paid to limiting signal amplitude. FIR units, in contrast, are inherently stable, thus their popularity.

To emphasize in a different way the difference between the FIR and the IIR configurations, in the FIR configuration, only the error signal is fed back, which is not destabilizing, whereas in the IIR configuration, the error signal and also the predicted signal itself are fed back. The former is not destabilizing, but the latter is potentially destabilizing. Thus, it can be said that the IIR format provides better results, but with some risks. The same is true for an ASP used to duplicate the characteristics of a system having unknown characteristics (i.e., the determination of "plant" or system characteristics), which are considered below.

15.3.3. Prediction with FIR and IIR Adaptive Signal Processors

Results with IIR and FIR configured ASPs are shown in Figure 15.16. On the left side, the results for prediction at a series of predictor intervals are shown. The column on the left shows the results for the IIR configuration, and the column on the right shows the results for the FIR (selected values only). As the prediction interval increases, the prediction error increases, the more so for the FIR mode than for the IIR mode, as expected.

15.3.4. Increase of Prediction Error with Decrease of Number of Weights (Predictor Coefficients)

The impairment of prediction (FIR mode) resulting from progressive loss weights (prediction coefficients) is depicted in Figure 15.17. In *A*, the results for two originally

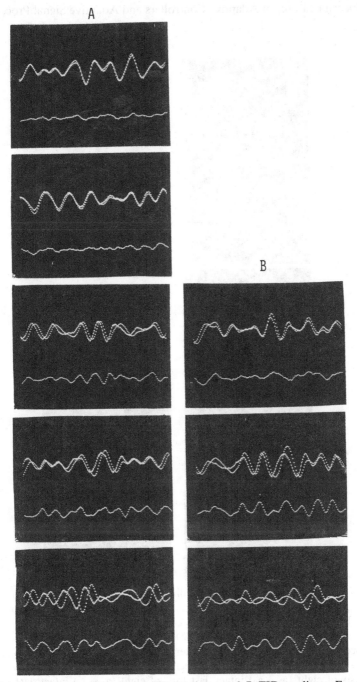

Figure 15.16. Prediction results with *A*: IIR predictor and *B*: FIR predictor. For each panel, the left one of the two superimposed upper traces is the predicted (output) signal, the right one is the input signal (i.e., the signal for prediction), and the lower trace is the error signal. For the IIR predictor (*A*), the predictions are for (from top down) 0, 1, 2, 4, and 8 sample intervals (i.e., 0, 4, 8, 16, and 32 milliseconds). For the FIR mode (*B*), the predictions are for 2, 4, and 8 sample times only (i.e., 8, 16, and 32 milliseconds). Note that as the prediction interval increases, the accuracy of the predicted signal diminishes in comparison with the input signal, and the error signal increases, the more so for the FIR (*B*) than for the IIR mode (*A*). Test signal: 10 Hz narrow-band (24 dB/octave roll-off) electronic noise.

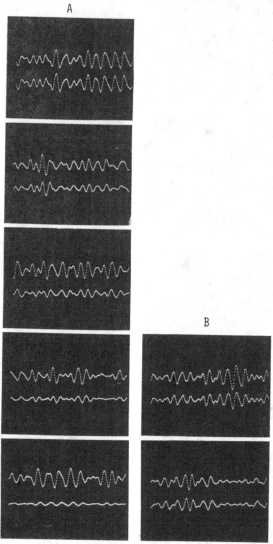

Figure 15.17. Degradation of fidelity of prediction resulting from decrease of the number of weights (predictor coefficients; equation 1). (Test signal: 10-Hz narrow band electronic noise, as in Fig. 15.16; prediction interval: 1 sample interval or 4 milliseconds.) The output of two predictors (both in FIR configuration) is shown in each panel. The upper trace in each instance shows the result from the unaltered predictor, and the lower trace, that for the altered one. In *A*, from top to bottom, respectively: eight out of eight coefficients ($a_1 - a_8$) intact; last six of eight ($a_3 - a_8$) intact; last four of eight ($a_5 = a_8$) intact; last two of eight ($a_7 = a_8$) intact; and no intact coefficients. Note that the prediction is progressively degraded as the number of lower numbered operative coefficients decreases. In *B*, from top down, the *first* four coefficients ($a_1, a_2, a_3,$ and a_4) and the first two coefficients (a_1, a_2), respectively, were left intact. Note the difference between the fourth panel down in *A* and the first panel in *B*, and between the bottom panel in *A* and the bottom panel in *B*, in that the lower numbered weights are more important for (short-lead) prediction than the higher numbered ones, as expected.

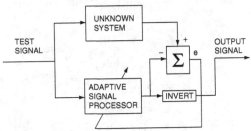

Figure 15.18. Schema of arrangement for modeling the forward characteristics of an unknown system. Both the ASP and the unknown system receive the same test signal (a swept-frequency sine wave or a random noise signal of the appropriate bandwidth) and the ASP receives the output of the unknown system as a training signal, matching its own characteristics to that of the unknown. The results were recorded after adaptation. (Modified from Barlow 1993; in Barlow, *The Electroencephalogram: Its Patterns and Origins*, copyright 1993, The MIT Press; reprinted by permission.)

identical predictors are shown in each panel, the top traces from the unaltered predictor, the bottom traces from the predictor in which the number of predictor coefficients is progressively decreased. It is evident that the prediction error increases (i.e., the accuracy of prediction decreases) as the number of higher order of intact coefficients decreases (Fig. 15.17A), but this effect is smaller for inoperative lower numbered coefficients (Fig. 15.17B).

15.4. Adaptive Modeling (System Characterization)

15.4.1. Forward Modeling

As noted in the previous chapter (Chapter 14), one of the applications of ASP that has been invoked in relation to the cerebellum is that of modeling or characterization of an unknown system (e.g., the control system for a limb). The principle is depicted in Figure 15.18. In brief, the ASP adjusts its own weights so its output matches that of the unknown system, in response to a test signal that is fed to both. It is from the difference between the two outputs that the error signal is obtained, from which in turn the weights are automatically adjusted. The term *adaptive filter* has sometimes been applied to the ASP functioning in this mode.

Illustrative examples of the determination of response characteristics of (i.e., forward modeling of) an unknown system by a FIR and an IIR ASP are shown in Figure 15.19. It is evident that in this case also, the performance of the IIR configuration (Fig. 15.19B) is superior to that of the FIR configuration (Fig. 15.19A). Note the delay and the poorer frequency response for the FIR configuration. Difficulties with instability of the IIR configuration were avoided by using relatively low levels of the test signal.

Additional examples of characterization or modeling of unknown systems (i.e., systems whose response characteristics are unknown) by means of an ASP of the IIR type are shown in Figure 15.20 for band-reject and band-limited signals.

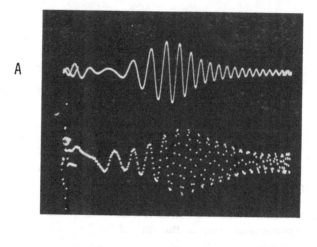

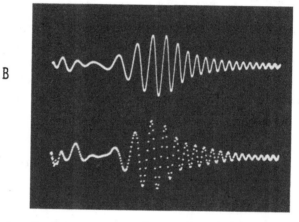

Figure 15.19. Modeling the response characteristics of an unknown system (a narrow-band filter 10 Hz center frequency, 18 dB/octave roll-off electronic filter) by means of *A*, an FIR ASP (Fig. 15.11), and *B* an IIR ASP (Fig. 15.15), each in the configuration of Figure 15.18. For both *A* and *B*, trace 1: output of the electronic filter for an input 1–20 Hz swept sine wave of constant amplitude; trace 2: output of ASP. The replication by the IIR ASP is superior to that by the FIR ASP; note the delay of the peak and the poorer output waveform for the FIR model. (From Barlow 1993; in Barlow, *The Electroencephalogram: Its Patterns and Origins*, copyright 1993, The MIT Press; reprinted by permission.)

15.4.2. Inverse Modeling (Inverse Characteristics)

The inverse characteristics or inverse dynamics of a system are defined as the non-linear system whose input and output are inverted. For example, in the case of the musculoskeletal system, the trajectory is the input and the motor command is the output, the inverse or opposite of the usual order. Thus, once an inverse dynamics model is acquired by motor learning, it can compute an appropriate motor command T_i directly from the desired trajectory.

A schema for obtaining the inverse characteristic or inverse-dynamics (as opposed to the forward characteristic or forward dynamics as in Figs. 15.18 to 15.20) of an

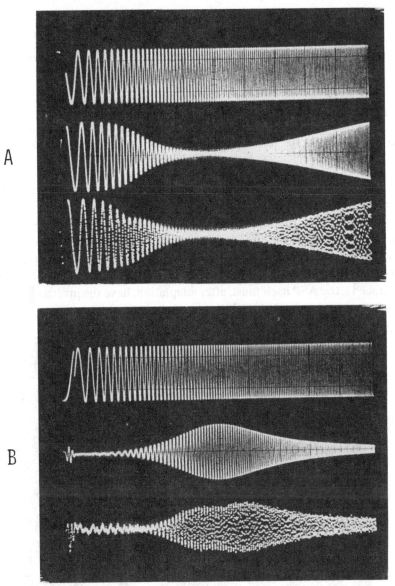

Figure 15.20. Modeling the response characteristics of two unknown systems: in *A*, a band-reject electronic filter; in *B*, a band-pass filter, both centered at 10 Hz with 24 dB/octave roll-off), by means of an IIR type of ASP (Fig. 15.15), using the configuration of Figure 15.18. Trace 1: 1–20 Hz swept sine wave test signal; trace 2: output of the electronic filter, which is the training signal input for the ASP; trace 3: output of the ASP, which has mimicked the response characteristic of the unknown system (i.e., the electronic filter).

unknown system is shown in Figure 15.21. The ASP and the unknown system are cascaded or placed in series (in principle, the order for the two is immaterial). Because the test signal is also the teaching signal, the ASP adjusts its coefficients such that, after adaptation, its characteristic is the inverse of the unknown system. (Correspondingly,

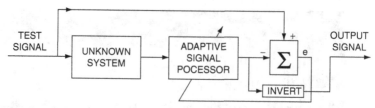

Figure 15.21. Schema for inverse modeling of an unknown system (i.e., for obtaining the inverse characteristic of an unknown system). The test signal serves as both the input signal and the teaching signal. The ASP is placed in series with the unknown system; the order of the two is in principal immaterial. Figure 15.22 shows an example.

the cascaded characteristics of the two yield a unity transformation, comparable to differentiation followed by integration or vice versa.)

An example of determination of inverse dynamics is shown in Figure 15.22. The test signal is shown at the top, the characteristic of the unknown system (an electronic filter set for band reject centered at 10 Hertz) is shown as the middle trace, and the output of the ASP is shown as the bottom trace. Because the latter reproduces the test signal (trace 1), the ASP itself must, after adaptation, have the inverse characteristic of trace 2 (i.e., the form of Fig. 15.20B, trace 3).

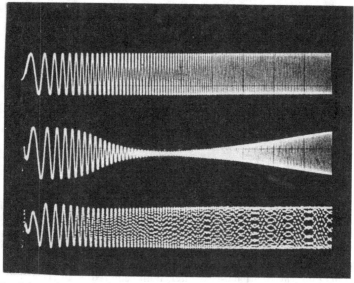

Figure 15.22. Adaptation to the inverse of a system characteristic. The input signal (trace 2) for the ASP is obtained from the band-reject electronic filter centered at 10 Hz, the input for which is a 1–20 Hz swept sine wave (trace 1). The latter signal also serves as the training signal for the ASP. Because the latter converts its input (trace 2) to be the same as the input to the electronic filter (trace 1), after adaptation, the transfer characteristic (i.e., frequency response) of the ASP is the inverse of the filter output (i.e., it resembles the middle trace of Fig. 15.20B, third trace). Stated in another way, the cascaded sequence of Figure 15.20A, trace 2, and Figure 15.20B, trace 2 (or trace 3 in each) is equivalent to a unity transform (i.e., is the same, except possibly for a scale factor; the output of the cascaded units becomes the same as the test signal input, that is, a swept sine wave of constant amplitude).

It is useful to reiterate that, in the configuration of an ASP to compute forward (predictive) characteristics, the ASP is interfaced in parallel with the unknown system (Fig. 15.18), whereas in the configuration of an ASP to compute inverse characteristics, the ASP is interfaced in series (tandem) with the unknown system (Fig. 15.21).

15.5. Summary of Features of Adaptive Signal Processors

From the topics discussed in this chapter, it is appropriate to gather a list of characteristics of ASPs.

1. For a particular task (e.g., forward modeling, inverse modeling), there is self-adjustment of parameters, or better, self-optimization of parameters (i.e., of weights or multiplying coefficients) by ASPs, a process that is carried out simultaneously for all parameters.
2. There is basically one type of ASP, the linear combiner, which comprises multiple parallel inputs (Fig. 15.8). Some, or all, of the individual inputs can, however, be in the form of a time series (voltage/time graph), multiple representations of which can be derived from a tapped delay line (Figs. 14.9, 15.10, and 15.12).
3. ASPs have two basic inputs. For successive prediction of the next sample point, these are identical (Fig. 15.11), the prediction being based on the most recent values of the time series. If one time series (the input) is to be made to resemble another (the teaching signal), separate input and training signals are used (Fig. 15.12).
4. The coefficients, or weights, in an ASP are optimized by generating an error signal (Fig. 15.2A) in the form of a difference signal between the training signal and a scaled version of the input signal, the scaling factor (coefficient, weight) being determined by the sign and magnitude of the running integral (summation) of the product of the error signal and the input signal. The running integral of the product of the error signal and the input signal is a slowly varying signal (i.e., the coefficient or weight, which can assume either positive or negative values), in contrast to the (much) higher frequencies (e.g., by a factor of 100) of the input (and the training) signals.
5. There is a component in the error signal for each component in the input signal and the training signal (Figs. 14.9 and 15.8), from which the weights are derived.
6. The integrator time constant (Fig. 15.2A) is an important parameter. Too high a value will result in a slow rate of adaptation, whereas too low a value will result in a noisy output signal from the ASP (Fig. 15.5).
7. The rate of adaptation is related to the size of the product of the amplitudes of the input signal and the training signal (Fig. 15.4). To minimize this effect, signal compression (Figs. 14.1B, 14.2, and 14.3) or (negative) feedback stabilization of amplitude of the input signal and the training signal may be necessary. In this connection, there are several negative (and also some positive) feedback loops in the cerebellar system.

8. In the most general case, the input signals for an ASP (and also a neural-net configured ASP) comprise a mixture of fan-in or convergence (Fig. 15.8; Fig. 15.11, bottom row) and fan-out or divergence (Fig. 15.11, top row). For a neural network model, Figure 13.7 shows both fan-out (on the left) and fan-in, on the right.

9. For a FIR ASP, signals propagate through the ASP only once, yielding stability (i.e., lack of spurious oscillations) but with somewhat less than optimal performance. In an IIR ASP, the predicted signal may circulate through the ASP multiple times and, by such positive feedback, disabling oscillations can occur if careful attention is not given to limiting the amplitudes.

10. Overall malfunction of an ASP can occur because of malfunction at several points (Fig. 15.1A): the differencer (upper right); the input signal; one or the other of the two multipliers, the integrator of which or the input for which could be interrupted, or zeroed; the weight (output of the integrator); and the inverter for the output signal. In short, malfunction can occur as a result of a defect at any one of several sites.

11. Failure of prediction could occur as a result of a defect in the initial elements of the tapped delay line (Fig. 15.12).

15.6. Comment

From the foregoing, it is evident that ASP (and, correspondingly, adaptive controllers, in which there is a specifically controlled object such as a limb) are extremely powerful and flexible devices. Prior to a detailed examination of cerebellar anatomy and mechanisms in the light of features of ASPs, some additional, adaptive control models of the cerebellum of increasing sophistication are surveyed.

SIXTEEN

Adaptive Control Models

16.1. Some Additional Terminology

In this chapter, which can be considered a continuation of Chapter 14, the emphasis is entirely on adaptive control. To reiterate the definition, an adaptive control system has been defined as one that automatically changes its parameters in accordance with detected or measured changes in its environment. Such changes affect only the values of the parameters but not the structure of the system (Kalman and Bucy 1961); thus, the term *optimal filter* is sometimes used. By definition, an adaptive system is free of the requirement of stationarity (i.e., constancy of statistical characteristics) of its input signals. The term *self-optimizing*, implying that a system organizes itself, has also been used (Gibson 1963; Widrow 1963).

In brief, *adaptive controller* has been defined as a controller with adjustable parameters and a mechanism for automatically adjusting the parameters.

Accounts of the history of adaptive control can be found in Gibson (1963), Åström and Wittenmark (1995), and Isermann, Lachmann, and Matko (1992).

16.1.1. Adaptive Control vs. Adaptive Signal Processing

To make the distinction between the two clearer, adaptive control and adaptive signal processing have strong similarities; that is, similar mathematical models and techniques are used in the two fields (Åström and Wittenmark 1995). However, there are also some significant differences. For example, the time scales can be different. Thus, adaptive signal processing often deals with rapidly varying (higher frequency) signals, as in acoustics, in which sampling rates of tens of kilohertz are needed, and hence more emphasis is given in signal processing to fast algorithms. In adaptive control applications, it is often, but not always, possible to work with much slower sampling rates.

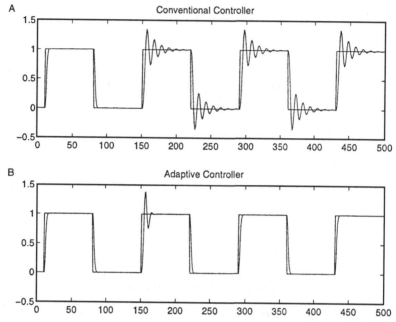

Figure 16.1. Schema of comparison of a conventional controller having fixed parameters (A) with an adaptive controller (B). Note the recurrent "ringing" (resulting from inadequate damping) in the conventional controller that results from a change of plant parameters, but which is eliminated in the adaptive controller after a single transient. (From Landau, Lozano, and M'Saad 1998; *Adaptive Control*, copyright 1998, Springer-Verlag; reprinted by permission of publisher and author.)

A more significant difference is that time delays play a minor role in signal processing. It is often permissible to delay a signal without any noticeable difficulty. Because control systems deal with feedback, even small time delays can result in drastic deterioration in performance, a difference that can be considered to be related to the inertia of the controlled object (e.g., a limb).

A third difference is in the settings for the respective technologies. Adaptive control is used to design control systems that work well in an unknown or changing environment. Adaptive signal processing, however, is used to process signals whose characteristics are unknown or changing. Although there have been attempts to bring the fields closer together, the view has been expressed that much more effort is needed in this direction (Åström and Wittenmark 1995).

16.1.2. Adaptive Control vs. Conventional Control

Consider, as an example, the case of a conventional feedback control loop designed to have a given damping. When a disturbance acts upon the controlled variable, the return of the controlled variable toward its nominal value will be characterized by the desired damping if the plant parameters have their known nominal values (i.e., have the specified damping). If the plant parameters change, however, the damping will change. This effect is shown in Figure 16.1. In Figure 16.1A, a conventional controller

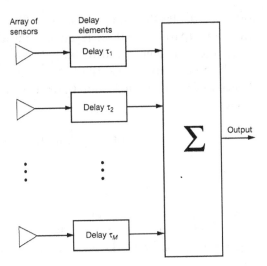

Figure 16.2. Delay-and-sum beamformer. Explanation in text. (From Haykin 1996; in Haykin, *Adaptive Filter Theory*, copyright Prentice-Hall, Inc.; reprinted by permission of the publisher.)

with fixed parameters is used; a change of the plant (model) parameters occurring at $t = 150$ results in poor performance as manifested in the repetitive "ringing." In Figure 16.1B, an adaptive controller is used, from which it is evident that, after an adaptation transient, the nominal performance is recovered.

Thus, whereas the design of a conventional feedback control system is oriented first toward the elimination of the effect of disturbances on the controlled variables, the design of adaptive control systems is oriented first toward the elimination of the effect of parameter disturbances on the performance of the control system (Landau, Lozano, and M'Saad 1998).

16.1.3. Adaptive Beamforming in Signal Processing

In connection with the preceding discussion, one aspect of signal processing may have some relevance to cerebellar-like structures, as mentioned previously. In beamforming, or spatial filtering, a device termed a beamformer may be used for the purpose of increasing the signal-to-noise ratio of a desired signal arriving from a specific direction, relative to the background noise, the latter being received omnidirectionally. In a primitive beamformer, termed a delay-and-sum beamformer (Fig. 16.2), the members of the series of output signals of an array of sensors are progressively delayed so the array "points" in the direction of the origin of the signal. In an adaptive beamformer, this process is carried out automatically (electronically), and the "pointing" can become "tracking" (Haykin 1996).

16.1.4. State-Space Models for Adaptive Systems

Adaptive control models are sometimes termed state-space models, associated with which there are three multidimensional vectors each with real elements: (1) the state of the system, (2) the input variable or control input of the system, and (3) the output variables that can be measured. (The three real elements can be considered the counterpart of the three layers in a three-layer neuronal network [Fig. 14.1C]). Each vector is considered to be defined in its respective space, the dimensions of which need not necessarily be the same. The output of the system can be obtained by formal multiplication (more exactly, convolution) of the input by the state vector:

$$\text{output} = (\text{input}) \times (\text{transfer function}).$$

16.1.5. Adaptive Control and Neural Networks

According to Landau, Lozano, and M'Saad (1998), neural networks have begun to be used in adaptive control, although generally their use has been limited to one-layer neural networks because the network parameters in that case appear linearly.

16.1.6. Complex Adaptive Systems

The more general topic of *complex adaptive systems*, which characteristically employ internal models – that is, built-in rule-governed procedures that allow for the anticipation of consequences to direct their behavior (Singer 1995) – is the subject of brief surveys by Gell-Mann (1995) and Holland (1995).

16.2. Internal Models

Kawato (1999) defined internal models as neural mechanisms that can mimic the input–output characteristics, or their inverses, of the motor apparatus. Forward internal models can predict sensory consequences from efference copies of issued motor commands, whereas inverse internal models can calculate necessary feedforward motor commands from desired trajectory information. According to Kawato, the internal model concept had its origin in control theory and robotics. Ito (1970) proposed that the cerebellum contains forward models of the limbs and other brain regions. Ito (1990) and Kawato (1999) foresaw the extension of the concepts concerning internal models beyond purely sensory motor control to higher cognitive domains such as language; data implicating involvement of the cerebellum in the latter continue to accumulate (Chapter 9).

Kawato (1995) listed the necessary characteristics of the representation in the brain (in the first instance, in the cerebellum) of internal models of the motor apparatus: (1) adaptive capability (essential for acquisition and continuous updating of the internal models); (2) a broad range of sensory inputs and a sufficiently high capacity to approximate complex dynamics (to match the many degrees of freedom and complicated nonlinear dynamics of the controlled objects, e.g., arms, speech articulators, torso). Thus, the internal models are systems that mimic – within the central nervous system (CNS) – the behavior of the controlled systems (Jordan and Wolpert 2000).

16.2.1. Combining Multiple Internal Models

In testing two general hypotheses concerning internal models of sensorimotor transformations, (1) the composition hypothesis (which holds that the CNS can effectively combine internal models of two previously learned sensorimotor transformations when dealing with a novel environment in which both transformations are present), and (2) the decomposition hypothesis (which holds that, when encountering a complex environment featuring more than one sensory transformation, the CNS can effectively decompose the environment into separate internal models appropriate for the separate transformations), Flanagan et al. (1999) reported clear support for the composition hypothesis. Thus, movement performance in the combined transformation was superior if subjects had previously learned the separate transformations. For their experiments, the authors used a kinematic transformation (visuomotor rotation), a dynamic transformation (viscous curl field), and a combination of these transformations.

Doya (1999) concluded that there is enough anatomical, physiological, and theoretical evidence to support the hypotheses that the cerebellum is a specialized organism for supervised learning (as are the basal ganglia for reinforcement learning and the cerebral cortex for unsupervised learning). Specialized learning modules are envisaged for each structure. In the case of the cerebellum, the specialized learning modules are assumed to be used as "internal models" of the environment and correspondingly, the teaching signals that guide learning in supervised learning in the cerebellum are directional error vectors. (Correspondingly, for reinforcement learning, i.e., for the basal ganglia, the teaching signals are taken to be scalar rewards or reinforcement signals, and no teaching signals are assumed in unsupervised learning, i.e., for the cerebral cortex.)

16.2.2. Forward Models

Forward (dynamic) models predict the next state (e.g., position and velocity) on the basis of the current state and the motor command (compare Fig. 15.18), whereas forward output models predict the sensory feedback (Jordan and Wolpert 2000). Wolpert and Kawato (1998) pointed out that forward models have been proposed for motor learning, state estimation (prediction), and motor control. For example, a forward dynamic model of an arm predicts the next state (e.g., position and velocity), given the current state and motor command. The authors proposed that multiple predictors exist with at least one able to provide an accurate prediction of the next state for any given context. (Miall and Wolpert [1996] consider forward models for physiological motor control such as limb movement and the cerebellum as their probable site.)

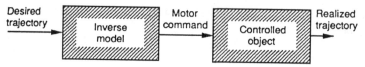

Figure 16.3. An inverse neural model used as a feedforward controller. (From Kawato and Gomi 1993; in Mano, Hamada, and DeLong; *Role of the Cerebellum and Basal Ganglia in Voluntary Movement*, copyright 1993, Elsevier Science; reprinted by permission.)

Starting from the premise (Miall et al. 1993) that the cerebellum provides predictive estimates based on (efferent) copies of motor commands, Miall (1998) reiterated the view of the cerebellum as a "forward model" such that, in mimicking the forward, causal responses of the motor effectors of the motor command, its output becomes a sensory prediction, a signal estimating the outcome of movement (i.e., the sensory consequences of the motor commands). Thus, the cerebellum as a forward model was considered to require sensory inputs to update its knowledge of the current state of the motor system, a copy of the motor commands that are being sent to the motor system, and a learning mechanism to ensure the forward model accurately reflects the motor system behavior and adapts over a long time scale (minutes or hours) to its changes.

16.2.3. Inverse Models

Inverse model means a neural representation (Fig. 16.3) such that the motor commands required to attain a given movement (the actual trajectory) are derived from the desired trajectory (compare Fig. 15.21). Ideally, the transfer function (i.e., the input–output characteristic of the inverse model) is the inverse of that of the controlled object (e.g., limb). Hence, as indicated in Figure 16.4A, feeding the representation of the desired trajectory into the inverse model (after learning has occurred), thence to the controlled object, results in a realized trajectory that is ideally the same as the desired trajectory. The feedback controller has the role of an approximation of the inverse model of the controlled object, and converts the trajectory error into the motor command error. The feedforward controller (i.e., the inverse model) does not mimic the feedback controller, rather it acquires the fully nonlinear inverse model by minimizing the feedback motor command. A recasting of this approach, in neural net format, appears in Figure 16.4B (Kawato 1996a; Kawato and Gomi 1993).

Thus, once the inverse dynamics (inverse transfer characteristic) is acquired by motor learning, it can compute an appropriate motor command directly from the desired trajectory. In testing the model with a robotic manipulator used as a controlled system, it was found that both the (forward) dynamics and the inverse dynamics model were acquired during control of movements. As motor learning proceeded, the inverse dynamics model gradually took the place of external (sensorimotor) feedback as the main controller (thus, the characterization, "hierarchical"). Further, the neural network was able to generalize (i.e., once having learned to control some movements, it could control quite different and faster ones).

A

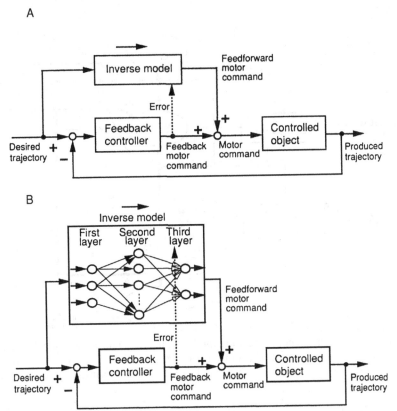

B

Figure 16.4. A. Feedback error learning scheme to acquire the inverse model of the controlled object. B. The same learning scheme using a three-layer feedforward neural network model as the inverse dynamics model. In A and B, the broken lines indicate information used for training. (From Kawato 1996a; in Bloedel, Ebner, and Wise (eds.), *The Acquisition of Motor Behavior in Vertebrates*, copyright 1996, The MIT Press; reprinted by permission of the publisher.)

16.3. Adaptive Control Models of the Cerebellum

16.3.1. A Hierarchical Neural Network Model

Kawato, Furukawa, and Suzuki (1987) and Kawato (1990a, 1990b) described a hierarchical neural network model (Fig. 16.5) for control and learning of voluntary movement. This model consisted of three parts: (1) the main descending motor pathway from the motor cortex (to which the original motor command is sent by association cortex) and the somatosensory (proprioceptive) feedback pathway to the motor cortex, (2) the spinocerebellum-magnocellular red nucleus system as an internal model of the (forward) dynamics of the musculoskeletal system, and (3) the lateral or cerebrocerebellum-parvocellular red nucleus system as an internal neural model of inverse dynamics of the musculoskeletal system. (Synaptic plasticity in the cerebellar cortex is included in the inverse model.)

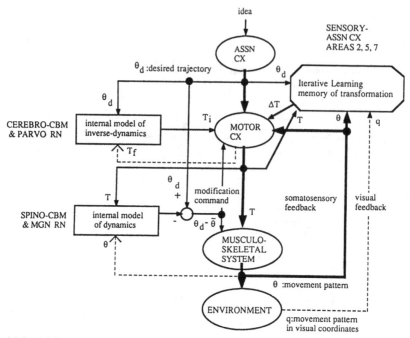

Figure 16.5. A hierarchical neural network model for learning and control of voluntary movement. (For explanation see text.) (From Kawato 1990a; in Miller, Sutton, and Werbos (eds.), *Neural Networks for Control*, copyright 1990, The MIT Press; reprinted by permission of the publisher.)

In this hierarchical neural network (Fig. 16.5), the association cortex sends the desired movement pattern θ, expressed in body coordinates, to the motor cortex where the motor command T (i.e., the torque to be generated by muscles is then computed by some means). The actual movement pattern θ is measured by proprioceptors and is returned to the motor cortex via the transcortical loop. Then feedback control can be performed using error in the movement trajectory. However, both feedback delays and small gains limit the controllable speeds of motions.

The cerebrocerebellum and the parvocellular part of the red nucleus system (Fig. 16.5) receive synaptic inputs from wide areas of the cerebral cortex, but they do not receive peripheral sensory input. That is, they monitor both the desired trajectory and the motor command but do not receive information about the actual movement. Within the cerebrocerebellum-parvocellular red nucleus system, an internal neural model of the inverse dynamics of the musculoskeletal system is acquired. The inverse dynamics of the musculoskeletal system is defined as the nonlinear system whose input and output are inverted; that is, the desired trajectory is the input and the motor command is the output (compare Figs. 15.21 and 15.22). Once the inverse dynamics model is acquired by motor learning, it can compute an appropriate motor command T_i directly from the desired trajectory θ_d.

16.3.2. Ito's General Functional Model

Ito (1990) proposed a general functional model of the cerebellum based on the then recently developed anatomical and physiological concept of the cerebellar microcomplex (Fig. 16.6A). As previously described, the latter consists of a cortical microzone and a small cell group in a cerebellar or vestibular nucleus acting as an adaptive controller (Ito 1984), the adaptability arising from the synaptic plasticity of long-term depression (LTD) in Purkinje cells. The magnitude of the LTD is determined by control error signals of climbing fibers, which originate in the inferior olive. Such microcomplexes were envisaged as being inserted in reflex arcs, command systems for voluntary motor control, and probably even cortical systems performing certain mental activities (Fig. 16.6B), providing adaptive learning capabilities to these systems (Ito 1990).

16.3.3. Kawato and Gomi's Feedback Error Learning Model

Subsequently (Gomi and Kawato 1992; Kawato 1993; Kawato and Gomi 1992a, 1992b), the model of feedback error learning (as it was now called), in conjunction with the acquiring by the cerebellum of the inverse of the controlled object (e.g., a limb), was extended to include not only the lateral cerebellum (the cerebrocerebellum) but also the intermediate zone and the vermis (jointly, the spinocerebellum), and the flocculus (vestibulocerebellum), as shown in Figure 16.7. At the same time, the model was imbedded into the known anatomy and physiology of the cerebellum (e.g., that climbing fiber responses represent motor command errors, and including microcomplexes as a functional unit). Because the inverse model is a model system whose input and output correspond to the output and input, respectively, of the controlled object, it makes an ideal feedforward controller and can also serve the purpose of coordinate transformation and trajectory planning. A schema for the feedback error learning model for voluntary movement is shown in Figure 16.7d. Figure 16.8 shows a schematic diagram of the counterpart components and interconnections in the brain.

In this schema (Kawato and Gomi 1992a), it is assumed that the sensorimotor learning required for movement takes place first in the cerebral cortex and then in the cerebellum. The coordinate transformation required for computing motor commands is learned first in the cerebral cortex, probably in the parietal association area, premotor area, and motor area. The resultant initially learned movement is still clumsy. The feedback motor command (i.e., error) is next sent to the cerebellum as climbing fiber input. Procedural motor learning then occurs, and smooth, fast, subconscious movements then become possible. Climbing fiber responses are assumed to represent motor command errors (including both amplitude and direction) generated by premotor networks, such as the feedback controllers at the spinal, brain stem, and cerebral levels, so the motor errors reported by the climbing fiber are in motor command coordinates rather than in sensory coordinates. By LTD in Purkinje cells, each corticonuclear microcomplex learns to execute predictive and

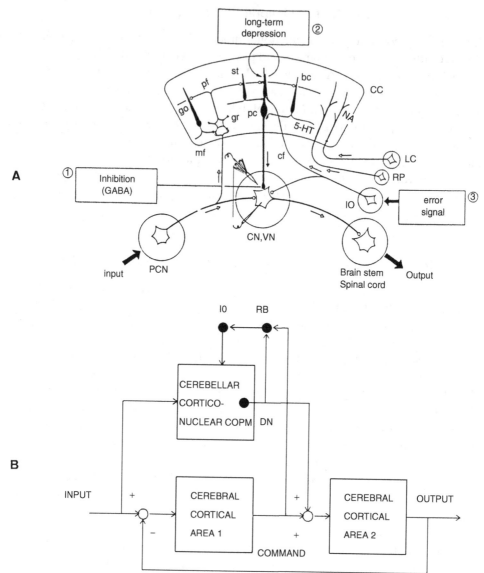

Figure 16.6. A. Structure of a cerebellar corticonuclear microcomplex. CC: cerebellar cortical microzone; CN, VN: cerebellar and vestibular nuclei; PCN: precerebellar nuclei; IO: inferior olive; LC: locus coeruleus; RP: raphe nucleus; NA: noradrenaline; 5-HT: serotonin; mf: mossy fiber; cf: climbing fiber; pc: Purkinje cell; bc: basket cell; st: stellate cell; gr: granule cell; go: Golgi cell; pf: parallel fiber; 1, 2, 3: major findings that suggest adaptive operation of the corticonuclear microcomplex. B. Modification of A for mental control. IO: inferior olive, RB: parvocellular red nucleus. DN: dentate nucleus. (From Ito 1990; in *Revue. Neurologique*, Vol. 146, copyright 1990, Editions Masson; reprinted by permission of the publisher and author.)

a. Adaptive Modification of Vestibulo-ocular Reflex

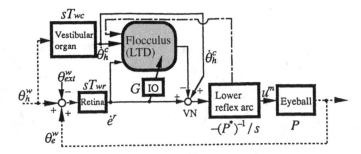

b. Adaptive Control for Posture

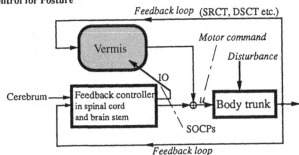

c. Adaptive Control for Locomotion

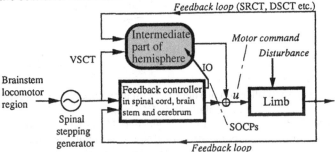

d. Learning Control for Voluntary Movement

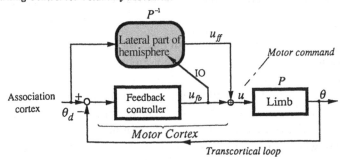

Figure 16.7. Functional roles played by different parts of the cerebellum interpreted according to the feedback error learning scheme. (a) Flocculus for adaptive modification of the VOR; (b) vermis, for adaptive control of posture; (c) intermediate zone for adaptive control of locomotion; and (d) lateral hemisphere for learning voluntary motor control. (From Kawato 1993; in Meyer and Kornblum (eds.), *Attention and Performance XIV. Synergies in Experimental Psychology, Artificial Intelligence, and Cognitive Neuroscience*, copyright 1993, The MIT Press; reprinted by permission of the publisher.)

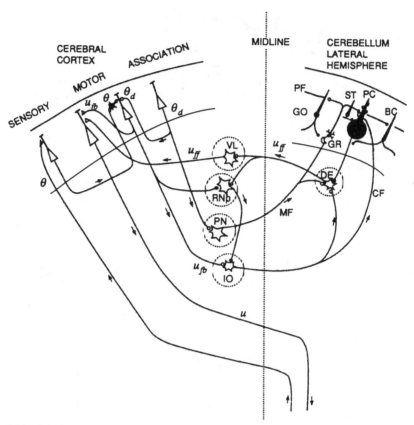

Figure 16.8. Schematic diagram of a neural circuit for voluntary movement learning control by a cerebrocerebellar loop. CF: climbing fiber; BC: basket cell; GO: Golgi cell; GR: granule cell MF: mossy fiber; PC Purkinje cell; PF: parallel fiber; ST: stellate cell; DE: dentate nucleus; IO: inferior olivary nucleus; PN: pontine nuclei, RNp: parvocellular red nucleus; VL: ventrolateral nucleus of the thalamus. (From Kawato and Gomi 1992a; *Biol. Cybern.* Vol. 68, copyright 1992, Springer-Verlag, Heidelberg; reprinted by permission of publisher and author.).

coordinate control of different types of movements. Ultimately, an inverse model of the controlled object is built up, making it an ideal feedforward controller (Kawato and Gomi 1992a).

Experimental support for the cerebellum as a site for inverse dynamics modeling of controlled movements in the form of slow tracking eye movements (to ramp stimuli) in monkeys was reported by these authors (Shidara et al. 1993; Kawano et al. 1996), who compared activity of Purkinje cells in the ventral paraflocculus of the cerebellum with eye velocity and acceleration. It was found that the complex temporal pattern of the firing frequency occurring during the ocular following response elicited by movements of a large visual scene could be reconstructed by an inverse dynamics representation, using position, velocity, and acceleration of the eye movements.

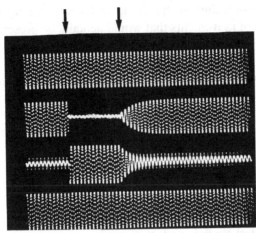

Figure 16.9. Idealized simulation with an ASP (Chapter 15) of the effect of sudden loss (first arrow), and recovery (second arrow) of cerebellar participation in voluntary motor control, based on the schema in Figure 16.4A. Top trace: a constant amplitude constant frequency sinusoid representing normal functioning of the desired movement. Trace 2: output of cerebellum as feedforward motor command. Trace 3: output of motor cortex into feedback controller. Trace 4: output to controlled object (limb). Note that the sum of the output of the cerebellum (trace 2) and of the motor cortex (trace 3) is constant (trace 4). The disablement of the "cerebellum" (trace 2) was actually accomplished by temporarily zeroing the weights in the adaptive signal processor (Chapter 15). Upon termination of the zeroing, the coefficients restore themselves, and the output of the cerebellum restores itself. (See Figure 15.6.)

16.3.4. Feedback Error Modeling of Temporary Immobilization of the Cerebellar Cortex and/or Nuclei

A temporary failure of the cerebellum or of a cerebellar nucleus (e.g., from injection of mucimol into the cerebellar nuclei) in a feedback error cerebellar learning model after learning has already been completed is schematized in Figure 16.9, based on the schema in Figure 16.4A. The signal pathway is from the cerebral cortex via the inverse model, the output of which is the feedforward motor command, in motor coordinates. The trajectory produced is essentially the same as the desired trajectory, and hence the output of the feedback controller is essentially zero, as is the error signal, the two being the same. In Figure 16.9, trace 1 simulates the input signal from the cerebral cortex to the cerebellum, and trace 2 simulates the output of the cerebellar nuclei to a summing point projecting to, for example, spinal motor centers; the other input to the summing point is the feedback motor command. When a sudden loss of function of the cerebellum (Fig. 16.9, trace 2) occurs (first arrow), the input from the motor cortex to the aforementioned summing point takes over entirely (trace 3). With (exponential) recovery of cerebellar output (trace 2, second arrow), the motor cortex contributes progressively less to the summing point (trace 3), so the output to the summing point (trace 4) remains essentially constant in amplitude. (This simulation is intended to show only that the cerebral cortex automatically substitutes for the disabled cerebellum and relinquishes control when the cerebellum recovers.

The depiction does not include such pathological manifestations as cerebellar ataxia and decomposition of movements that would actually be present during cerebellar disablement.)

Maintenance of Saccadic Accuracy. Dean, Mayhew, and Langdon (1994) proposed a combined cerebellar–brain stem model for learning and maintaining saccadic accuracy that incorporates Kawato's principle of feedback error learning in conjunction with Albus's (neural net) Cerebellar Model Arithmetic Computer (CMAC) to achieve adaptive control of saccades.

16.3.5. Modeling Adaptation to Prism Spectacles and Saccadic Adaptation

Arbib, Schweighofer, and Thach (1995) proposed a general model of the cerebellum applicable both to dart-throwing adaptation with prism spectacles (lateral cerebellum) and to saccadic adaptation (medial cerebellum), with the details for the two being different (Fig. 16.10). The basic model, which takes into account the concept of microzones (Ito 1984) and the long length of parallel fibers that overlap different microzones (Fig. 13.6), thus makes possible the coordination of modulation of different movement pattern generators (MPGs). The model includes the concepts of modifiable synapses and of synapse eligibility (Houk et al. 1990), the latter being a kind of delay to compensate for transit time of sensory information to the cerebellar cortex. The inferior olive outputs error signals via climbing fibers, and its effect on the cerebellar nuclei via climbing fiber collaterals is to nullify the strong inhibition caused by the complex spikes, which are the responses of the Purkinje cells to the climbing fibers themselves. Illustrative simulations of prism adaptation to throwing were reported to compare well with results from normal humans (Arbib, Schweighofer, and Thach 1995).

16.3.6. Feedback Error Models – An Update

Kawato (1996a) provided an overview of feedback error models of the motor apparatus. A more recent update (Wolpert, Miall, and Kawato 1998) is shown in Fig. 16.11 (compare with Fig. 16.4), on which certain of the corresponding presumptive cerebellar components (Fig. 16.11B; i.e., mossy fibers, granule cells, parallel fibers, simple spikes, and complex spikes) are indicated.

16.3.7. Distributed Inverse Dynamics Control

In computer modeling of visually guided reaching movements by humans, Schweighofer et al. (1998a) compared the virtual trajectory control hypothesis (in which the planned trajectory issued by a feedforward controller is fed directly to the muscles in terms of desired muscle equilibrium lengths; McIntyre and Bizzi 1993), and the inverse dynamics control hypothesis (in which a neural representation is made of the transformation from the desired movement to the corresponding

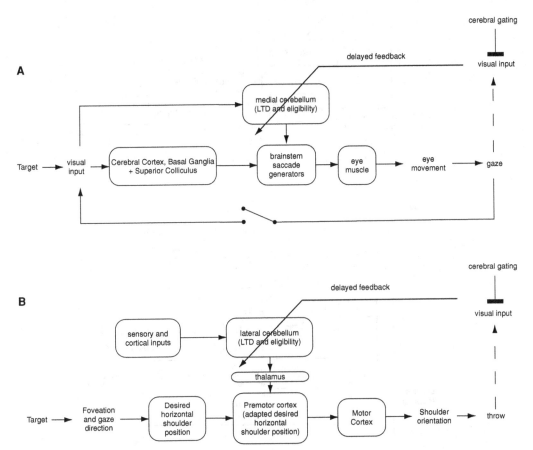

Figure 16.10. Systems views of cerebellar modulation of the saccadic system and in the adaptation of the throw to deviating prisms: (A) The saccadic system must be adaptive. Note that "delayed feedback" (which is relayed via the IO [not shown] is a form of visual input, but it is segregated from that which serves as input to the nonadaptive pathway. (B). Putative mechanisms of adjustment between eye position and synergy of the muscles in the trunk and arm involved in throwing. Afferent information on eye position arriving in intermediate zone lobulus simplex is carried over parallel fibers to Purkinje cells, which project to cells in the dentate nucleus with control eye, neck, arm, and hand muscle synergies. As the saccade model, the cerebellum provides a correction to the main pathway, but here the correction is further "upstream," via the premotor cortex. (From Arbib, Schweighofer, and Thach 1995; reprinted from Glencross and Pick (eds.), *Motor Control and Sensory Motor Integration: Issues and Directions*, copyright 1995, Elsevier Science; reprinted by permission of the publisher.).

motor commands; Kawato and Gomi 1993). The virtual trajectory model, extended to whole arm reaching movements, accurately reproduced slow movements (of the order of 1 second), but faster reaching movements deviated significantly from the planned trajectories faster reaching movements (of the order of 0.5 second) because the controllers operating for each joint are not coupled and hence this control system does not generate straight trajectories for rapid movements with large interaction forces. These results led the authors to propose a new distributed functional model

A

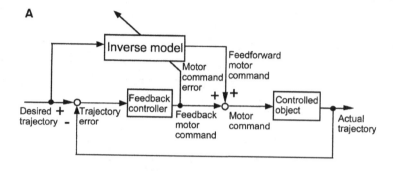

B

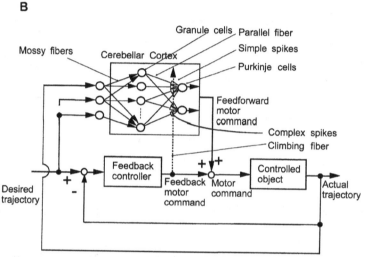

Figure 16.11. The cerebellar feedback error learning model (CBFELM). (This is a more recent version of Figure 16.5.) (A) The general feedback-error-learning model. (B) The CBFELM. The "controlled object" is a physical entity that is to be controlled by the CNS, such as the eyes, hands, legs, or torso. The controlled object can be considered as a cascade of transformations between motor command (e.g., joint torques or muscle activations) and linkage motions (e.g., joint angular position, velocity, acceleration), and between this linkage motion and the controlled object motion (e.g., spatial position, velocity, acceleration of the hand). Such transformations represent the system dynamics and kinematics, respectively. By "inverse model" is meant a neural representation of the transformation from the desired movement trajectory of the controlled object to the motor commands required to attain this movement goal. Because the inverse model possesses input transfer characteristics that are the inverse of those of the controlled object, the cascade of the two systems gives an approximate identity function. That is, if a desired trajectory is given to the inverse model, then at the end of the cascade the actual trajectory will be fairly close to the desired trajectory. Thus, accurate inverse models can be used as ideal feedforward controllers. An example of the trajectory error is retinal slip for the VOR and ocular following responses (OFR). In engineering, a proportional-integral-derivative controller is often used as a feedback controller. The component of the final motor command that is generated by a feedback controller is called the feedback motor command. (From Wolpert, Miall, and Kawato 1998; in *Trends in Cognitive Sciences*, Vol. 2, copyright 1998; reprinted by permission from Elsevier Science; illustration courtesy Dr. Daniel Wolpert.)

in which the CNS, using a basic feedforward/feedback controller, acquires, in the motor cortex and spinal cord (at the C3/C4 level), a distributed inverse dynamics model of the arm. The basic model was refined by having the cerebellum compensate for the interaction torques among the limb members by learning a portion of the inverse dynamics model. (Without the addition of the cerebellum, the results for the basic inverse model were similar to those for the expanded virtual trajectory model; both showed features in common with those encountered in cerebellar disease, including inaccurate trajectories and overshoots.) The latter thus becomes a three-part distributed inverse dynamics model: in the motor cortex, the spinal cord, and the cerebellum (but without its associated inferior olive, see below).

In a companion article (Schweighofer et al. 1998b), a biologically based detailed cerebellar neural network was added that comprised the major units (including the inferior olive, and cell types of the cerebellar system) and that learned that part of the inverse dynamics of the arm not provided by the basic feedforward/feedback controller (Fig. 16.12). Realistically based parameter selections resulted in performance that compared favorably (Fig. 16.13) with published results from humans (Holmes 1939). Among other points, the authors found that only long parallel fibers allowed proper learning (i.e., proper coordination of movement at two joints). If the parallel fibers were short, the Purkinje cell inputs originated mostly from the same joint, and many terms of the inverse dynamics equation could not be computed. Also, it was found that, during learning of a movement, two peaks of inferior olive activity occurred, at the beginning of the movement and at the end, whereas after learning, only remnants of the early peak remained. The authors concluded that their results with the model support the theory that the cerebellum is involved in motor learning.

16.3.8. Wolpert and Kawato's Multiple Paired Forward-Inverse Model

Kawato and Wolpert (1998) summarized findings that have provided strong support for the hypothesis that the CNS learns and maintains internal models of the sensorimotor system and of objects in the external environment. Internal models enable the CNS to predict the consequences of motor commands and to determine the motor commands required to perform specific tasks. To deal with a variety of behavioral paradigms associated with different objects and environments, specific sensorimotor transformations must be employed that are tailored to particular situations.

A reasonable inference, according to the authors, is that the CNS learns, maintains, and switches among multiple internal models of sensorimotor transformations. The authors illustrated this point with models for the ocular following response in monkeys. The models included the phylogenetically older simple feedback circuit of the cerebellar feedback error learning model (CBFELM; Wolpert, Miall, and Kawato 1998) comprising the retina, the accessory optic system (AOS) and the brain stem, and the phylogenetically newer, more sophisticated feedforward/feedback pathway and the inverse dynamics model of CBFELM, corresponding to the cerebral and cerebellar cortical pathway and to the cerebellar cortex, respectively.

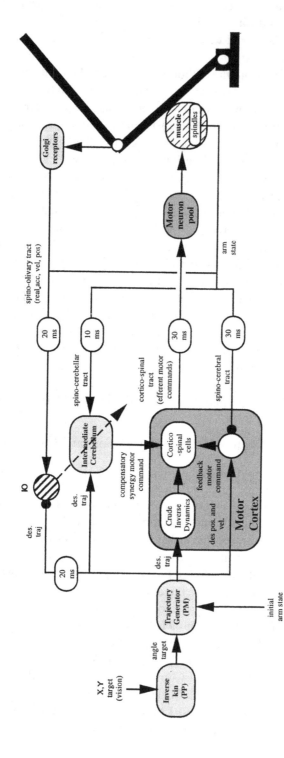

Figure 16.12. Functional diagram of a model for on-line control of arm movements with inclusion of the inferior olive (IO), which computes the feedback error. The delayed desired trajectory (position, velocity, and acceleration) forms the inhibitory inputs to the IO, whereas the actual delayed trajectory, sensed by muscle spindles and Golgi tendon receptors forms the excitatory input. PP, posterior parietal cortex; PM, premotor cortex. (From Schweighofer et al. 1998b; in *European Journal of Neuroscience*, Vol. 10, 1998, copyright by Blackwell Science Ltd; reprinted by permission of the publisher.)

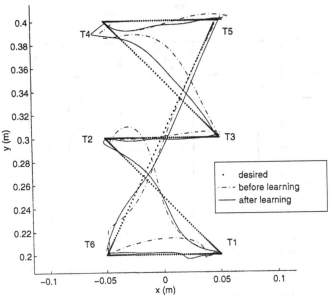

Figure 16.13. Arm trajectories before learning and after 2000 trials in a successive "zs" Holmes-like maneuver (Chapter 11) for movements lasting 750 milliseconds. Note that, after learning, the real trajectory is closer to the desired trajectory. (From Schweighofer et al. 1998b; in *European Journal of Neuroscience*, Vol. 10, 1998, copyright by Blackwell Science Ltd; reprinted by permission of the publisher.)

The authors (Haruno, Wolpert, and Kawato 1999; Kawato and Wolpert 1998; Wolpert and Kawato 1998; Wolpert, Miall, and Kawato 1998) then proposed a new computationally intense model in which each inverse (controller) model is augmented with a corresponding forward (predictive) model, the pair being tightly coupled during acquisition, motor learning, and use, through gating dependent on the behavioral context. Ensembles of such pairs were termed multiple forward inverse models (MPFIMs; Fig. 16.14). On the basis of simulations of object manipulation, the authors concluded that the MPFIM model of human motor learning and control, like the human motor system itself, can learn multiple tasks (e.g., reaching and grasping), show generalization to new tasks, and exhibit an ability to switch appropriately between tasks (Haruno, Wolpert, and Kawato 1999).

The following is taken from a detailed description of the MPFIM by the authors (Wolpert, Miall, and Kawato 1998). (Additional mathematical details are provided by Wolpert and Kawato [1998].)

Each module consists of three interacting parts. The first two, the forward model and the responsibility predictor, are used to determine the responsibility (extent of participation) of the module. This responsibility signal reflects the degree to which the module captures the current context and hence should participate in control. The aim is that the multiple forward models learn to divide experience so at least one forward model can predict the consequence of performed actions under any given context. The likelihood that a particular forward model captures

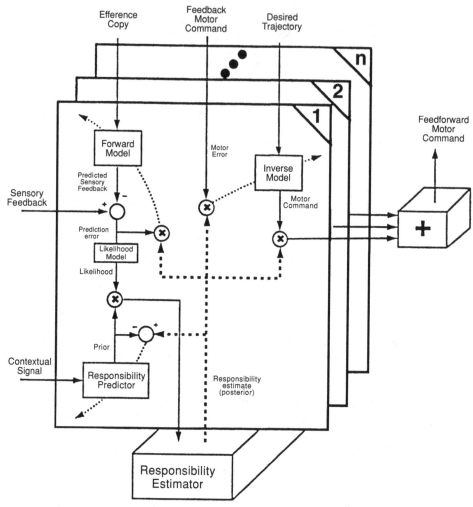

Figure 16.14. Schematic of the multiple paired forward-inverse model (MPFIM), including *n* paired modules that are depicted as stacked sheets (the dotted lines represent training signals and X indicates multiplication). The details of the first module are shown and interactions between modules take place through the Responsibility Estimator (bottom). Further description in text. (From Wolpert and Kawato 1998; in *Neural Networks*, Vol. 11, copyright 1998, Elsevier Science; reprinted by permission of the publisher.) (See also Wolpert, Miall, and Kawato [1998]).

the current behavior is determined from its prediction error. The smaller this error, the more likely the sensory feedback and efference copy are consistent with the context captured by the forward model, and hence the higher the module's responsibility. However, the forward model can only be used to estimate responsibility once a movement has been initiated and the results of action are known. To allow sensory contextual signal to alter the responsibility prior to movement, a responsibility predictor estimates the responsibility before movement onset using sensory contextual cues and is trained to approximate the final responsibility estimate. By multiplying this estimate (a priori estimate) by the likelihood derived from the forward models, and normalizing across the modules using the responsibility estimator (with soft-max [normalization], for example), an estimate of the module's responsibility (a posteriori estimate) is achieved.

This responsibility signal represents the extent to which each forward model/responsibility predictor accounts for the behavior of the system. It ensures that the smaller the prediction error, the higher the forward module's responsibility and vice versa. The responsibilities are then used to control the learning within the forward models, with those models having high responsibilities receiving proportionately more of their error signal than modules with low responsibility. By weighting the errors by the responsibility, we ensure competitive learning so forward models will learn to divide the system dynamics experienced and the responsibilities will reflect the extent to which each forward model captures the current behavior of the system.

For each behavior captured by a forward model, a controller is to learn it. Hence, the third component of the model is the inverse model, which generates a motor command given a desired trajectory. Each module has an inverse model that learns to provide suitable control signals under the context for which the paired forward model provides accurate predictions. Again, the responsibilities are used to weight the error signal (the feedback motor command previously mentioned in connection with inverse models) for each inverse model, thereby ensuring that the inverse model and forward model within a module are rigidly coupled during learning. If one forward model's prediction is good, its corresponding inverse model receives the major part of the motor error signal. Finally, the responsibilities are used to determine the extent to which each inverse model's output contributes to the final feedforward motor command. (Reprinted from *Trends Cogn. Sci.* Vol. 2. by Wolpert, D. M., Miall, R. C., and Kawato, M., "Internal models in the carebellum." pp. 338–347. Copyright 1998, with permission from Elsevier Science.)

Wolpert and Kawato (1998) indicated that the model assumes that the desired motor command is available to train multiple inverse models; an assumption, however, that they pointed out is implausible for biological motor learning. For a more sophisticated physiological computational model, they used the feedback error learning model (Kawato, Furawaka, and Suzuki 1987; Kawato and Gomi 1992a) in conjunction with the just-described simple model. In this more sophisticated version, the total motor command fed to the motor apparatus is the summation of the total feedforward motor command and the feedback motor command. The latter can be calculated from the difference between the desired movement pattern and the actual pattern, in which the feedback motor command is used as the error signal for the motor command (Wolpert and Kawato 1998).

It was assumed by the authors (Wolpert and Kawato 1998) that the cerebellum is the most logical site for the location of the forward and inverse models and that a pair of forward and inverse models were localized within a microzone or functional unit of the cerebellar context. It was also assumed that both forward and inverse models are used in mental simulation of movement, as follows. Forward models would be used (instead of the motor apparatus) to simulate the results of nonperformed actions on an imaginary controlled object, and inverse models would be required to generate the motor command.

16.3.9. Modeling of Objects in External World by Cerebellar Hemispheres

Imamizu et al. (2000) proposed a computational theory in which the phylogenetically newer part of the cerebellum (i.e., the lateral cerebellar hemispheres) acquires internal models of objects in the external world, in a manner analogous to that in which the cerebellar cortex acquires internal models through motor learning to control movements accurately. The authors cited their earlier proposal (see above; Wolpert and Kawato 1998) that multiple internal models exist and that they compete to learn new environments and tools. During the learning, all these multiple internal models receive a copy of the error signal but only one or a few learn the new transformation, thereby reducing the error signal and localizing the new activity to a distinct region of the cerebellum. The two types of cerebellar activity representing the error signals in the internal model were predicted to occur in specific spatiotemporal patterns.

To test the theory, the authors carried out functional magnetic resonance imaging (fMRI) studies while human subjects learned to use a new tool (a computer mouse with a novel rotational transformation). Two types of activity were found. The first was spread over wide areas of the cerebellum and is taken to reflect that phase in which all the multiple internal models receive a copy of the error signal, but only a few learn the new transformation, thus reducing the error signal. The other type of activity was confined to the area near the posterior superior fissure and remained even after learning was complete; this activity was taken to reflect, probably, an acquired internal model of the new tool.

In an accompanying commentary on the above-cited paper of Imamizu et al. (2000), Ito (2000) suggested that complex body movements can probably be carried out so easily and accurately because the cerebellum provides a model of what is to be moved. The particular reference model in Ito's discussion was the two-degree of freedom adaptive control system with feedback error learning described by Kawato and Gomi (1992a; see above). This system combines a feedback control by the cerebral cortex and a feedforward system controlled by the cerebellum. The cerebral cortex compares the instructed, desired movement with an actually realized movement by sensory feedback, whereas the cerebellum receives only the instruction. For a desired movement to occur without feedback of the actually realized movement, the cerebellum must form an inverse model of the hand/arm system. Ito (2000) pointed out that the report of Imamizu et al. (2000) provided the first evidence of the actual formation in the cerebellum of the resulting inverse model. In turn, the mechanism of learning of the model itself was attributed by Ito to LTD at the parallel fiber–Purkinje cell synapse, under the influence of an error signal conveyed by the climbing fibers from the inferior olive (Ito 1998).

In his commentary, Ito (2000) also described the basic function of an adaptive control system in relation to the corresponding cerebellar microcomplex components,

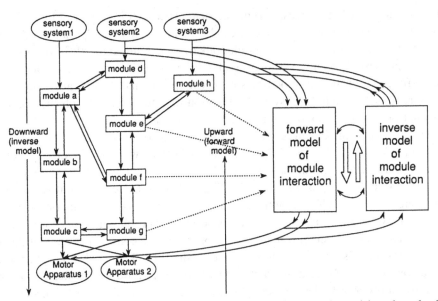

Figure 16.15. Schematic diagram showing how self-consciousness is envisioned as the forward and inverse models of interactions between parallel sensorimotor modules. (From Kawato 1997; in Ito, Miyashita, and Rolls (eds.), *Cognition, Computation, and Consciousness*, copyright 1997, Oxford University Press; reprinted by permission of publisher and author.) (Compare with Ito's schema in Fig. 16.6B.)

and pointed out that, if LTD is the only synaptic plasticity that underlies the learning mechanism of the cerebellar circuitry, then the learning is unlikely to be accompanied by an increase in rate of discharge of Purkinje cells (which may be reflected as increased local blood flow by fMRI). Therefore, although the original authors (Imamizu et al. 2000) assumed that both excitatory and inhibitory synaptic transmission to the Purkinje cells are facilitated, and hence that discharge rates of the Purkinje cells increase, Ito (2000) pointed out that there may be other possibilities (e.g., the release of nitric oxide, which relaxes blood capillaries).

16.3.10. Kawato's Bidirectional Theory Approach to Consciousness

In connection with the question of mechanisms of cognitive activity, Kawato (1997) proposed extending the concept of paired internal forward and inverse (i.e., bidirectional) models to sensorimotor integration and beyond that to the question of consciousness. As a starting point in the proposal, it is assumed that the brain consists of a number of modules that roughly correspond to different (cerebral) cortical areas, and that these modules are organized in a hierarchical yet parallel manner (Fig. 16.15). Thus, the downward information flow implemented by the feedforward connection constitutes an approximated inverse model of some physical process outside the brain such as a kinematics (movement only) transformation, dynamics (movement plus forces) transformation, or optics (image generation process). However, the upward information flow implemented by the feedback connection provides a forward model of the corresponding physical process. It is a tenet of the proposal that coherent perception and behavior can be achieved only if the parallel and multiple sensorimotor transformation modules talk to each other and settle into a coherent state in the sense of von der Malsburg (1997; i.e., that the essence of coherence is successful collaboration of modalities in solving problems). In Kawato's view, such a coherent state is achieved by fast relaxation computation through bidirectional information flow between different levels of the hierarchy.

The extension of Kawato's proposal to self-consciousness then proceeds as follows. If the brain has the capability of acquiring both forward and inverse models of the external world, it should be easier for some part of the brain to acquire internal models of some other part of the brain (Fig. 16.15, right side). Then, it is proposed that some portion of self-consciousness and self-awareness can be understood as forward and inverse modeling of interactions between multiple sensorimotor modules. To obtain a coherent perception of a scene or to adopt a consistent behavioral plan, many brain regions or sensorimotor modules should talk to each other and settle into a coherent equilibrium in which the state of every module satisfies constraints given by all other modules connected to it. Yet further acceleration of this convergence could be acquired if a model of these dynamics of module interactions could be acquired through frequent observations of this convergence process. Here it is proposed to view the forward model of module interactions as an approximate model of the other brain regions (Fig. 16.15, right side). In this sense, self-consciousness would be just a very rough and imperfect model of all the complicated dynamical interactions of many brain modules always working subconsciously to solve the most difficult ill-posed (i.e., an arbitrarily large number of solutions) sensorimotor interaction problems. Overall, the forward model of the brain itself makes transformations from sensory signals to motor outputs. Thus, it is closer to some inverse model of the external world. However, the inverse model of the brain can be classified as the forward model of the external world. By relaxation computation through these forward and inverse models, emulation of oneself, prediction of one's behavior in interaction with the environment, and retrospection can be made possible. (Correspondingly, a completely unconscious state of mind is one in which there is a very low level of coherence between subsystems, to the extent that one cannot talk of a functional state at all [i.e., the brain not capable of reacting to any event altogether, von der Malsburg 1997]).

PART FOUR

SUMMARY AND CONCLUSIONS

SEVENTEEN

The Cerebellum as an Adaptive Controller

17.1. Introduction

In this final chapter, a brief retrospective is presented on the history of the cerebellum as an adaptive controller, a term used as an inclusive term also for adaptive signal processor (ASP) and adaptive filter, to refer to a system having the capability to adjust or optimize its own parameters automatically. An alternative but equivalent view of the cerebellum as a three-layer neural net follows. Then, the significance of the basic uniformity of the structure of the cerebellar system is briefly reviewed, as a preliminary to several other topics. (As previously in this book, the term *cerebellar system* refers to the cerebellar cortex, cerebellar nuclei, and the inferior olive [the olivary nucleus], together with their interconnections.) The significance of the two principal afferent fiber systems of the cerebellum is then considered in relation to their features and to their counterparts in adaptive controllers.

Next, the vestibulo-ocular reflex (VOR), which is based on the vestibulocerebellum, is viewed as the simplest and most straightforward manifestation of an adaptive controller model of the cerebellum. The VOR is then used as a model for the functions of the remaining parts of the cerebellum, the spinocerebellum and the cerebrocerebellum, including the controversial question of the cerebellum and cognition. Then, some remaining problems are considered, such as the functions of the cerebellar nuclei and especially the inferior olive, and the function of negative and positive feedback circuits.

Major questions that arise from an examination of cerebellar anatomy from the perspective of adaptive controllers are then considered, including the question of whether the cerebellum functions only in a scaling (multiplicative) mode in contrast to a fully predictive mode, which necessitates a precise time-delay capability (i.e., a tapped delay line) and the related question of whether the cerebellum stores motor patterns as opposed to scaling coefficients. A final conclusion is reached that the cerebellar system functions as a scaling device but not as a predictor alone.

17.2. A Brief History of the Cerebellum as an Adaptive Controller

From the reviews presented in Chapters 13, 14, and 16, it is evident that the view of the cerebellum as an adaptive controller extends back to the late 1960s, to the publication of the papers of Grossberg (1969), Marr (1969), Ito (1970), Albus (1971), Robinson (1976), Seijnowski (1977), Optican and Robinson (1980), and Fujita (1982a). The engineering literature on adaptive control began to appear somewhat earlier (Chapter 14): Widrow and Hoff (1960), Widrow (1963), the review by Widrow and Lehr (1990). Further, adaptive control has become used with increasing frequency since the early 1990s. The closely related neural net model, which shares with adaptive controllers the ability to adjust its own parameters automatically, had its origins in the visual pattern-recognition device of Rosenblatt (1958, 1961), the Perceptron. This device can be traced back (Arbib and Amari 1985) to the modeling by Pitts and McCulloch (1947) of the superior colliculus as a distributed controller of eye movements. More recently, neural net models have become increasingly used as a model for the cerebellum (Chapter 16).

17.3. Modeling the VOR with an Adaptive Controller

In the VOR (in which, upon turning the head, the direction of gaze is maintained constant by virtue of counter-rotation of the eyes), the gain is normally somewhat less than 1.0, so eye velocity compensates rather closely for head velocity during movements of the head. The relevant corrective signal for this purpose is derived from retinal slip (i.e., displacement of the visual image on the retina), which stimulates motion detectors of the retina. The retinal slip signal carries information about both velocity and direction.

Figure 17.1A, a schema for the VOR (same as Fig. 8.1), is redrawn schematically in Figure 17.1B, with the components of the latter in approximately the same arrangement as those in Figure 17.1A. Of essential importance is to note that, from the semicircular canal (SCC, taken for simplicity to be a horizontal semicircular canal that is responsive to head-turning about the vertical axis), there are two pathways to the (lateral) vestibular nucleus (VN): a direct path, A, constituted of mossy fiber collaterals, and an indirect path, B, via the vestibulocerebellum, that is, via the granule cell (gc), parallel fibers (pf), Purkinje cell (Pc), and finally, via the axon of the Purkinje cell to the VN. In the indirect path (B), the effect of activity of the climbing fiber (conjointly with the parallel fibers) is to induce LTD in the Purkinje cell, which has the effect of decreasing the rate of its simple spike output, so there is less inhibition of the vestibular nucleus, the firing rates of neurons of which thus increase. This phenomenon of scaling, which occurs irrespective of the impulse (firing) rate of the mossy fiber input from the semicircular canals, is the basic operation throughout the entire cerebellum, it appears. The Purkinje cell shown in Figure 17.1A and a group of other Purkinje cells and their associated granule, Golgi, basket, and stellate cells, together with their afferent mossy fibers and climbing fibers, constitute a microzone, which together with the associated cells in the inferior olive and the vestibular nuclei (or cerebellar nuclei), constitute a microcomplex (in the sense of Ito), the basic computational unit of the cerebellar system (Chapter 5).

The remainder (right side) of Figure 17.1A is concerned with oculomotor nuclei (*OMN*) and eye movement (*EM*), and is of such a nature as to compensate for head turning so the direction of gaze (arrow at the extreme right) remains constant. If this is not the case, displacement of the visual image on the retina (i.e., retinal slip) results, and generates an error signal that is transmitted via the accessory optic tract (*aot*) and the nucleus of the accessory optic tract, the inferior olive (*IO*), and the Purkinje cells via the climbing fibers (*cf*). It is the conjoint action of climbing fibers and parallel fibers that results in a change in the gain (rate of Purkinje cell simple spikes) presumably through the action of a change in the LTD and LTP at the parallel fiber–climbing fiber–Purkinje cell dendritic tree interface (Chapter 7) that results in a change of gain $(\alpha - \beta)$ (Fig. 17.1A) for the VOR reflex.

Thus, if the eye movement compensatory to head movement is inadequate and the eye lags behind, the retinal slip error, conveyed by the climbing fibers via the IO, results in an altered LTD/LTP level at the Purkinje cells, which in turn induces a decrease in Purkinje cell inhibitory output, so the resultant diminished inhibition (i.e., disinhibition) of the VN yields an increased output to the oculomotor nuclei and a greater velocity of compensatory eye movement, which in turn diminishes the error signal (i.e., retinal slip).

Turning now to the engineering detail of the schema of the basic adaptive control model depicted in Figure 17.1C (same as Fig. 15.1A), the counterpart of the semi-circular canal output is the input signal (upper left in Fig. 17.1C), the amplitude of which is to be made to be the same as that of a training signal (upper left). To carry out the match, the scaled input signal (multiplier on the right with scale factor, *a*) is subtracted from the training signal (differencer at the upper right) to generate an error signal, *e*. Actually, the error signal has a magnitude as well as a phase, relative to the training signal (i.e., the error signal is either of the same phase as, or opposite in phase to, the training signal, depending on the relative amplitudes of the training signal and the scaled input signal). In the schema of Figure 17.1C, the phase, or polarity, is established by multiplication of the error signal by the input signal (multiplier on the lower left), and the resultant positive (or negative, depending on the above-mentioned relative amplitudes) signal is integrated (i.e., fine-grain summated – box with integration sign) to yield the scale or multiplication factor, *a*. Assuming that *a* begins with a value of zero, it builds up to approach a limit, and the error signal, *e*, approaches zero as a decaying exponential. (The input signal, now matched in amplitude to the training signal, is fed to the differencer in inverted form for the subtraction; therefore, it is inverted to constitute the output signal [right, in Fig. 17.1C], as a replica of the training signal).

In the engineering version of the adaptive controller shown in Figure 17.1C, both multipliers can accept either positive or negative inputs, and consequently their outputs can be either positive or negative. However, such an arrangement is not

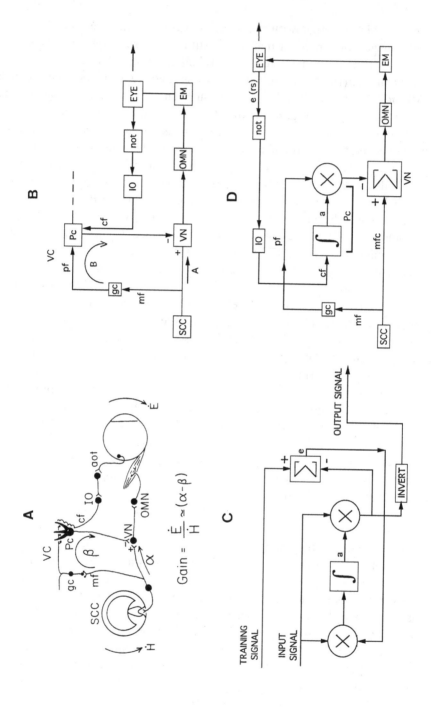

A

SCC · gc · mf · VC · Pc · β · cf · IO · aot · $\dot{E}$

$-$VN$+$ · α · OMN · $\dot{H}$

$$\text{Gain} = \frac{\dot{E}}{\dot{H}} \simeq (\alpha - \beta)$$

B

SCC → gc → mf · B · pf · Pc · cf · IO · not · EYE · EM

VC · VN $-$ $+$ · A · OMN

C

TRAINING SIGNAL · $+$ · e · $-$ · OUTPUT SIGNAL

INPUT SIGNAL · ⊗ · ∫ a · ⊗ · INVERT

D

SCC → gc → mf · pf · cf · ∫ a · Pc · ⊗ · IO · not · e (rs) · EYE

mfc · VN $+$ $-$ · OMN · EM

feasible biologically because the biological signals are pulse trains of varying frequency, which can have only positive values. Revamping the basic adaptive controller as depicted in Figure 17.1D overcomes this difficulty, and at the same time, more closely approximates the actual VOR circuit of Figure 17.1B, the labeling terms of which have been transferred to Figure 17.1D. As in Figure 17.1B, the input signal (from the SCC in Fig. 17.1D), is split into two pathways to the vestibular nuclei (VN): a direct one, via mossy fiber collaterals (mfc), and an indirect one, via mf, gc, pf, Pc, and inhibitory Pc axons. The scaled signal via the indirect Path B is subtracted from that via the direct Path A to generate, in the oculomotor nucleus (OMN), the eye movement (EM) signal. As in Figure 17.1B, if the eye movement does not compensate exactly for head movement (thus maintaining the direction of gaze constant – arrow at the upper right in Figure 17.1D), an error signal is generated from retinal slip ($e(rs)$), transmitted via the accessory optic tract, the IO, and climbing fibers, and then, in the Purkinje cell–parallel fiber–climbing fiber complex (indicated by the horizontal bracket below the lettering Pc, the scaling factor, a, is altered in such a way as to decrease the rate of retinal slip (i.e., so eye movement velocity matches [is equal and opposite to] that of the head movement, and consequently the error signal progressively decreases). Figure 17.1D is thus a combination of Figure 17.1B and Figure 17.1C.

It should be noted that the two inputs to the multiplier in Figure 17.1D (i.e., the scaling constant, a, and the pf [parallel fiber] rate) are both nominally positive, so the output of the multiplier itself will be positive. However, because the Purkinje cell has an inhibitory output, the multiplier output will be subtracted from the input arriving from the mf collaterals in the VN.

Figure 17.1. Comparison of VOR with ASP. *A*. (same as Fig. 8.1). Simplified version according to Robinson (1976) for Ito's (1972) hypothesized basis of adaptability of gain of the VOR. Output of semicircular canal (SCC) projects directly to vestibular nucleus (VN) with gain α, and indirectly via mossy fibers (mf), to granule cells (gc), parallel fibers, and Purkinje cells (Pc) in the vestibulocerebellum (VC) with gain β. Retinal image slip signal is conveyed from retina via accessory optic tract (aot) through nucleus of optic tract (not labeled) and inferior olive (IO) to Purkinje cells via climbing fibers (cf). If cf activity could change mf-Pc synaptic gain β, the gain of the entire reflex could be changed to eliminate retinal slip during head movements. $\dot{E}$: eye velocity; $\dot{H}$: head velocity (gain $= \alpha - \beta$); OMN: oculomotor nucleus. (From Robinson 1976; in *Journal of Neurophysiology*, Vol. 39, copyright 1975 American Physiological Society, reprinted by permission of the publisher and author.) *B*. Schematized redrawing of *A*. *C*. Basic adaptive signal processor (same as Fig. 15.1A). *D*. Combination of *B* and *C* to show direct and indirect pathway for the training signal. Labels as in *C*, except mfc: mossy fiber collaterals; a: scaling factor; e(rs): error signal (retinal shift). Note that the scaling factor for the indirect pathway is determined by the conjunctive activity on the Purkinje cells (Pc) of the integrated climbing activity and the parallel fibers, and that the scaled activity in the indirect pathway, arising from Purkinje cells, which are inhibitory, is subtracted from the input to the vestibular nuclei arising from the direct pathway from the SCC.

Further, it is important to note that the adaptability of the gain $(\alpha - \beta)$ in Figure 17.1A of the VOR is such as to compensate, within limits, either for changes in the gain of the indirect pathway, or for changes in the gain of the direct pathway, or for changes in both (e.g., with age, etc.). This feature of adaptability of the VOR arises from the fact that the directionally sensitive error signal (e, in Figs. 17.1C and 17.1D) is generated whenever the counter-rotation of the eye does not completely compensate for the underling head rotation, whatever the origin of the discrepancy.

Not shown in Figures 17.1B and 17.1D is a hypothetical "freezing" or "locking" mechanism whereby a newly altered coefficient, a, is retained on a long-term basis, for example, because of a decrease of the rate of firing of climbing fibers or of parallel fibers, or both, below some minimum (compare Fig. 15.7).

It is useful to note the difference in the manner in which the error signals in Figures 17.1C and 17.1D are generated. In Figure 17.1C, the error signal, e, is generated by comparing (subtracting) the output of the adaptive controller with an external training signal, but the error signal so generated must be processed further before being used to generate the scaling coefficient, a. Also, because the output (scaled) signal has no effect on the training signal, the configuration of Figure 17.1C can be considered to be open-loop. In contrast, in Figure 17.1D, the error signal originates from the eye itself, as part of a closed loop. It is the latter that will be taken as a model for the operation of the spinocerebellum and the cerebrocerebellum.

Although the diagram in Figure 17.1A for the VOR appears simple, the totality of the VOR becomes quite complex when compensatory eye movements must be made for the myriad of possible head movements.

In summary, it seems evident that the VOR can be considered as a basic adaptive controller (Fig. 17.1C), modified (Fig. 17.1D) to have two pathways (A and B) for the input signal from the semicircular canal (Fig. 17.1D), rather than a single pathway as in the standard engineering adaptive controller. This feature permits a simpler but equally effective automatic scaling procedure for the VOR, in comparison with the standard engineering format. In this view, as far as the VOR is concerned, the vestibulocerebellum and its associated component is purely a scaling device with automatic adjustment of the scaling coefficients (i.e., an adaptive controller). It is also important to note that the signal source in Figures 17.1A, 17.1B, and 17.1D (i.e., the SCC) lies external to the scaling mechanism. Thus, the scaling mechanism itself generates no signals such as motor patterns; the latter, however, of external (i.e., noncerebellar) origin, may be scaled by the adaptive controller. To reiterate, an adaptive controller does not itself generate patterns or signals; it only modifies the input signals that are fed into it.

Later in this chapter, the vestibulocerebellum, because of its particularly simple form that makes it relatively easy to analyze, is taken as a model for the function of the spinocerebellum and the cerebrocerebellum as adaptive controllers, possibly including a role in cognition.

17.4. Comparison of the Directionally Sensitive Error Signal of an Adaptive Signal Processor with the VOR Retinal Slip Signal

Figure 15.3 can be viewed in relation to the retinal slip error signal of the VOR as follows. Let trace 1 of Figure 15.3 be considered to represent alternating periods of impaired strength of the ocular muscles (induced, for example, by temporary partial paralysis), responding to sinusoidal alternations through a constant angle of head movements in the horizontal plane, displayed on a compressed time scale. Trace 3 of Figure 15.2 is the basic error signal, e, of the adaptive signal processor, and trace 2 of Figure 15.3 is the directionally sensitive error signal, which can be compared with the directionally sensitive retinal slip signal in the adaptation of the VOR, including reversals of direction (polarity) with each change of strength of the extraocular muscles. The integrated (summated) error signal (trace 3 of Fig. 15.3) is the counterpart of the overall gain of the VOR and can be considered to be an indication of the level of LTD. Trace 4 can be considered to represent the successive adaptations of the horizontal eye movement to the succession of periods of normal and impaired ocular muscle strength.

17.5. The Optokinetic Reflex and Smooth Pursuit Eye Movements

In light of the preceding discussion concerning mechanisms of the VOR, it may be suggested that, in the case of the optokinetic reflex (OKR), the head-turning velocity-dependent output of the semicircular canal is replaced by a constant impulse-rate generator, the output of which is scaled in response to retinal slip error, the latter conveyed to the cerebellum via the IO and the climbing fibers, the error being driven to a minimum by matching of the eye movement velocity with the target movement velocity. Such a mechanism would be essentially the same as that in Figure 17.1, except for an eye movement rate generator replacing the semicircular canal (SCC).

17.6. An Alternative View: The Cerebellum as a Three-Layer Neural Net

In the preceding sections, the cerebellum is viewed as an adaptive controller. However, it is also useful to view the cerebellum from the complementary perspective of a neural network (Figs. 14.1 and 14.4). If the cerebellum is viewed as a three-layer neural net (Fig. 17.2), then the first layer would include the granule cells, the granule cell axons, and their branched parallel fibers as the connections between the first layer and the second layer. The second layer (the "hidden" layer) would consist of the layer of Purkinje cells (of which the weights are an integral part), and the Purkinje cell axons would constitute the interconnections between the second layer and the cerebellar nuclear cells as the third layer. (In this schema, the parallel fiber–Golgi cells and the axons of the latter would constitute a negative feedback system to the rosettes (glomeruli) of the granule cells (Fig. 17.3; i.e., in parallel with the first layer but apart from it). (Compare the single-layer feedback neural

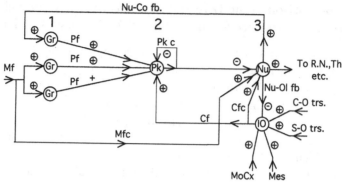

Figure 17.2. Schema (greatly simplified) for the cerebellum (spinocerebellum) based on a combination of adaptive controller and three-layer neural network configurations. Granular cells (layer 1), Purkinje cells (layer 2), and cerebellar nuclear cells (layer 3). Fan-out and fan-in between second and third layers not indicated. Abbreviations: excitatory connections: +; inhibitory connections: −; Mf: mossy fibers; Mfc: mossy fiber collaterals to the nuclei; Gr: granule cells; Pf: parallel fibers (vertical segment of granule cell axons not shown); Pk: Purkinje cells; Pk c: Purkinje cell recurrent collateral; IO: inferior olive; C-O: cerebrocortical-olivary tracts; S-O: spino-olivary tracts; MoCx: motor cortex; Mes: mesencephalon; Cf: climbing fibers; Cfc: climbing fiber collaterals; Nu: cerebellar nuclear cell; Nu-Ol fb: nuclear-olivary feedback; R.N.: red nucleus; Th.: thalamus. In the schema, the inferior olive is considered to be a part of the weight-determining mechanism, and therefore strictly speaking, not part of the third layer. (The excitatory nucleo-olivary feedback is not shown.)

network of Figure 14.4.) Similarly, the stellate and basket cells would represent a negative feedforward system to the Purkinje cells. Optionally, the mossy fiber–glomeruli (rosette) system could constitute a preliminary layer prior to the first layer described previously.

The neural net model shown in Figure 17.2, which is greatly simplified, depicts the cerebellum (specifically, the cerebrocerebellum) and is based on combined considerations of adaptive controllers and neural nets, specifically, of three layers. The schema includes, in particular, the most important common feature of neural nets and adaptive controllers (i.e., self-adjustment of weights; via the climbing fibers). (In the case of the vestibulocerebellum, the schema would require some modification because the counterparts of some of the mechanisms are located in the vestibular nuclei rather than in the cerebellar nuclei.) The schema includes the cerebellar nuclei and the inferior olive, as well as the nucleo-olivary and the nucleocortical feedback paths.

In Figure 17.2, the mossy fiber signal input (extreme left) originates, for example, from the periphery (e.g., muscle spindles in the limbs after preprocessing in the spinal cord) and from the cerebral cortex, and is distributed in a relatively widespread manner among the Purkinje cells via the granule cells and parallel fibers. The nucleocortical feedback pathway is shown at the top in Figure 17.2. A large divergence (fan-out), not shown because only one Purkinje cell is depicted, and convergence (fan-in) thus occurs between the first and second layers of the cerebellar cortex viewed as a neural net, of which the Purkinje cells constitute the second or "hidden"

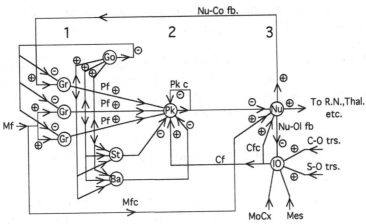

Figure 17.3. Same as Figure 17.2, but with the addition (on the left side) of a schema of the inhibitory Golgi (Go), stellate (St), and basket (Ba) cells.

layer. Changes in the strength of the synapses (entailing changes of long-term depression of Purkinje cells) between parallel fibers and Purkinje cell dendrites (i.e., the weights) are determined by the conjoint action of parallel fibers and climbing fibers from the inferior olive probably acting as an error detector.

The inferior olive also receives an important (inhibitory) input from the cerebellar nuclei (Fig. 17.2), as previously mentioned in Chapter 6. This input appears to have the effect of controlling not only the rate of firing of olivary neurons, but also the degree of electrotonic spread among olivary neurons, and hence controlling the number of inferior olivary cells activated and, in turn, the size of the group of Purkinje cells activated.

A schema in which the two feedback networks within the cerebellar cortex, namely, the inhibitory (negative feedback) Golgi cell–granule cell network, and the stellate cell-basket cell–Purkinje cell network (Chapter 3) have been added, is shown in Figure 17.3. For this discussion, it is assumed that both of these networks serve the purpose of maintaining the cerebellar cortex in an appropriate (i.e., optimum) dynamic operating range, as suggested previously by other authors. It seems likely that the recurrent collaterals of the (inhibitory) Purkinje cell, which may synapse onto the soma and proximal dendrites of the same and other Purkinje cells (Brodal 1981) also participate in automatic-level control.

At the conclusion of this section on neural networks as models for the cerebellum, it is relevant to reiterate the view expressed by Robinson (1992a, 1992b), previously mentioned in Chapter 14, that experience with neural networks indicates that attempts to explain how any biological neural network works on a cell-by-cell (i.e., reductionist) basis may be futile, and that one may have to be content with attempting to understand the brain at higher levels of organization. In a word, it could be said that the main work in neural networks is done not at the input and output levels (layers) but by the "hidden units" of the intermediate layers, and although the self-organization that characterizes the neural net accomplishes the desired task (e.g., of modeling a certain brain system), the details of this distributed, internal organization "may be impenetrable and incomprehensible and even meaningless from the outside, and, in the biological case, even with microelectrodes" (Robinson 1992a, 1992b).

The above characterization of neural net modeling is also true of adaptive control modeling. Once there is some redundancy in the number of weights in relation to the complexity (bandwidth) of the signal being processed in an adaptive controller, the problem of the value of the individual weights can have more than one solution.

17.7. The Uniformity of Cerebellar Structure

An important aspect of the microscopic anatomy of the cerebellum is that its structure (i.e., its basic organization) appears to be essentially the same throughout. (Perhaps the only exception is the presence, in the vestibulocerebellum and spinocerebellum, but not in the cerebrocerebellum, of unipolar brush cells [UBCs; Chapter 3], which may have a function as a kind of intensifier of the mossy fiber input for those parts of the cerebellum in which they are found.) Accordingly, whatever type of computation or data processing is performed by the cerebellum, it appears to be the same in the above-mentioned three major divisions of the cerebellum. It follows, then, that the functions of the different parts of the cerebellum are principally dependent on their input and output connections rather than on variations in local anatomy, as is the case for the cerebral cortex

17.8. The Two Major Input Systems to Cerebellar Cortex and Their Counterparts in Adaptive Controllers

The two major input systems to the cerebellar cortex comprise (1) the mossy fiber system, derived from peripheral sources (e.g., muscle spindles, tendon organs), which, after modification by the granule cells, is fed to the distal apical dendritic tree of the Purkinje cells via the parallel fibers, and (2) the climbing fiber system, which originates in the inferior olive, a presumptive differencing structure in which an error signal is derived.

The latter error signal, conveyed to the Purkinje cells via the climbing fibers, is of a relatively low frequency (1–10 Hertz), modulates or scales the firing rate of the Purkinje cell output (as simple spikes, at 50–500 Hertz) to the cerebellar nuclei in response to the parallel fiber input to the Purkinje cells. Just such a two-signal (a fast "throughput" signal and a slow modulating or scaling signal) arrangement also obtains in an adaptive controller (see below). It is an essential feature of modeling the cerebellum as an adaptive controller that the error signal be integrated (summed or accumulated) by the Purkinje cells to derive the scaling factor; long-term depression (LTD) and long-term potentiation (LTP) provide just such mechanisms. In the cerebellar nuclei, the indirect, Purkinje cell-scaled mossy fiber inhibitory output is subtracted from the direct mossy fiber input, conveyed to the nuclei via the collaterals of the mossy fibers, and constitutes the output from the nuclei. The details of this arrangement are now summarized comparatively.

17.9. The Relative Rates of Purkinje Cell Simple and Complex Spikes and Their Counterparts in Adaptive Controllers

Linear combiners and linear predictors share certain important signal characteristics that are also found in the biological adaptive controllers. Thus, an important characteristic of both the circuit of the VOR (Fig. 17.1A) and of the basic adaptive controller (Fig. 17.1C) is the difference between the operating frequencies of the adaptive control mechanism (i.e., the scaling mechanism) and the signal frequencies. For the basic adaptive controller, the frequencies of the control or scaling mechanism (i.e., of the output of the integrator [Fig. 15.1A], which constitutes the scaling coefficient, a) are much lower than the frequencies of the signal being controlled or modulated (compare trace 3 with trace 4 of Fig. 15.3). In the VOR circuit, these are manifested respectively in the complex spike rate and the simple spike rate of the Purkinje cell. The frequency range of the former is of the order of 1 to 10 Hertz, much lower than the simple spike rate of 50 to 500 Hertz. There are corresponding differences for the respective afferent fibers to the cerebellar cortex: the higher firing rate mossy fibers (which, via the parallel fibers, and in conjunction with the climbing fiber-induced Purkinje cell complex spikes, give rise to Purkinje cell simple spikes) are thick and heavily myelinated (permitting higher conduction velocities and faster rates), whereas the climbing fibers of lower firing rate are myelinated but thinner. The faster complex spike rates (i.e., in the range of 10 Hertz) tend to be associated with a change (an increase or decrease) in the simple spike rate, whereas the slower complex spike rates tend to be associated with relatively unchanging simple spike rates, perhaps even fixed ("locked") rates, commensurate with long-term storage. (At the level of the cerebellar nuclei, complex spikes have only a minimal effect because of their relative infrequency as compared with simple spikes.)

Expressed in a different manner, the signal with the lower frequencies can be viewed as a modulating signal, the (output) signal with the higher frequencies as the modulated signal. From this perspective, an important corollary arises: adaptive controllers do not themselves generate new patterns of activity; they only modulate the amplitude (or frequency) of existing patterns of activity.

17.10. The Three Major Cerebellar Divisions from the Perspective of an Adaptive Controller

The three divisions of the cerebellar cortex – the vestibulocerebellum, spinocerebellum, and cerebrocerebellum (Fig. 3.1) – are now considered, in turn, in relation to adaptive control.

17.11. The Vestibulocerebellum

The vestibulocerebellum is the oldest and the simplest of the neuronal systems of the cerebellum. There are no inputs from the trunk, the limbs, or the cerebral cortex. Further, its nucleus is the lateral vestibular (Deiter's) nucleus rather than one of the cerebellar nuclei proper. The vestibulocerebellum has been considered in some detail in Chapter 8, particularly as concerns the VOR, and comparison of it with the adaptive controller is relatively straightforward.

17.12. The Spinocerebellum as an Adaptive Controller

In the VOR, the basic signal generator is the semicircular canal, the mossy fibers of which feed directly to the vestibular nuclei and also indirectly to the vestibular nuclei via the vestibulocerebellum after scaling in the latter. As already mentioned, the error signal to control the scaling is generated as retinal slip resulting from disparity between head movement and eye movement, the retinal slip in turn controlling the scaling by the vestibulocerebellum.

For the spinocerebellum, however, the manner of generating the error signal is rather less clear than for the VOR. The following is offered speculatively. The basic signal generators for the spinocerebellum include postural reflex centers and centers for locomotion. Their mossy fibers feed directly (as mossy fiber collaterals) and indirectly (via the spinocerebellar cortex) to the cerebellar nuclei, where the two branches are differenced or subtracted before being fed to spinal centers. The generation of the error signal (upon which scaling by the spinocerebellar cortex is dependent) can be presumed to be analogous to, in principle, but of course different, in detail, from that for the VOR.

The spinocerebellum has peripheral and brain stem connections. Its mossy fibers are derived from sensors for position and movement (e.g., tendon organs and muscle spindles reporting the tension in muscles and joint receptors). The climbing fibers of the spinocerebellum are usually believed to derive their correctional signals from an error-detecting comparator located primarily, but perhaps not exclusively, in the inferior olive, and for which the input training signals include those from the brain stem motor centers, "status" signals (e.g., joint receptors) from the periphery, and "interrupt" signals (e.g., tactile receptors reporting encounters and obstructions in the path of intended movement).

Brain stem centers for maintenance of stance and for engendering locomotion, in addition to their descending signals to spinal centers, may convey a "corollary discharge" to the inferior olive in the capacity of signaling an "intended" reflex movement. Report of the actual motion itself, sensed by joint and tendon (i.e., proprioceptive) receptors, or tactile or pressure contact resulting from movement, could be conveyed via the spino-olivary tracts to the IO. At the same time, the corresponding motive forces (muscle activity) are sensed by (e.g., muscle spindle fibers) and conveyed to the cerebellar cortex via spinocerebellar pathways.

The error signal, evaluated as the difference between the intended movement (as conveyed by the corollary discharge) and the actual movement (conveyed by the spino-olivary pathways) is assumed to be generated in the IO. (It should be mentioned that, in this formulation, the corollary discharge should arise from an inhibitory source, or at least, be inhibitory as it arrives at the IO, if the spino-olivary signals are excitatory.) The error signal is then assumed to be conveyed to the cerebellar cortex via the climbing fibers and employed to scale the report of the mossy fibers, thus, with repetition, correcting the actual movement to agree with the intended movement. (It should be mentioned that some interaction may occur in the spinal cord between the spinocerebellar pathways and the spino-olivary pathways via their respective spinal nuclei.) An additional input, presumably ultimately inhibitory, from the motor cortex to the IO would in principle permit voluntary modification of reflex spinocerebellar activity.

Thus, if for the VOR, retinal slip, as an error signal, e, can be viewed as resulting from a mismatch between head turning and eye turning (in the opposite direction), then for the spinocerebellum, the counterpart error signal can be viewed as resulting from a mismatch between the intended movement (represented by, e.g., a corollary discharge from descending pathways from brain stem spinal reflex centers to the IO) and the actual movement (as reported to the IO by spino-olivary pathways), the error being employed by the Purkinje cells to rescale the report of the mossy fibers, thus tending to diminish the error as the cerebellar nuclear output is fed to brain stem spinal reflex centers.

17.13. The Cerebrocerebellum as an Adaptive Controller

17.13.1. Adaptive Control of Voluntary Movement

If attempting to extrapolate mechanisms of adaptive control from the VOR to the mechanisms of the spinocerebellum encounters complexities and difficulties, further extension to the level of the cerebrocerebellum encounters even more complexities and difficulties. Reiteration (from Chapters 3 and 9) of some basic aspects of the cerebrocerebellum may be appropriate.

The cerebrocerebellum makes up by far the largest part of the cerebellum. Its mossy fiber projections from the cerebral cortex, via the pontine nuclei, number some 40 million for the two sides. Its climbing fibers, like all climbing fibers, arise from the inferior olivary nucleus, which in turn receives direct and indirect projections from the cerebral cortex (Chapter 9).

For that part of the cerebrocerebellum that interconnects with the motor cortex (i.e., the part of the cerebrocerebellum involved with planning and execution of voluntary movements, perhaps involving transformations among coordinate systems), the consideration of adaptive control could proceed much as for the spinocerebellum, except that instead of primary signals arising from brain stem motor centers, they arise from the motor cortex. Thus, such architectural details as the interrelationships among the inferior olive, the cerebellar cortex (in this case, the lateral cerebellum), the cerebellar nuclei (in the case of the cerebrocerebellum, the dentate or lateral nucleus), and the subtractive function of the dentate nucleus are in principle the same as for the spinocerebellum. (On a small scale, it is a question of the components of the microcomplexes: small regions of cerebellar cortex [the microzones], cerebellar nuclei, and inferior olive.) The same point can be made, it would seem, in relation to the manner of derivation of the error-correcting signal via the climbing fibers.

17.13.2. Adaptive Control and Cognition

As mentioned in Chapter 16, Ito (1990) proposed that the cerebellum could participate in cognitive activity as follows (Fig. 16.6B). Let it be assumed that cerebral cortical area 1 acts as a controller for another cortical area 2 that serves as a control object, for example, Wernicke's area would act on Broca's area. Such a corticocortical system would initially operate in a feedback mode, but after learning, the cerebellum would intervene to replace the control role of cerebral area 1. By analogy with Figure 16.6A, the elements of such a cerebellar–cerebral interconnection could include (1) fibers from the lower cerebrocortical layers passing to the pontine nuclei, thence as mossy fibers to the cerebrocerebellar cortex with collaterals to the dentate nucleus; (2) fibers from the dentate nucleus back to the respective cerebrocortical area via the superior cerebellar peduncle (brachium conjunctivum) and the ventrolateral nucleus of the thalamus to the upper layers of the same cerebrocortical area (in a manner similar to the interconnections among different cerebrocortical areas); and (3) an error-detecting mechanism of unclear site (but possibly cerebrocortical in part) and nature, except that its final output would be from the inferior olive, the error progressively diminishing to zero as the appropriate scaling (of impulse rates) is attained. The question might further be raised as to whether such a cerebral–cerebellar interaction could have a part in the phenomenon of binding or resonance, in the vicinity of 40 Hertz, among cortical sites, perhaps assisting in the communication of different cerebrocortical areas of differing intrinsic structures or architechtonics.

17.14. Organization and Functions of the Inferior Olive

There are several outstanding questions about the structure and function of the inferior olive, perhaps more so than among the other components of the cerebellar system.

The inferior olive receives projections from a number of sources (Fig. 5.2), including the spinal cord and the cerebral cortex, which appear to be excitatory. In contrast, the direct nucleo-olivary projection is inhibitory and regulates, via the dendritic lamellar bodies (DLBs), the olivary gap junctions, which in turn appear to recruit Purkinje cells. It now appears (Chapter 5) that these inhibitory fibers from the cerebellar nuclei do not terminate on the same olivary neurons as do the excitatory fibers.

Oscarsson (1980), in his schema of the inferior olive as a comparator (Fig. 5.10), included three sources of inputs: from peripheral receptors, lower motor centers, and collaterals of commands (corollary discharges) from higher to lower motor centers. In relation to Oscarsson's concept, it was considered unlikely that the signals of intention and of achievement are conveyed only through the descending and ascending projections, respectively, to the inferior olive, because these inputs generally do not converge on the same olivary neurons (De Zeeuw et al. 1998). Rather, a comparison was considered much more likely to occur between the ascending and descending inputs (which are all excitatory), on the one hand, and the inhibitory projection from the hindbrain, on the other hand. Thus, each dendritic spine of an olivary neuron receives both an inhibitory input from a hindbrain center (i.e., cerebellar nuclei, vestibular nuclei, nucleus prepositus hypoglossi, solitary nucleus, dorsal column nuclei) and an excitatory input from the spinal cord, brain stem, mesodiencephalic junction, or cerebral cortex.

The combination of relatively large receptive surfaces of the dendritic trees of olivary neurons (Fig. 5.3, cells 2–5), in combination with bushy terminals of afferent fibers (Fig. 5.4) would seem appropriate to receive and propagate axonal terminations conveying a great diversity of signals, any one of which may give rise to an error signal indicating necessary modification of one or another parameter of movement (e.g., a tactile or pressure encounter with an object or surface in the course of a movement). Such a divergence (fan-out) and convergence (fan-in) in the inferior olive is reminiscent of that of the parallel fibers and Purkinje cells of the cerebellar cortex itself.

It was pointed out in Chapter 5 (De Zeeuw et al. 1990) that at least one third of labeled glomeruli (rosettes, Fig. 5.4B) in the inferior olive appeared to contain both direct cerebellar nucleo-olivary (i.e., inhibitory) terminals, and mesodiencephalic (nucleus of Darkschewitsch and reticular tegmental nucleus [of Bechterew]; i.e., excitatory terminals). In many cases the terminals from both afferent systems contacted the same dendritic spines. It has been suggested that such excitatory–inhibitory terminations may form the basis of the differencing or subtraction, from which an error signal could be generated in the form of an increased climbing fiber discharge rate.

17.15. The Significance of Similarities Between Structures of the Inferior Olive and Cerebellar Nuclei

Parent (1996) pointed out the obvious similarity between the macroscopic form of the dentate nucleus (as having the shape of a folded bay with the opening or hilus directed medially and dorsally) and the inferior olivary nucleus; both present a corrugated appearance in transverse section, thus tending to maximize surface area for a given volume. As previously noted, Chan-Palay (1977) stressed the similarity between the microscopic structure of the inferior olive (Figs. 5.3–5.6) and the dentate nucleus (Figs. 6.1–6.4), in that both include terminal fibers that synapse with larger numbers of cells and other fibers that synapse with a smaller number of cells. (However, there appear to be no small interneurons in the inferior olive as there are in the cerebellar nuclei.)

It will be recalled that the inhibitory nucleo-olivary fibers modulate (i.e., shunt) the gap junctions of the dendrites of inferior olivary cells, thereby decreasing the links among them, as well as perhaps inhibiting the individual olivary neurons themselves. This feedback loop from the inferior olive to cerebellar nuclei back to the inferior olive could be a way of increasing the dynamic range of groupings (via gap junctions) of olivary neurons. The question then arises as to whether this similarity may be of some special significance in view of the special interconnectedness of these structures (Fig. 5.9), both of which contain components of the microcomplex (Chapter 3) and are associated with small cerebellar cortical regions (microzones). However, no evident answer appears to be immediately forthcoming.

It seems clear that a principal function of the cerebellar nuclei is that of subtracting the Purkinje inhibitory input from the excitatory input arriving via the mossy fiber collaterals. The function of the climbing fiber collaterals to the cerebellar nuclei is less clear, but it has been suggested that their purpose could be to minimize the inhibitory effect of Purkinje complex spikes on excitatory activity arriving at the cerebellar nuclei via the mossy fiber collaterals (but see below).

In an adaptive controller, the error-detecting component is as important as the scaling (multiplicative) component. It seems abundantly clear that the Purkinje cell serves the latter function. That the inferior olive serves as the error-detecting mechanism has been suggested for some time, and no other candidates for this function have been forthcoming, save for the possible partial contributions from spinal and brain stem nuclei. It seems highly likely that the inferior olive functions as an error detector (of the difference between the desired and the actual effect (e.g., of movement). The accumulating evidence appears to substantiate this conclusion. In a sense, the cerebellar cortical microzone can be considered to be the multiplicative component, and the cerebellar nuclei to be the subtractive component, of an arithmetic computing unit.

17.16. Further Considerations of Cerebellar Nuclei Structure

As noted in Chapter 3, the excitatory mossy and climbing fibers, on their way to the cerebellar cortex, give off collaterals to the cerebellar nuclei (see also Figs. 6.3 and 6.4; NC fibers). These fibers appear to synapse with multiple large cerebellar nuclear cells, whereas the Purkinje cell conelike axonal terminations evidently contact fewer of these same large nuclear cells. This difference arises as a consequence of the fact that the mossy and climbing fiber collaterals course obliquely with respect to the large nuclear cells, whereas the axis of the Purkinje cell terminal axonal cones tends to coincide with that of the large nuclear cells (Fig. 6.4). Functionally, this arrangement perhaps suggests that the "collateral" information distributed to the cerebellar nuclei by the mossy fiber collaterals is distributed relatively diffusely, in contrast to the more localized distribution of information via the Purkinje axons, thus permitting a larger region of the nuclei in which the differencing could potentially take place. As for collaterals of climbing fibers, it has been shown (De Zeeuw et al. 1997) that these fibers contact small neurons in the cerebellar nuclei that provide an inhibitory feedback to the inferior olive.

The output (to the red nucleus, thalamus, etc.) of the large cerebellar nuclear cells is excitatory. They are disinhibited (i.e., their firing rate increases) when there is a decrease of inhibitory influence resulting from, for example, LTD of the Purkinje cells (Fig. 17.2).

17.17. The Cerebellum: Linear Predictor or Linear Combiner?

In Chapter 15, the distinction was made between two types of adaptive controllers: the linear combiner (Fig.14.5) and the linear predictor (Fig. 14.9). In a linear combiner, a series of signals (having different amplitude and different frequency components) are fed to the respective inputs simultaneously. Then, if a signal consisting of the same frequency components but of different amplitude is used as a "training signal," the linear combiner will automatically adjust the weighting coefficient, a_i, for each of the several input signals so the output signal becomes a replica of the "training signal."

In a linear predictor (Figs. 14.9 and 15.11), there are also multiple input signals, but these signals are all the same except that the series of inputs is taken from the successive taps of a tapped delay line (Fig. 14.9). In this case, the training signal is taken from a tap on the delay line one or more steps ahead of the series of input signals, and the output signal from the linear predictor becomes a replica of the training signal, within the limits of the accuracy of prediction. The earlier the tap for the training signal, the poorer the prediction (Fig. 15.16).

In the cerebellum, a given parallel fiber does indeed synapse with the palisade-like dendritic trees of a succession of Purkinje cells (Fig. 3.2), but the total delay possible in half the length of a bifurcated parallel fiber is only about 20 milliseconds, for a 10-millimeters long parallel fiber, as indicated by Braitenberg (1987). (Braitenberg indicated that such small time differences could be expected to occur in the execution of complex movements, such as playing a violin.) Such short intervals would hardly seem to suffice, however, for a wide range of delays that may be encountered in movements executed at different speeds. Because prediction is contingent upon the presence of tapped delay lines (i.e., the prediction of the next point in a series of values of a signal is made on the basis of the immediate past sample points), it would seem that, in general, linear prediction is not feasible for the cerebellum.

However, the combination of parallel fibers and Purkinje dendritic tree, especially when combined with arrays of granule cells from which the parallel fibers arise, would appear to constitute almost an idealized design for an adaptive combiner (Fig. 14.5). Thus, the depiction of cerebellar circuitry in Figure 13.6, with mossy fiber inputs on the lower right, the Purkinje cells in the middle (multiplying or scaling according to the level of LTD and/or LTP determined by the integral of the climbing fibers) can be taken as a basic wiring diagram for a linear combiner, in which delay line function of the parallel fibers is not an essential feature, rather than for a linear predictor, for which delay lines are an essential feature. Thus, the parallel fibers are viewed basically as a distribution system over the entire extent of the representation in the cerebellum of an extremity (Fig. 13.6), rather than as tapped delay lines. (The essential function served by the mossy fiber collaterals to the cerebellar nuclei is not depicted in Figure 14.5 [compare Figs. 8.1 or 17.1A, for the VOR].

17.18. The Valvula of Mormyrid Fish as an Idealized Tapped Delay Line (Delay Device)

In contrast to the cerebellum proper of mormyrid fish, which is a conventional cerebellar cortex, the valvula of this species (Chapter 12) appears specifically suited to perform the function of a tapped delay line (compare Fig. 12.3 with top row of boxes in Figs. 15.12 and 16.2). In contrast to the somewhat irregular relative arrangement of Purkinje cell dendritic tree and parallel fibers in the mammalian cerebellum (Fig. 3.2), the arrangement in the valvula is extremely regular or palisade-like, inviting attributes of precise time measurement, and spatial tuning as in a directional array (Chapter 12; Fig. 16.2). Moreover, in contrast to the region of synapses of climbing fibers onto the mammalian cerebellum extending over the proximal third of its dendritic tree, in the valvula, the extent is essentially confined to the cell body of the Purkinje cell and its immediate vicinity (compare middle and bottom parts of Fig. 12.6). The mammalian arrangement permits much more interplay between effects of climbing fibers and parallel fibers than does the mormyrid arrangement, the latter idealized as a delay device for coincidence detection of time differences (Meek 1992b).

17.19. Can the Cerebellum Alone Function as a Linear Predictor?

If the mammalian cerebellum is not optimized to function (in part) as a tapped delay line, it follows that the characterization of the cerebellum as a linear predictor (as contrasted with a linear combiner) must be questioned because linear prediction of necessity implicates the existence of the equivalent of a tapped delay line system. The implication is that for such complex processes as forward modeling (Fig. 15.18) and inverse modeling (Fig. 15.21), the necessary time delays (i.e., tapped delay line) must lie outside the cerebellum itself. As previously noted, however, no such candidate is immediately apparent.

It can be argued that, for the vestibulocerebellum, no tapped delay line is necessary, but it is difficult to make this argument for the spinocerebellum. For the cerebrocerebellum, the question could be raised as to whether the cerebral cortex could have this capability, but no corroborative evidence is immediately apparent in its structure. In addition, for the spinocerebellum, the answer is perhaps equally unclear.

Thus, the question of whether the cerebellar system (including cerebral cortex, and inferior olive) can alone function as a linear predictor (i.e., including a tapped delay line capability) must be left open.

17.20. Does Cerebellum Store Movement Commands? Or Only Weights?

As indicated in Chapter 7, this question has been much debated since Marr (1969) originally proposed plasticity at the parallel fiber–Purkinje cell dendritic tree interface under the influence of activity in the climbing fiber. There would seem to be little remaining doubt that there is indeed such plasticity.

From the perspective of neural networks and adaptive controllers, the question may be posed in a somewhat different way. That is, are weights (coefficients) within the cerebellar cortex (i.e., synaptic efficacy at the above-mentioned synapses) modified and retained for a long time, but subject to modification? The answer would seem to be yes, even if some details are still lacking. However, a given movement pattern cannot be reconstituted from stored weights because weights modify.

They are not themselves signals for movement. Thus, it is only when the stored weights operate on an input and generate an output that a movement is generated. In this sense, the cerebellum cannot be considered to be a (movement) pattern generator.

In the case of voluntary movements, the original source of commands appears to be the cerebral cortex, not the cerebellum. It is upon this cerebral signal, and sensory information from the periphery associated with it, that the cerebellum, with its existing or altered weights (the latter according to error or modifying signals from the inferior olive) carries out its transactions (i.e., its remapping operations or transformations), sculpting signals for dispatch to lower (brain stem/spinal cord) and/or to higher (motor) centers for further execution. In this sense, the cerebellum can be said to have the function of "proportioning" the muscular response, as Wiener (1948, 1961) suggested.

It should be noted that, in this view, the cerebellum is in continuous operation, regardless of whether the ensemble of weights (coefficients) remains fixed or undergoes change, continuously modifying its mossy fiber input to generate the signals for fine control of movements. Evidently, it is only when, for whatever reason, a new trajectory must be made that the inferior olive–climbing fiber system becomes active, and the weights become altered.

In the latter connection, a more complete understanding of mechanisms of alterations of weights is contingent on further clarification of mechanisms of modification of synaptic efficacy (e.g., in terms of LTD/LTP and perhaps other processes).

17.21. The Cerebellum as an Adaptive Controller: Final Conclusions

In considering this topic, it is again convenient to divide the cerebellum into its major parts:

1. *The vestibulocerebellum.* It can be considered as well established that the vestibulocerebellum functions as an adaptive controller.
2. *The spinocerebellum.* It appears highly probable that the spinocerebellum functions as an adaptive controller, but the manner in which the error signal is evaluated has not been fully clarified.
3. *The cerebrocerebellum.* In relation to voluntary movement, it appears reasonable to say that the assertion that the cerebrocerebellum functions as an adaptive controller is perhaps as valid as the same assertion for the spinocerebellum. For cognitive activity, it appears reasonable to suggest that the cerebrocerebellum functions as an adaptive controller (the use of ASP is perhaps better in this context) is speculative. Nonetheless, the fact that cerebellar structure is essentially the same throughout, as is also the case for the inferior olive and the cerebellar nuclei, strongly suggests that the basic cerebellar transaction of scaling is also implicated in cognitive processes.

Finally, it seems evident that the cerebellar system, including the cerebellar cortex, the cerebellar nuclei, and the inferior olive, functions only as a scaling device (i.e., as a multiplier) and that the additional capability for time delay (e.g., tapped delay lines), which would be required to perform such complex functions as prediction and inverse transformations, lies outside the cerebellar system proper, for example, in brain stem nuclei (cf. Moore, Desmond, and Berthier 1989). Such a capability is found in a highly specialized part of the cerebellum of certain species (i.e., the valvula of mormyrid fish), the structure of which is uniquely suited to enable the generation of precise time delays.

A Hybrid Analogue/Digital Multiplexer/Multiplier-Based Adaptive Signal Processor

The implementation of the adaptive signal processors (ASPs) depicted in Figures 15.11, 15.12, and 15.15, with some modifications, was as follows. In the case of the linear predictor of Figure 15.11 (in which the training signal is identical with the input signal), the processor consists basically of a 16-tap delay line (Fig. A.1), the outputs of taps 9–16 of which are fed, respectively, to eight amplitude-matching units, each of the type shown in Figure 15.1A. (If the 16 taps of such a delay line are summed by means of precision (1%) resistors, linear interpolation results [compare traces 1 and 2 of Fig. A.2]. If two such units are cascaded, a sigmoid [actually a double parabolic] curve can be generated from a step function [compare traces 1 and 3 of Fig. A.2].)

As indicated in Figure A.1, the analog tapped delay line itself (which has a DC response) consists of two synchronously driven 16-channel analogue multiplexers, which serially transfer, via their interconnected common terminals, the stored voltages between adjacent condenser-based storage (sample-and-hold) units (Barlow 1993, pp. 313–315). The outputs are available both in individual form and in multiplexed form, the latter from the interconnected common terminals of the multiplexers (Fig. A.1). In essence, the unit operates as a "bucket brigade," as does a charge-transfer device. In the present unit, however, it is voltage rather than charge that is transferred. Figure 15.10 shows a sine wave read out from the tapped delay line at four successively increasing delays.

For the ASP depicted in Figures 15.11 and 15.12, eight coefficients were used, which, with individual components for each of the eight units, would have required a total of 16 individual multipliers (note the 2 multipliers in Fig. 15.1A). The circuit was enormously simplified (Fig. A.3), however, by using only two multipliers (of the same type as for Fig. 15.1A; Analog Devices Type 534), in combination with sample-and-hold circuits and four 8-channel multiplexers (Analog Devices Type 1706), so the multipliers were timeshared among the eight amplitude-matching units. The result is that the complete linear predictor solves eight linear equations simultaneously. The output (predicted) signal and the error signal (both in sampled form) are available

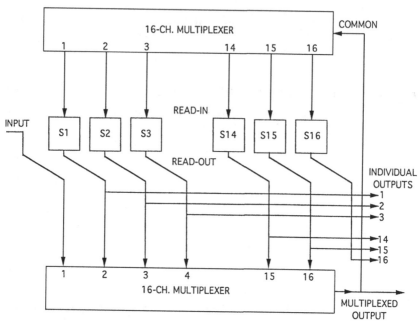

Figure A.1. Schema of a 16-tap analog delay line made up of two interfaced synchronously driven 16-channel analogue multiplexers interconnected by sample-and-hold circuits (S1–S16). The outputs are available in either individual form or multiplexed form. (From Barlow 1993; in Barlow, *The Electroencephalogram: Its Patterns and Origins*, copyright 1993, The MIT Press; reprinted by permission.)

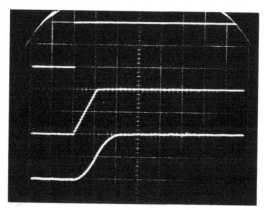

Figure A.2. Use of the summated individual outputs of two cascaded 16-tap analogue multiplexers used as an interpolator. Top trace: step function; middle trace: output of the first multiplexer showing linear interpolation; bottom trace, output of second multiplexer with resultant quadratic interpolation. Further explanation in text. (From Barlow 1993; in Barlow, *The Electroencephalogram: Its Patterns and Origins*, copyright 1993, The MIT Press; reprinted by permission.)

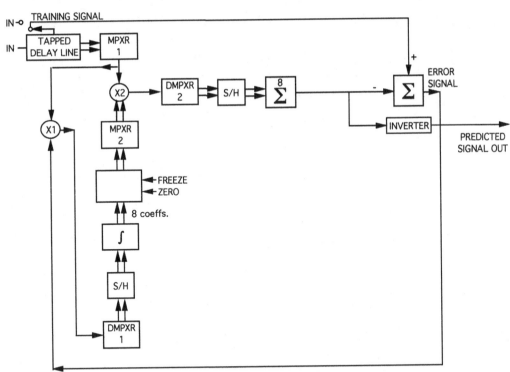

Figure A.3. Schema of a hybrid analogue/digital multiplexer/multiplier-based ASP. X1, X2: analogue multipliers; MPXR 1, 2: multiplexers; DMPXR 1, 2: demultiplexers; S/H: sample-and-hold units; $\sum$: differencer; $\int$: integrators (8); FREEZE: freeze (predictor) coefficients; ZERO make all predictor coefficients zero; eight coeffs.: the eight predictor coefficients; single arrows: single line or eight-channel multiplexed line; double arrows: eight parallel lines. MPXRs and DMPXRs are identical eight-channel chips (Analog Devices Type 7506); multipliers are Analog Devices Type 534). The switch at the upper left permits either an independent Training Signal (as in system characterization), or an earlier tap on the tapped delay line to be used, as in prediction.

as outputs (e.g., Figs. 16.13, traces 2 and 3, respectively), as are the weights (predictor coefficients; Figs. 15.13A and 15.14).

Basically, the ASP uses the second 8 taps of the 16-tap delay line to obtain eight successive sample values (as though through a window), four 8-channel analogue multiplexers, and 2 analogue multipliers, in combination with eight of the units depicted in Figure 15.1A, to generate a predicted signal (Fig. A.3, upper right). (The first 8 taps of the 16-tap delay line enabled a selectable initial delay [one to eight steps] against which the predicted output of the ASP can be compared [Fig. 15.16].) By varying the configuration of the ASP, forward dynamics (prediction), inverse dynamics, and "plant" characterization, as illustrated in Chapter 15 (Figs. 15.18 and 15.21) can be carried out. Both finite response impulse response (FIR) (Fig. 15.11) and infinite response impulse response (IIR) (Fig. 15.15) configurations are possible (Chapter 15), although the IIR configuration in effect requires the equivalent of a second ASP essentially identical with the first (including an independent delay line) because of the feedback path (Fig. 15.15, lower part).

Author's Note

The origins of this book, in a sense, go back to the mid-1940s, because it was then, at the MIT Navy Radar School, that I encountered "hunting" or oscillation as a manifestation of maladjustment of the control system of radar antennae. In reading Norbert Wiener's *Cybernetics* as a first-year medical student, I again encountered mention of this phenomenon, which Wiener compared with cerebellar tremor. As I was learning about the elegance of the anatomy of the cerebellum, the choice of a career in what was later to become known as neuroscience seemed almost assured.

Serious exploration of the cerebellum in relation to movement control was, however, to wait quite a number of years, because soon after arriving in Boston in the early 1950s I had the good fortune to join a small group at the Massachusetts General Hospital and the Massachusetts Institute of Technology, including James Casby, Mary Brazier, Walter Rosenblith, and Norbert Wiener, who were exploring applications of Wiener's time-series analysis (Wiener 1950) to the electroencephalogram (EEG). These activities on my part ranged from the design of equipment to tutorials by Wiener on time-series analysis, including prediction theory, the concept of which I found slightly ethereal at the time. More or less at the same time, I was gaining some experience in clinical neurology, including manifestations of cerebellar disease such as ataxia (loss of muscular coordination) and tremor, particularly under the tutelage of Dr. Raymond D. Adams, chief of neurology at the Massachusetts General Hospital.

An important part of the EEG studies during those years was equipment of my own design and construction, some of it related to artifact suppression or elimination (e.g., eye movement, and electrocardiographic or EKG artifact), in the form of an automatic nulling device. Another device constructed was a tapped delay line, for introducing a series of steadily increasing time delays (e.g., for an EEG signal). One day in the mid-1980s, it occurred to me that, if I combined these two devices, a predictor similar to the type Wiener had mentioned years earlier should result – and indeed, that was the case. Some early results and basic schema appear as an appendix in *The Electroencephalogram: Its Patterns and Origins* (MIT Press, 1993). But a predictor is one of the formats of a more general adaptive controller, a device that, at times, can seem almost alive.

Almost immediately, the circuit of the predictor reminded me of the anatomy of the cerebellar cortex, of the Purkinje cells, in particular, and I wondered if the cerebellum were an adaptive controller or, more exactly, could be modeled as an adaptive controller. I soon found that this was not a new idea, but in the interim, evidence from multiple sources has accumulated and the time seemed ripe to assemble it. After more than 15 years of incubation, this book is the result.

References

Wiener, N. (1948). *Cybernetics or Control and Communication in the Animal and the Machine.* Cambridge, Mass.: MIT Press.

Wiener, N. (1950). *Extrapolation, Interpolation, and Smoothing of Stationary Time Series.* Cambridge, Mass.: MIT Press.

Bibliography

Adams, J.C. (1986). Neuronal morphology in the human cochlear nucleus. *Arch. Otolarnyngol.* 112: 1253–1261.

Aiba, A., Kano, M., Chen, C., Stanton, M.E., Fox, G.D., Herrup, K., Zwingman, T.A., and Tonegawa, S. (1994). Deficient cerebellar long-term depression and impaired motor learning in mGluR1 mutant mice. *Cell* 79: 377–388.

Akshoomoff, N.A., and Courchesne, E. (1992). A new role for the cerebellum in cognitive operations. *Behav. Neurosci.* 106: 731–738.

Albus, J.S. (1971). A theory of cerebellar function. *Math. Biosci.* 10: 25–61.

Albus, J.S. (1975a). A new approach to manipulator control: the cerebellar model articulation controller (CMAC). *J. Dyn. Sys. Meas. Contr.* 97: 220–227.

Albus, J.S. (1975b). Data storage in the cerebellar model articulation controller (CMAC). *J. Dyn. Sys. Meas. Cont.* 97: 228–233.

Allen, G.I., and Tsukahara, N. (1974). Cerebrocerebellar communication systems. *Physiol. Rev.* 54: 957–1006.

Altman, J., and Bayer, S.A. (1997). *Development of the Cerebellar System in Relation to Its Evolution, Structure, and Functions.* New York: CRC Press, pp. 20–22.

Anastasio, T.J. (1992). Simulating vestibular compensation using recurrent back-propagation. *Biol. Cybern.* 66: 389–397.

Anastasio, T.J., and Robinson, D.A. (1989a). The distributed representation of vestibulo-oculomotor signals by brain-stem neurons. *Biol. Cybern.* 61: 79–88.

Anastasio, T.J., and Robinson, D.A. (1989b). Distributed parallel processing in the vestibulo-oculomotor system. *Neural Comput.* 1: 230–241.

Anastasio, T.J., and Robinson, D.A. (1990). Distributed parallel processing in the vertical vestibulo-ocular reflex: learning networks compared to tensor theory. *Biol. Cybern.* 63: 161–167.

Andersen, R.A., Snyder, L.H., Li, C.-S., and Stricanne, B. (1993). Coordinate transformation in the representation of spatial information. *Curr. Opin. Neurobiol.* 3: 171–176.

Andersson, G., and Oscarsson, O. (1978). Climbing fiber microzones in cerebellar vermis and their projection to different groups of cells in the lateral vestibular nucleus. *Exp. Brain Res.* 32: 565–579.

Apps, R. (2000). Gating of climbing fibre input to cerebellar cortical zones. *Progr. Brain Res.* 124: 199–211.

Apps, R., and Garwicz, M. (2000). Precise matching of olivo-cortical divergence and cortico-nuclear convergence between somatotopically corresponding areas in the medial C1 and medial C3 zones of the paravermal cerebellum. *Eur. J. Neurosci.* 12: 205–214.

Apps, R., and Lee, S. (1999). Gating of transmission in climbing fibre paths to cerebellar cortical C1 and C3 zones in the rostral paramedian lobule during locomotion in the cat. *J. Physiol.* 5163: 875–883.

Arbib, M.A. (ed.). (1998). *Handbook of Brain Theory and Neural Networks.* Cambridge, MA: MIT Press.

Arbib, M.A., and Amari, S.-I. (1985). Sensori-motor transformations in the brain (with a critique of the tensor theory of cerebellum). *J. Theoret. Biol.* 112: 123–155.

Arbib, M.A., Schweighofer, N., and Thach, W.T. (1995). Modeling the cerebellum: from adaptation to coordination. In: D.J. Glencross and J.P. Pick (eds.), *Motor Control and Sensory Motor Integration: Issues and Directions.* Amsterdam: Elsevier, pp. 11–36.

Ariëns Kappers, C.U., Huber, G.C., and Crosby, E.C. (1960). *The Comparative Anatomy of the Nervous System of Vertebrates, Including Man,* 3 vols. New York: Hafner.

Armstrong, D.M. (1974). Functional significance of connections of the inferior olive. *Physiol. Rev.* 54: 358–417.

Arnold, D.B., and Robinson, D.A. (1991). A learning network model of the neural integrator of the oculomotor system. *Biol. Cybern.* 64: 447–454.

Arnold, D.B., and Robinson, D.A. (1992). A neural network model of the vestibular-ocular reflex using a local synaptic learning rule. *Philos. Trans. R. Soc. Lond. B, Biol. Sci.* 337: 327–330.

Arnold, D.B., and Robinson, D.A. (1997). The oculomotor integrator: testing of a neural network model. *Exp. Brain Res.* 113: 57–74.

Asanuma, H. (1996). Neuronal mechanisms subserving the acquisition of new skilled movements in mammals. In: J.R. Bloedel, T.J. Ebner, and S.P. Wise (eds.), *The Acquisition of Motor Behavior in Vertebrates.* Cambridge, MA: MIT Press, pp. 387–390.

Asanuma, C., Thach, W.T., and Jones, E.G. (1983a). Distribution of cerebellar terminations and their relation to other afferent terminations in the ventral lateral thalamic region of the monkey. *Brain Res. Rev.* 5: 237–265.

Asanuma, C., Thach, W.T., and Jones, E.G. (1983b). Brainstem and spinal projections of the deep cerebellar nuclei in the monkey, with observations on the brainstem projections of the dorsal column nuclei. *Brain Res. Rev.* 5: 299–322.

Åström, K.J. (1995). Adaptive control: general methodology. In M.A. Arbib (ed.), *The Handbook of Brain Theory and Neural Networks.* Cambridge, MA: MIT Press, pp. 66–69.

Åström, K.J., and Wittenmark, B. (1995). *Adaptive Control* (2nd ed.). Reading, MA: Addison-Wesley.

Azizi, S.A., and Woodward, D.J. (1987). Inferior olivary nuclear complex of the rat: morphology and comments on the principles of organization within the olivocerebellar system. *J. Comp. Neurol.* 263: 467–484.

Baker, R., and Gilland, E. (1996). The evolution of hindbrain visual and vestibular innovations responsible for oculomotor function. In J.R. Bloedel, T.J. Ebner, and S.P. Wise (eds.), *The Acquisition of Motor Behavior in Vertebrates.* Cambridge, MA: MIT Press, pp. 29–55.

Balaban, C.D., and Beryozkin, G. (1994). Organization of vestibular nucleus projections to the caudal dorsal cap of Kooy in rabbits. *Neuroscience* 62: 1217–1236.

Balaban, C.D., Kawaguchi, Y., and Watanabe, E. (1981). Evidence of a collateralized climbing fiber projection from the inferior olive to the flocculus and vestibular nuclei in rabbits. *Neurosci. Lett.* 22: 23–29.

Barinaga, M. (1996). The cerebellum: movement coordinator or much more? *Science* 272: 482–483.

Barlow, J.S. (1964). Inertial navigation as a basis for animal navigation. *J. Theoret. Biol.* 6: 76–117.

Barlow, J.S. (1966). Inertial navigation in relation to animal navigation. *J. Inst. Navigation* (*Lond.*) 19: 302–316.

Barlow, J.S. (1985). Methods of analysis of nonstationary EEGs, with emphasis on segmentation techniques: a comparative review. *J. Clin. Neurophysiol.* 2: 267–364.

Barlow, J.S. (1993). *The Electroencephalogram: Its Patterns and Origins*. Cambridge, MA: MIT Press.

Barto, A.G., Buckingham, J.T., and Houk, J.C. (1996). In D.S. Touretsky, M.C. Mozer, and M.E. Hasselmo (eds.), *Advances in Neural Information Processing Systems 8*. Cambridge, MA: MIT Press, pp. 138–144.

Barto, A.G., Fagg, A.H., Sitkoff, N., and Houk, J.C. (1999). A cerebellar model of timing and prediction in the control of reaching. *Neural Comput.* 11: 565–594.

Bastian, A.J., and Thach, W.T. (1995). Cerebellar outflow lesions: a comparison of movement deficits resulting from lesions at the levels of the cerebellum and thalamus. *Ann. Neurol.* 38: 881–892.

Bastian, A.J., Martin, T.A., Keating, J.G., and Thach, W.T. (1996). Cerebellar ataxia: abnormal control of interaction torques across multiple joints. *J. Neurophysiol.* 76: 492–509.

Bastian, A.J., Zackowski, K.M., and Thach, W.T. (2000). Cerebellar ataxia: torque deficiency or torque mismatch between joints? *J. Neurophysiol.* 83: 3019–3030.

Bastian, J. (1993). Descending control of electroreception in gymnotid fish: contrasting properties of direct and indirect feedback pathways. *J. Comp. Physiol. A.* 173: 670–673.

Batini, C., Buisseret-Delmas, C., Compoint, C., and Daniel, H. (1989). The GABAergic neurones of the cerebellar nuclei in the rat: projections to the cerebellar cortex. *Neurosci. Lett.* 99: 251–256.

Batini, C., Compoint, C., Buisseret-Delmas, Daniel, H., and Guegan, M. (1992). Cerebellar nuclei and the nucleocortical projections in the rat: retrograde tracing coupled to GABA and glutamate immunohistochemistry. *J. Comp. Neurol.* 315: 74–84.

Bäurle, J., Helmchen, C., and Grüsser-Cornehls, U. (1997). Diverse effects of Purkinje cell loss on deep cerebellar and vestibular nuclei neurons in Purkinje cell degeneration mutant mice: a possible compensatory mechanism. *J. Comp. Neurol.* 384: 580–596.

Bell, C., Bodznick, D., Montgomery, J., and Bastian, J. (1997). The generation and subtraction of sensory expectations within cerebellum-like structures. *Brain Behav. Evol.* 50 (suppl. 1): 17–31.

Bell, C., Cordo, P., and Harnad, S. (1996). Controversies in neuroscience IV: motor learning and synaptic plasticity in the cerebellum: introduction. *Behav. Brain Sci.* 19: v–vi.

Bell, C.C. (1986). Electroreception in mormyrid fish: central physiology. In: T.H. Bullock and W. Heiligenberg (eds.), *Electroreception*. New York: Wiley, pp. 423–452.

Bell, C.C. (1993). The generation of expectations in the electrosensory lobe of mormyrid fish. *J. Comp. Physiol. A.* 173: 677–680.

Bell, C.C., and Szabo, T. (1986). Electroreception in mormyrid fish: central anatomy. In: T.H. Bullock and W. Heiligenberg (eds.), *Electroreception*. New York: John Wiley, pp. 375–421.

Bell, C.C., Han, V.Z., Sugawara, Y., and Grant, K., (1997). Synaptic plasticity in a cerebellum-like structure depends on temporal order. *Nature* 387: 278–281.

Bennett, M. (1969). Discussion of Oscarsson (1969), In R. Llinás (ed.), *Neurobiology of Cerebellar Evolution and Development*. Chicago: American Medical Association Educational and Research Foundation, p. 536.

Berkley, K.J., and Worden, I.G. (1978). Projections to the inferior olive of the cat: comparisons of input from the dorsal column nuclei, the lateral cervical nucleus, the spino-olivary pathways, the cerebral cortex and the cerebellum. *J. Comp. Neurol.* 180: 237–252.

Berrebi, A.S., and Mugnaini, E. (1991). Distribution and targets of the cartwheel cell axon in the dorsal cochlear nucleus of the guinea pig. *Anat. Embryol.* 183: 427–454.

Berrebi, A.S., and Mugnaini, E. (1993). Alterations in the dorsal cochlear nucleus of cerebellar mutant mice. In M.A. Merchán, J.M. Juiz, D.A. Godfrey, and E. Mugnaini (eds.), *The Mammalian Cochlear Nuclei: Organization and Function*. New York: Plenum, pp. 107–119.

Berrebi, A.S., Morgan, J.I., and Mugnaini, E. (1990). The Purkinje cell class may extend beyond the cerebellum. *J. Neurocytol.* 19: 643–654.

Berthier, N.E., Singh, S.P., and Barto, A.G. (1993). Distributed representation of limb motor programs in arrays of adjustable pattern generators. *J. Cogn. Neurosci.* 5: 56–78.

Berthier, N.E., Singh, S.P., Barto, A.G., and Houk, J.C. (1992). A cortico-cerebellar model that learns to generate distributed motor commands to control a kinematic arm. In J.E. Moody, S.J. Hanson, and R.P. Lippmann (eds.), *Advances in Neural Information Processing Systems 4*. San Mateo, CA: Morgan Kaufmann, pp. 611–618.

Blakemore, S.-J., Frith, C.D., and Wolpert, D.M. (1999). Spatio-temporal prediction modulates the perception of self-produced stimuli. *J. Cogn. Neurosci.* 11: 551–559.

Blakemore, S.-J., Wolpert, D.M., and Frith, C.D. (1999). The cerebellum contributes to somatosensory cortical activity during self-produced tactile stimulation. *Neuroimage* 10: 448–459.

Bloedel, J.R. (1992). Functional heterogeneity with structural homogeneity: how does the cerebellum operate? *Behav. Brain Sci.* 15: 666–678.

Bloedel, J.R. (1993). 'Involvement in' versus 'storage of.' *Trends Neurosci.* 16: 451–452.

Bloedel, J.R., and Bracha, V. (1995). On the cerebellum, cutaneomuscular reflexes, movement control and the elusive engrams of memory. *Behavi. Brain Res.* 68: 1–44.

Bloedel, J.R., and Bracha, V. (1998). Current concepts of climbing fiber function. *Anat. Rec.* 253: 118–126.

Bloedel, J.R., and Courville, J. (1981). Cerebellar afferent systems. In V.B. Brooks (ed.), *Handbook of Physiology Vol. II, Motor Control, Part 2*. Bethesda: American Physiological Society, pp. 735–829.

Bloedel, J.R., and Kelly, T.M. (1992). The dynamic selection hypothesis: a proposed function for cerebellar sagittal zones. In: R. Llinás and C. Sotelo (eds.), *The Cerebellum Revisited*. New York: Springer-Verlag, pp. 267–282.

Bloedel, J.R., and Roberts, W.J. (1971). Action of climbing fibers in cerebellar cortex of the cat. *J. Neurophysiol.* 34: 17–31.

Bloedel, J.R., Bracha, V., and Larson, P.S. (1993). Real time operations of the cerebellar cortex. *Can. J. Neurol. Sci.* 20(suppl. 3): S7–S18.

Bloedel, J.R., Bracha, V., and Milak, M.S. (1993). Role of the cerebellar nuclei in the learning and performance of forelimb movement in the cat. In N. Mano, I. Hamada, and M.R. De-Long (eds.), *Role of the Cerebellum and Basal Ganglia in Voluntary Movement*. Amsterdam: Elsevier, pp. 21–31.

Bloedel, J.R., Bracha, V., Shimansky, Y., and Milak, M.S. (1996). The role of the cerebellum in the acquisition of complex volitional forelimb movements. In J.R. Bloedel, T.J. Ebner, and S.P. Wise (eds.), *The Acquisition of Motor Behavior in Vertebrates*. Cambridge, MA: MIT Press, pp. 320–330.

Blomfield, S., and Marr, D. (1970). How the cerebellum may be used. *Nature* 227: 1224–1228.

Blond, O., and Crépel, F. (1996). Letter to the editor. *Trends Neurosci.* 19: 11.

Bodznick, D., and Montgomery, J.C. (1993). The physiology of the dorsal nucleus of elasmobranchs and its descending control. *J. Comp. Physiol. A.* 173: 680–682.

Boose, A., Dichgans, J., and Topka, H. (1999). Deficits in phasic muscle force generation explain insufficient compensation for interaction torque in cerebellar patients. *Neurosci. Lett.* 26: 53–56.

Botez, M.I. (1992). The neuropsychology of the cerebellum: an emerging concept. *Arch. Neurol.* 49: 321–324.

Bower, J.M. (1995). The cerebellum as sensory acquisition controller: commentary on the underestimated cerebellum by Leiner et al. *Hum. Brain Mapp.* 2: 255–256.

Bower, J.M. (1997). Is the cerebellum sensory for motor's sake, or motor for sensory's sake: the view from the whiskers of a rat. *Progr. Brain Res.* 114: 463–496.

Box, G.E.P., and Jenkins, G.M. (1970). *Time Series Analysis: Forecasting and Control*. San Francisco: Holden Day.

Boxall, A.R., Lancaster, B., and Garthwaite, J. (1996). Tyrosine kinase is required for long-term depression in the cerebellum. *Neuron* 16: 805–813.

Boylls, C.C. (1975a). *A Theory of Cerebellar Function with Applications to Locomotion. I. The Physiological Role of Climbing Fiber Inputs in Anterior Lobe Operation*. Amherst: University of Massachusetts (COINS Tech. Rep. 75C-6).

Boylls, C.C. (1975b). *A Theory of Cerebellar Function with Applications to Locomotion. II. The Relation of Anterior Lobe Climbing Fiber Function to Locomotor Behavior in the Cat*. Amherst: University of Massachusetts (COINS Tech. Rep. 76-1).

Boylls, C.C. (1980). Cerebellar strategies for movement coordination. In G.E. Stelmach and J. Requin (eds.), *Tutorials in Motor Behavior*. Amsterdam: North Holland, pp. 83–94.

Braak, H., and Braak, E. (1984). Local circuit neurons in the cerebellar dentate nucleus of man. In J.R. Bloedel, J. Dichgans, and W. Precht (eds.), *Cerebellar Functions*. New York: Springer-Verlag, pp. 324–325.

Bracha, V., Zhao, L., Wunderlich, D.A., Morrissy, S.J., and Bloedel, J.R. (1997). Patients with cerebellar lesions cannot acquire but are able to retain conditioned eyeblink reflexes. *Brain* 120: 1401–1413.

Braitenberg, V. (1961). Functional interpretation of cerebellar histology. *Nature* 190: 539–540.

Braitenberg, V. (1967). Is the cerebellar cortex a biological clock in the millisecond range? *Progr. Brain Res.* 25: 334–346.

Braitenberg, V. (1977). *On the Texture of Brains* (Chapter 7: Analysis of the cerebellum). New York: Springer-Verlag.

Braitenberg, V. (1983). The cerebellum revisited. *J. Theor. Neurobiol.* 2: 237–241.

Braitenberg, V. (1987). The cerebellum and the physics of movement: some speculations. In M. Glickstein, C. Yeo, and J. Stein (eds.), *Cerebellum and Neuronal Plasticity*. New York: Plenum, pp. 193–207.

Braitenberg, V. (1990). Reading the structure of brains. *Network: Comput. Neural Syst.* 1: 1–11.

Braitenberg, V. (1993). The cerebellar network: attempt at a formalization of its structure. *Network* 4: 11–17.

Braitenberg, V., and Atwood, R.P. (1958). Morphological observations on the cerebellar cortex. *J. Comp. Neurol.* 109: 1–27.

Braitenberg, V., and Preissl, H. (1992). Why is the output of the cerebellum inhibitory? *Behav. Brain Sci.* 15: 715–717.

Braitenberg, V., Heck, D., and Sultan, F. (1997). The detection and generation of sequences as a key to cerebellar function: experiments and theory. *Behav. Brain Sci.* 20: 229–245.

Brand, S., Dahl, A.-L., and Mugnaini, E. (1976). The length of parallel fibers in the cat cerebellar cortex. An experimental light and electron microscopic study. *Exp. Brain Res.* 26: 39–58.

Bravin, M., Rossi, F., and Strata, P. (1995). Different climbing fibers innervate separate dendritic regions of the same Purkinje cell in hypogranular cerebellum. *J. Comp. Neurol.* 357: 395–407.

Brazier, M.A.B. (1988). *A History of Neurophysiology in the 19th Century*. New York: Raven Press, pp. 131–133.

Brindley, G.S. (1964). The use made by the cerebellum of the information that it receives from sense organs (report on symposia and meetings). *IBRO Bull.* 3(3): 80.

Brodal, A. (1967). Anatomical studies of cerebellar fibre connections with special reference to problems of functional localization. *Progr. Brain Res.* 25: 135–173.

Brodal, A. (1981). *Neurological Anatomy in Relation to Clinical Medicine* (3rd ed.). Oxford, England: Oxford University Press.

Brodal, A., and Drabløs, P.A. (1963). Two types of mossy fiber terminals in the cerebellum and their regional distribution. *J. Comp. Neurol.* 121: 173–187.

Brodal, A., and Jansen, J. (1954). Structural organization of the cerebellum. In J. Jansen and A. Brodal (eds.), *Aspects of Cerebellar Anatomy*. Oslo: Johan Grundt Tanum Forlag, pp. 285–395.

Brodal, A., and Kawamura, K. (1980). Olivocerebellar projections: a review. *Adv. Anat. Embryol. Cell Biol.* 64: 1–140.

Brodal, P. (1998). *The Central Nervous System: Structure and Function* (2nd ed.). Oxford, England: Oxford University Press.

Brodal, P., and Bjaalie, J.G. (1997). Salient anatomic features of the cortico-ponto-cerebellar pathway. *Progr. Brain Res.* 114: 227–247.

Buisseret-Delmas, C., and Angaut, P.E. (1989). Anatomical mapping of the cerebellar nucleocortical projections in the rat: a retrograde labeling study. *J. Comp. Neurol.* 288: 297–310.

Bullock, D., Fiala, J.C., and Grossberg, S. (1994). A neural model of timed response learning in the cerebellum. *Neural Netw.* 7: 1101–1114.

Bullock, T.H. (1969). Discussion of Oscarsson (1969), In R. Llinás (ed.), *Neurobiology of Cerebellar Evolution and Development*. Chicago: American Medical Association and Research Foundation, p. 536.

Bullock, T.H. (1986). Significance of findings on electroreception for general neurobiology. In: T.H. Bullock and W. Heiligenberg (eds.), *Electroreception*. New York: John Wiley, pp. 651–674.

Buonomano, D.V., and Mauk, M.D. (1994). Neural network model of the cerebellum: temporal discrimination and the timing of motor responses. *Neural Comput.* 6: 38–55.

Butler, A.B., and Hodos, W. (1996). *Comparative Vertebrate Neuroanatomy: Evolution and Adaptation.* (Chapter 12: The cerebellum.) New York: Wiley-Liss, pp. 180–197.

Cabeza, R., and Nyberg, L. (2000). Imaging cognition II: an empirical review of 275 PET and fMRI studies. *J. Cogn. Neurosci.* 12: 1–47.

Calne, D.B. (1959). Pathways converging upon Purkinje cells in the frog's cerebellum. *J. Physiol.* 146: 459–464.

Calvert, T.W., and Meno, F. (1972). Neural systems modeling applied to the cerebellum. *IEEE Trans. Sys. Man Cybern.* SMC-2: 363–374.

Cant, N.B. (1992). The cochlear nucleus: neuronal types and their synaptic organization. In: D.B. Webster, A.N. Popper, and R. R. Fay (eds.), *The Mammalian Auditory Pathway: Neuroanatomy*. New York: Springer, pp. 66–116.

Caroni, P. (1997). Overexpression of growth-associated proteins in the neurons of adult transgenic mice. *J. Neurosci. Methods* 71: 3–9.

Casini, L., and Ivry, R.B. (1999). Effects of divided attention on temporal processing in patients with lesions of the cerebellum or frontal lobe. *Neuropsychology* 13: 10–21.

Caston, J., Vasseur, F., Stelz, T., Chianale, C., Delhaye-Bouchaud, N., and Mariani, J. (1995). Differential roles of cerebellar cortex and deep cerebellar nuclei in the learning of the equilibrium behavior: studies in intact and cerebellectomized lurcher mutant mice. *Brain Res. Dev. Brain Res.* 86: 311–316.

Catalan, M.J., Honda, M., Weeks, R.A., Cohen, L.G., and Hallett, M. (1998). The functional neuroanatomy of simple and complex sequential finger movements: a PET study. *Brain* 121: 253–264.

Chan-Palay (1982). Discussion of Tolbert, D.L. (1982). The cerebellar nucleocortical pathway. In S.L. Palay and V. Chan-Palay (eds.), *The Cerebellum – New Vistas*, Berlin: Springer-Verlag, pp. 296–319.

Chan-Palay, V. (1977). *Cerebellar Dentate Nucleus*. New York: Springer-Verlag.

Chapeau-Blondeau, F., and Chauvet, G. (1991). A neural network model of the cerebellar cortex performing dynamic associations. *Biol. Cybern.* 65: 267–279.

Chen, C., Kano, M., Abeliovich, A., Chen, L., Bao, S., Kim, J.J., Hashimoto, K., Thompson, R.F., and Tonegawa, S. (1995). Impaired motor coordination correlates with persistent multiple climbing fiber innervation in PKC_{gamma} mutant mice. *Cell* 83: 1233–1242.

Chen, G., Hanson, C.L., and Ebner, T.J. (1998). Optical responses evoked by cerebellar surface stimulation *in vivo* using neutral red. *Neurosciences* 84: 645–668.

Clark, H.B., and Orr, H.T. (2000). Spinocerebellar ataxia Type 1 – modeling the pathogenesis of a polyglutamine neurodegenerative disorder in transgenic mice. *J. Neuropathol. Exp. Neurol.* 59: 265–270.

Clarke, E., and O'Malley, C.D. (1968). Chapter 11: The cerebellum. In *The Human Brain and Spinal Cord: A Historical Study Illustrated by Writings from Antiquity to the Twentieth Century*. Berkeley Los Angeles: University of California Press, pp. 628–707.

Coenen, O. (1999). Learning to make predictions in the cerebellum may explain the anticipatory modulation of the vestibulo-ocular reflex (VOR) with vergence. In *Modeling the Vestibulo-Ocular Reflex and the Cerebellum: Analytical & Computational Approaches*. Ph.D. Dissertation, University of California, San Diego, pp. 74–95.

Coenen, O., Seijnowski, T.J., and Lisberger, S.G. (1992). Biologically plausible local learning rules for the adaptation of the vestibulo-ocular reflex. In S.J. Hanson, J.D. Cowan, and C.L. Giles (eds.), *Advances in Neural Information Processing Systems 5*. San Mateo, CA: Morgan Kaufmann Publishers, pp. 961–968.

Cohen, B., Reisine, H., Yokota, J.-I., and Raphan, T. (1992). The nucleus of the optic tract: its function in gaze stabilization and control of visual-vestibular interaction. *Ann. N. Y. Acad. Sci.* 656: 277–296.

Cohen, D., and Yarom, Y. (2000). Unraveling cerebellar circuitry: an optic imaging study. *Progr. Brain Res.* 124: 107–114.

Cole, J.D. (1991). *Pride and a Daily Marathon*. London: Duckworth Reprinted (1995), Cambridge, MA: MIT Press.

Contreras-Vidal, J.L., Bloedel, J.R., and Stelmach, G.E. (1995). A network model of the sagittal olivo cerebellar complex. *Soc. Neurosci.* 21: 216.

Contreras-Vidal, J.L., Grossberg, S., and Bullock, D. (1997). A neural model of cerebellar learning for arm movement control: cortico-spino-cerebellar dynamics. *Learn. Mem.* 3: 475–502.

Courchesne, E., and Allen, G. (1997). Prediction and preparation, fundamental functions of the cerebellum. *Learn. Mem.* 4: 1–35.

Courville, J., de Montigny, C., and Lamarre, Y. (1980). (Eds.) *The Inferior Olivary Nucleus: Anatomy and Physiology*. New York: Raven Press.

Courville, J., and Otabe, S. (1974). The rubro-olivary projection in the macaque: an experimental study with silver impregnation methods. *J. Comp. Neurol.* 158: 479–494.

Cowan, J.D., and Sharp, D.H. (1988a). Neural nets. *Q. Rev. Biophys.* 21: 365–427.

Cowan, J.D., and Sharp, D.H. (1988b). Neural nets and artificial intelligence. *Daedalus* 117(1): 85–121.

Crépel, F., Audinat, E., Daniel, H., Hemart, N., Jaillard, D., Rossiter, J., and Lambolez, B. (1994). Cellular locus of the nitric oxide-synthase involved in cerebellar long-term depression induced by high external potassium concentration. *Neuropharmacology* 33: 1399–1405.

Crépel, F., Hemart, N., Jaillard, D., and Daniel, H. (1996). Cellular mechanisms of long-term depression in the cerebellum. *Behav. Brain Sci.* 19: 347–353.

Crick, F. (1984). Function of the thalamic reticular complex: the searchlight hypothesis. *Proc. Natl. Acad. Sci. USA* 81: 4586–4590.

Crispino, L., and Bullock, T.H. (1984). Cerebellum mediates modality-specific modulation of sensory responses of midbrain and forebrain in rat. *Proc. Natl. Acad. Sci. USA* 81: 2917–2920.

Crosby, E.C. (1969). Comparative aspects of cerebellar morphology. In R. Llinás (ed.), *Neurobiology of Cerebellar Evolution and Development.* Chicago: American Medical Association Educational and Research Foundation, pp. 19–41.

Cummings, C.J., Orr, H.T., and Zoghbi, H.Y. (1999). Progress in pathogenesis studies of spinocerebellar ataxia type 1. *Philos. Trans. R. Soc. Lond. B Biol. Sci.* 354: 1079–1081.

D'Angelo, E., Rossi, P., Armano, S., and Taglietti, V. (1999). Evidence for NMDA and mGlu receptor-dependent long-term potentiation of mossy fiber–granule cell transmission in rat cerebellum. *J. Neurophysiol.* 81: 277–287.

Daniel, H., Levenes, C., and Crépel, F. (1998). Cellular mechanisms of cerebellar LTD. *Trends Neurosci.* 21: 401–407.

Davis, K.A., and Young, E.D. (1997). Granule cell activation of complex-spiking neurons in dorsal cochlear nucleus. *J. Neurosci.* 17: 6798–6806.

Davis, K.A., Miller, R.L., and Young, E.D. (1996). Effects of somatosensory and parallel-fiber stimulation on neurons in dorsal cochlear nucleus. *J. Neurophysiol.* 76: 3012–3024.

Day, B.L., Thompson, P.D., Harding, A.E., and Marsden, C.D. (1998). Influence of vision on upper limb reaching movements in patients with cerebellar ataxia. *Brain* 121: 357–372.

De Schutter, E. (1995). Cerebellar long-term depression might normalize excitation of Purkinje cells: a hypothesis. *Trends Neurosci.* 18: 291–295.

De Schutter, E. (1996). Reply. *Trends Neurosci.* 19: 12.

De Schutter, E. (1997). A new functional role for cerebellar long-term depression. *Progr. Brain Res.* 114: 529–542.

De Schutter, E., and Bower, J.M. (1994a). An active membrane model of the cerebellar Purkinje cell. I. Simulation of current clamps in slice. *J. Neurophysiol.* 71: 375–400.

De Schutter, E., and Bower, J.M. (1994b). An active membrane model of the cerebellar Purkinje cell. II. Simulation of synaptic responses. *J. Neurophysiol.* 71: 401–419.

De Schutter, E., Vos, B., and Maex, R. (2000). The function of cerebellar Golgi cells revisited.*Progr. Brain Res.* 124: 81–93.

De Zeeuw, C., and Ruigrok, T.J.H. (1994). Olivary projecting neurons in the nucleus of Darkschewitsch in the cat receive excitatory monosynaptic input from the cerebellar nuclei. *Brain Res.* 653: 345–350.

De Zeeuw, C.I., and Berrebi, A.S. (1995). Postsynaptic targets of Purkinje cell terminals in the cerebellar and vestibular nuclei of the rat. *Eur. J. Neurosci.* 7: 2322–2323.

De Zeeuw, C.I., and Berrebi, A.S. (1996). Individual Purkinje cell axons terminate on both inhibitory and excitatory neurons in the cerebellar and vestibular nuclei. *Ann. N. Y. Acad. Sci.* 781: 607–610.

De Zeeuw, C.I., and Koekkoek, S.K.E. (1997). Signal processing in the C2 module of the flocculus and its role in head movement control. *Progr. Brain Res.* 114: 299–320.

De Zeeuw, C.I., Gerrits, N.M., Voogd, J., Leonard, C.S., and Simpson, J.I. (1994). The rostral dorsal cap and ventrolateral outgrowth of the rabbit inferior olive receive a GABAergic input from dorsal group y and the ventral dentate nucleus. *J. Comp. Neurol.* 341: 420–432.

De Zeeuw, C.I., Hansel, C., Bian, F., Koekkoek, S.K.E., van Alphen, A.M., Linden, D.J., and Oberdick, J. (1998). Expression of a protein kinase C inhibitor in Purkinje cells blocks cerebellar LTD and adaptation of the vestibulo-ocular reflex. *Neuron* 20: 495–508.

De Zeeuw, C.I., Hertzberg, E.L., and Mugnaini, E. (1995). The dendritic lamellar body: a new neuronal organelle putatively associated with dendrodendritic gap junctions. *J. Neurosci.* 15: 1587–1604.

De Zeeuw, C.I., Holstege, J.C., Ruigrok, T.J.H., and Voogd, J. (1989). Ultrastructural study of the GABAergic, cerebellar, and mesodiencephalic innervation of the cat medial accessory olive: anterograde tracing combined with immunocytochemistry. *J. Comp. Neurol.* 284: 12–35.

De Zeeuw, C.I., Holstege, J.C., Ruigrok, T.J.H., and Voogd, J. (1990). Mesodiencephalic and cerebellar terminals terminate upon the same dendritic spines in the glomeruli of the cat and rat inferior olive: an ultrastructural study using a combination of [³H]leucine and wheat germ agglutinin coupled horseradish peroxidase anterograde tracing. *Neuroscience* 34: 645–655.

De Zeeuw, C.I., Koekkoek, S.K.E., Wylie, D.R.W., and Simpson, J.I. (1997). Association between dendritic lamellar bodies and complex spike synchrony in the olivocerebellar system. *J. Neurophysiol.* 77: 1747–1758.

De Zeeuw, C.I., Ruigrok, T.J.H., Holstege, J.C., Jansen, H.G., and Voogd, J. (1990). Intracellular labeling of neurons in the medial accessory olive of the cat: II. Ultrastructure of dendritic spines and their GABAergic innervation. *J. Comp. Neurol.* 300: 478–494.

De Zeeuw, C.I., Ruigrok, T.J.H., Holstege, J.C., Schalekamp, M.P.A., and Voogd, J. (1990). Intracellular labeling of neurons in the medial accessory olive of the cat: III. Ultrastructure of axon hillock and initial segment and their GABAergic innervation. *J. Comp. Neurol.* 300: 495–510.

De Zeeuw, C.I., Simpson, J.I., Hoogenraad, C.C., Galjart, N., Koekkoek, S.K.E., and Ruigrok, T.J.H. (1998). Microcircuitry and function of the inferior olive. *Trends Neurosci.* 21: 391–400.

De Zeeuw, C.I., van Alphen, A.M., Hawkins, R.K., and Ruigrok, T.J.H. (1997). Climbing fibre collaterals contact neurons in the cerebellar nuclei that provide a GABAergic feedback to the inferior olive. *Neuroscience* 80: 981–986.

De Zeeuw, C.I., Wentzel, O.P., and Mugnaini, E. (1993). Fine structure of the dorsal cap of the inferior olive and its GABAergic and non-GABAergic input from the nucleus prepositus hypoglossi in rat and rabbit. *J. Comp. Neurol.* 327: 62–82.

De Zeeuw, C.I., Wylie, D.R., DiGiorgi, P.L., and Simpson, J.I. (1994). Projections of individual Purkinje cells of identified zones in the flocculus to the vestibular and cerebellar nuclei in the rabbit. *J. Comp. Neurol.* 349: 428–447.

Dean, P. (1995). Modelling the role of the cerebellar fastigial nuclei in producing accurate saccades: the importance of burst timing. *Neuroscience.* 68: 1059–1077.

Dean, P., Mayhew, J.E., and Langdon, P. (1994). Learning and maintaining saccadic accuracy: a model of brainstem-cerebellar interactions. *J. Cogn. Neurosci.* 6: 117–138.

Decety, J., Sjöholm, H., Ryding, E., Stenberg, G., and Ingvar, D.H. (1990). The cerebellum participates in mental activity: tomographic measurements of regional cerebral blood flow. *Brain Res.* 535: 313–317.

Denk, W., Sugimori, M., and Llinás, R. (1995). Two types of calcium response limited to single spines in cerebellar Purkinje cells. *Proc. Natl. Acad. Sci. USA* 92: 8279–8282.

Desmond, J.E., and Fiez, J.A. (1998). Neuroimaging studies of the cerebellum: language, learning and memory. *Trends Cogn. Sci.* 2: 355–362.

Desmurget, M., Pélisson, D., Urquizar, C., Prablanc, C., Alexander, G.E., and Grafton, S.T. (1998). Functional anatomy of saccadic adaptation in humans. *Nat. Neurosci.* 1: 524–528.

de'Sperati, C., Montarolo, P.G., and Strata, P. (1993). Effects of inferior olive inactivation and lesion on the activity of medial vestibular neurons in the rat. *Neuroscience* 53: 139–147.

Diener, H.C., Dichgans, J., Guschlbauer, B., Bacher, M., and Langenbach, P. (1989). Disturbances of motor preparation in basal ganglia and cerebellar disorders. *Progr. Brain Res.* 880: 481–488.

Dietrichs, E., and Walberg, F. (1979). The cerebellar corticonuclear and nucleocortical projections in the cat as studied with anterograde and retrograde transport of horseradish peroxide. *Anat. Embryol.* 158: 13–39.

Dietrichs, E., and Walberg, F. (1989). Direct bidirectional connections between the inferior olive and the cerebellar nuclei. In P. Strata (ed.), *The Olivocerebellar System in Motor Control (Exp. Brain Res. Ser. 17)*, pp. 61–81.

Diño, M.R., Nunzi, M.G., Anelli, R., and Mugnaini, E. (2000). Unipolar brush cells of the vestibulocerebellum: afferents and targets. *Progr. Brain Res.* 124: 123–137.

Donoghue, J.P., Hess, G., and Sanes, J.N. (1996). Substrates and mechanisms for learning in motor cortex. In J.R. Bloedel, T.J. Ebner, and S.P. Wise (eds.), *The Acquisition of Motor Behavior in Vertebrates.* Cambridge, MA: MIT Press, pp. 363–386.

Dow, R.S. (1949). Action potentials of cerebellar cortex in response to local electrical stimulation. *J. Neurophysiol.* 12: 245–256.

Dow, R.S., and Moruzzi, G. (1958). *The Physiology and Pathology of the Cerebellum.* Minneapolis: University of Minnesota Press.

Doya, K. (1999). What are the computations of the cerebellum, the basal ganglia and the cerebral cortex. *Neural Netw.* 12: 961–974.

Droulez, J., and Cornilleau-Pérès, V. (1993). Application of the coherence scheme to the multisensory fusion problem. In: A. Berthoz (ed.), *Multisensory Control of Movement.* Oxford, England: Oxford University Press, pp. 485–501.

du Lac, S., Raymond, J.L., Seijnowski, T.J., and Lisberger, S.G. (1995). Learning and memory in the vestibulo-ocular reflex. *Annu. Rev. Neurosci.* 18: 409–441.

Dunin-Barkowski, W.L., and Larionova, N.P. (1985a). Computer simulation of a cerebellar compartment. I. General principles and properties of a neural net. *Biol. Cybern.* 51, 399–406.

Dunin-Barkowski, W.L., and Larionova, N.P. (1985b). Computer simulation of a cerebellar cortex compartment. II. An information learning and its recall in the Marr's Memory Unit. *Biol. Cybern.* 51: 407–415.

Dunn, M.E., Vetter, D.E., Berrebi, A.S., Krider, H.M., and Mugnaini, E. (1996). The mossy fiber–granule cell–cartwheel cell system in the mammalian cochlear nuclear complex. In W.A. Ainsworth, E.F. Evans, and C.M. Hackney (eds.), *Advances in Speech, Hearing and Language Processing*, Vol. 3, Part A. London: JAI Press, pp. 63-87.

Ebner, T.J. (1998). A role for the cerebellum in the control of limb movement velocity. *Curr. Opin. Neurobiol.* 8: 762–769.

Ebner, T.J., and Chen, G. (1995). Use of voltage-sensitive dyes and optical recordings in the central nervous system. *Progr. Neurobiol.* 46: 463–506.

Ebner, T.J., Flament, D., and Shanbhag, S.J. (1996). In J.R. Bloedel, T.J. Ebner, and S.P. Wise (eds.), *The Acquisition of Motor Behavior in Vertebrates.* Cambridge, MA: MIT Press, pp. 235–260.

Eccles, J.C. (1966). Functional organization of the cerebellum in relation to its role in motor control. In: R. Granit (ed.), *Muscular Afferents and Motor Control* (Proceedings of the First Nobel Symposium, 1965). Stockholm: Almqvist and Wiksell; New York: John Wiley. pp. 19–36.

Eccles, J.C. (1967). Circuits in the cerebellar control of movement. *Proc. Natl. Acad. Sci. USA* 58: 336–343.

Eccles, J.C. (1973). The cerebellum as a computer: patterns in space and time. *J. Physiol.* 229: 1–32.

Eccles, J.C. (1977a). An instruction-selection theory of learning in the cerebellar cortex. *Brain Res.* 127: 327–352.

Eccles, J.C. (1977b). Cerebellar functions in the control of movement (with special reference to the pioneer work of Sir Gordon Holmes). In F.C. Rose (ed.), *Physiological Aspects of Clinical Neurology.* Oxford, England: Blackwell, pp. 157–178.

Eccles, J.C. (1982). The future of studies on the cerebellum. In: S.L. Palay and V. Chan-Palay (eds.), *The Cerebellum – New Vistas.* New York: Springer, pp. 607–620.

Eccles, J.C., Ito, M., and Szentágothai, J. (1967). *The Cerebellum as a Neuronal Machine.* New York: Springer-Verlag.

Eccles, J.C., Llinás, R., and Sasaki, K. (1966). The excitatory synapse action of climbing fibres on the Purkinje cells of the cerebellum. *J. Physiol. (Lond.)* 182: 268-296.

Eccles, J.C., Sabah, N.H., Schmidt, R.F., and Táboríková, H. (1972). Mode of operation of the cerebellum in the dynamic loop control of movement. *Brain Res.* 40: 73–80.

Eisenman, L.M. (2000). Antero-posterior boundaries and compartments in the cerebellum: evidence from selected neurological mutants. *Progr. Brain Res.* 124: 81–93.

Ekerot, C.-F. (1999). Climbing fibers – a key to cerebellar function. *J. Physiol.* 516.3: 629.

Ekerot, C.-F., and Oscarsson, O. (1981). Prolonged depolarization elicited in Purkinje cell dendrites by climbing fiber impulses in the cat. *J. Physiol.* 318: 207–221.

Ekerot, C.-F., Garwicz, M., and Jörntell, H. (1997). The control of forelimb movements by intermediate cerebellum. *Progr. Brain Res.* 114: 423–429.

Ekerot, C.-F., Larson, B., and Oscarsson, O. (1979). Information carried by the spinocerebellar paths. *Progr. Brain Res.* 50: 79–90.

Elias, S.A., Yae, H., and Ebner, T.J. (1993). Optical imaging of parallel fiber activation in the rat cerebellar cortex: spatial effects of excitatory amino acids. *Neuroscience* 52: 771–786.

Eskandar, E.N., and Assad, J.A. (1999). Dissociation of visual, motor and predictive signals in parietal cortex during visual guidance. *Nat. Neurosci.* 2: 88–93.

Fahle, M., and Braitenberg, V. (1985). Some quantitative aspects of cerebellar anatomy as a guide to speculation on cerebellar functions. In J.R. Bloedel, J. Dichgangs, and W. Precht (eds.), *Cerebellar Functions.* Berlin: Springer, pp. 186–200.

Fetz, E.E. (1993). Dynamic neural network models of sensorimotor behavior. In: D. Gardner (ed.), *The Neurobiology of Neural Networks.* Cambridge, MA: MIT Press, pp. 164–190.

Fetz, E.E., and Shupe, L.E. (1990). Neural network models of the primate motor system. In: R. Eckmiller (ed.), *Advanced Neural Computers.* Amsterdam: North Holland, pp. 43–50.

Fiala, J.C., Grossberg, S., and Bullock, D. (1996). Metabotropic glutamate receptor activation in cerebellar Purkinje cells as substrate for adaptive timing of the classically conditioned eye-blink response. *J. Neurosci.* 16: 3760–3774.

Fiez, J.A., Petersen, S.E., Cheney, M.K., and Raichle, M.E. (1992). Impaired non-motor learning and error detection associated with cerebellar damage (a single case study). *Brain* 115: 155–178.

Finger, T.E., Bell, C.C., and Russell, C.J. (1981). Electrosensory pathways to the valvula cerebelli in mormyrid fish. *Exp. Brain Res.* 42: 23–33.

Flanagan, J.R., Nakano, E., Imamizu, H., Osu, R., Yoshioka, T., and Kawato, M. (1999). Composition and decomposition of internal models in motor learning under altered kinematic and dynamic environments. *J. Neurosci.* 19: RC34.

Flourens, P. (1824, 1842). Recherches experimentales sur less propriétés nerveux dans les animaux vertébrés. (Ed. 1), Paris; Crevot, 1824; ed. 2, Paris: Bailliere, 1842, pp. 4, 5, 12, 13, 14, 23.

Freeman, J.A. (1969). The cerebellum as a timing device: an experimental study in the frog. In R. Llinás (ed.), *Neurobiology of Cerebellar Evolution and Development.* Chicago: American Medical Association Educational and Research Foundation, pp. 397–413.

Freeman, J.A. (1970). Space-time transformation in the frog cerebellum through an intrinsic tapped delay line. *Nature (Lond.)* 226: 640–642.

Freeman, W.J. (1983). Dynamics of information formation by nerve cell assemblies. In E. Basar, H. Flohr, H. Haken, and A.J. Mandell (eds.), *Synergetics of the Brain.* New York: Springer-Verlag, pp. 102–121.

Frens, M.A., Mathoera, A.L., and Van der Steen, J. (2000). On the nature of gain changes of the optokinetic reflex. *Progr. Brain Res.* 124: 247–255.

Friston, K.J., Frith, C.D., Passingham, R.E., Liddle, P.F. and Frackowiak, R.S.J. (1992). Motor practice and neurophysiological adaptation in the cerebellum: a positron tomography study. *Proc. R. Soc. Lond. B. Biol. Sci.* 248: 223–228.

Fu, Q-G. Flament, D., Coltz, J.D., and Ebner, T.J. (1997). Relationship of cerebellar Purkinje cell simple spike discharge to movement kinematics in the monkey. *J. Neurophysiol.* 78: 478–491.

Fu, Q-G., Mason, C.R., Flament, D., Coltz, J.D., and Ebner, T.J. (1997). Movement kinematics encoded in complex discharge of primate cerebellar Purkinje cells. *Neuroreport* 8: 523–529.

Fuchs, A.F., Mustari, M.J., Robinson, F.R., and Kaneko, C.R.S. (1992). Visual signals in the nucleus of the optic tract and their brain stem destinations. *Ann. N. Y. Acad. Sci.* 656: 266–276.

Fuchs, A.F., Robinson, F.R., and Straube, A. (1994). Participation of the caudal fastigial nucleus in smooth-pursuit eye movements. I. Neuronal activity. *J. Neurophysiol.* 72: 2714–2728.

Fuhrman, Y., Piat, G., Thomson, M.A., Mariani, J., Delhaye-Bouchaud, N. (1995). Abnormal ipsilateral functional vibrissae projection onto Purkinje cells multiply innervated by climbing fibers in the rat. *Devel. Brain Res.* 87: 172–178.

Fujita, M. (1982a). Adaptive filter model of the cerebellum. *Biol. Cybern.* 45: 195–206.

Fujita, M. (1982b). Simulation of adaptive modification of the vestibulo-ocular reflex with an adaptive filter model of the cerebellum. *Biol. Cybern.* 45: 207–214.

Funabiki, K., Mishina, M., and Hirano, T. (1995). Retarded vestibular compensation in mutant mice deficient in $\delta2$ glutamate receptor subunit. *Neuroreport* 7: 189–192.

Gabor, D. (1954). Communication theory and cybernetics. *IRE Trans. Circuit Theory* CT-1(4): 19–31.

Gabor, D., Wilby, W.P.L., and Woodcock, R. (1961). A universal non-linear filter, predictor and simulator which optimizes itself by a learning process. *Proc. I.E.E. (London) B.* 108: 422–438.

Gao, J.-H., Parsons, L.M., Bower, J.M., Xiong. J-h, Li, J-Q. and Fox, P.T. (1996). Cerebellum implicated in sensory acquisition and discrimination rather than motor control. *Science* 272: 545–547.

Garwicz, M. (2000). Micro-organisation of cerebellar modules controlling forelimb movements. *Progr. Brain Res.* 124: 187–199.

Garwicz, M., and Andersson, G. (1992). Spread of synaptic activity along parallel fibres in cat cerebellar anterior lobe. *Exp. Brain Res.* 88: 615–622.

Gellman, R., Gibson, A.R., and Houk, J.C. (1985). Inferior olivary neurons in the awake cat: detection of contact and passive body displacement. *J. Neurophysiol.* 54: 40–60.

Gell-Mann, M. (1995). Complex adaptive systems. In H. Morowitz and J.L. Singer (eds.), *The Mind, The Brain, and Complex Adaptive Systems*. Reading, MA.: Addison-Wesley, pp. 11–23.

Ghez, C. (1991). The cerebellum. In E.R. Kandel, J.H. Schwartz, and T.M. Jessell (Eds.), *Principles of Neural Science* (3rd ed.). New York: Elsevier, pp. 627–646.

Ghez, C., Gordon, J., Ghilardi, M.F., Cristakos, C.N., and Cooper, S.E. (1990). Role of proprioceptive input in the programming of arm trajectories. *Cold Spring Harb. Symp. Quant. Biol.* 55: 837–847.

Ghez, C., and Thach, W.T. (2000). The cerebellum. In: E.R. Kandel, J.H. Schwartz, and T.M. Jessell (eds.), *Principals of Neural Science* (4th ed.). New York: McGraw-Hill, pp. 832–852.

Gibson, J.E. (1963). *Nonlinear Automatic Control.* New York: McGraw-Hill, pp. 491–547.

Gilbert, P.F.C. (1974). A theory of memory that explains the function and structure of the cerebellum. *Brain Res.* 709: 1–18.

Gilbert, P.F.C., and Thach, W.T. (1977). Purkinje cell activity during motor learning. *Brain Res.* 128: 309–328.

Gilbert, P.F.C., and Yeo, C.H. (1992). Cerebellar function: on-line control and learning. *Behav. Brain Sci.* 15: 743–744.

Gilman, S., Bloedel, J.R., and Lechtenberg, R. (1981). *Disorders of the Cerebellum.* Philadelphia: F.A. Davis.

Glickstein, M. (1993). Motor skills but not cognitive tasks. *Trends Neurosci.* 16: 450–451.

Glickstein, M. (1997). Mossy-fibre sensory input to the cerebellum. *Progr. Brain Res.* 114: 251–259.

Gluck, M.A., Reifsnider, E.S., and Thompson, R.F. (1990). Adaptive signal processing and the Cb: models of classical conditioning and VOR adaptation. In M.A. Gluck and D.E.

Rumelhart (eds.), *Neuroscience and Connectionist Theory*. Hillsdale, NJ: Lawrence Erlbaum Associates, pp. 131–185.

Goldberg, M.E., Musil, S.Y., Fitzgibbon, E.J., Smith, M., and Olson, C.R. (1993). The role of the cerebellum in the control of saccadic eye movements. In N. Mano, I. Hamada, and M.R. DeLong (eds.), *Role of the Cerebellum and Basal Ganglia in Voluntary Movement*. Amsterdam: Elsevier Science Publishers, pp. 203–211.

Goldman-Rakic, P.S. (1995). Neurobiology of mental representation. In H. Morowitz and J.L. Singer (eds.), *The Mind, The Brain, and Complex Adaptive Systems*. Reading, MA: Addison-Wesley, pp. 51–63.

Goldowitz, D., and Hamre, K. (1998). The cells and molecules that make a cerebellum. *Trends Neurosci.* 21: 375–382.

Gomi, H., and Kawato, M. (1992). Adaptive feedback control models of the vestibulocerebellum and spinocerebellum. *Biol. Cybern.* 68: 105–114.

Gomi, H., Shidara, M., Takemura, A., Inoue, Y., Kawano, K., and Kawato, M. (1998). Temporal firing patterns of Purkinje cells in the cerebellar ventral paraflocculus during ocular following responses in monkeys I. Simple spikes. *J. Neurophysiol.* 80: 818–831.

Gould, B.B. (1979). The organization of afferents to the cerebellar cortex in the cat: projections from the deep cerebellar nuclei. *J. Comp. Neurol.* 184: 27–42.

Gould, B.B., and Graybiel, A.M. (1976). Afferents to the cerebellar cortex in the cat: evidence for an intrinsic pathway leading from the deep nuclei to the cortex. *Brain Res.* 110: 601–611.

Graf, W., Simpson, J.I., and Leonard, C.S. (1989). A synthesis of input–output relationships of the rabbit flocculus. In: P. Strata (ed.), *The Olivocerebellar System in Motor Control*. New York: Springer-Verlag, pp. 338–344.

Gravel, C., Leclerc, N., Rafrafi, J., Sasseville, R., Thivierge, L., and Hawkes, R. (1987). Monoclonal antibodies reveal the global organization of the cerebellar cortex. *J. Neurosci. Methods* 21: 145–157.

Gray, C., Perciavalle, V., and Poppele, R. (1993). Sensory responses to passive hindlimb joint rotation in the cerebellar cortex of the cat. *Brain Res.* 622: 280–284.

Graybiel, A.M., Nauta, H.J.W., Lasek, R.J., and Nauta, W.J.H. (1973). A cerebello-olivary pathway in the cat: an experimental study using autoradiographic tracing techniques. *Brain Res.* 58: 205–211.

Green, J.T., and Woodruff-Pak, D.S. (2000). Eyeblink classical conditioning: hippocampal formation is for neutral stimulus associations as cerebellum is for association-response. *Psychol. Bull.* 126: 138–158.

Grinvald, A., Frostig, R.D., Lieke, E., and Hildesheim, R. (1988). Optical imaging of neuronal activity. *Physiol. Rev.* 68: 1285–1366.

Groenewegen, H.J., and Voogd, J. (1977). The parasagittal zonation within the olivocerebellar projection. I. Climbing fiber distribution in the vermis of cat cerebellum. *J. Comp. Neurol.* 174: 417–488.

Groenewegen, H.J., Voogd, J., and Freedman, S.L. (1979). The parasagittal zonation within the olivo-cerebellar projection. II. Climbing fiber distribution in the intermediate and hemispheric parts of cat cerebellum. *J. Comp. Neurol.* 183: 551–602.

Grossberg, S. (1969). On learning of spatiotemporal patterns by networks with ordered sensory and motor components 1. Excitatory components of the cerebellum. *Stud. Appl. Math* 48: 123–132.

Gupta, M.M., and Rao, D.H. (1994). *Neuro-Control Systems: Theory and Applications*. New York: The Institute of Electrical and Electronics Engineers, pp. 1–43.

Haines, D.E. (1989). HRP study of cerebellar corticonuclear-nucleocortical topography of the dorsal culminate lobule – lobule V – in a prosimian primate *(Galago)*: with comments on nucleocortical cell types. *J. Comp. Neurol.* 282: 274–292.

Haines, D.E., and Pearson, J.C. (1979). Cerebellar corticonuclear-nucleocortical topography: study of the tree shrew *(Tupaia)* paraflocculus. *J. Comp. Neurol.* 187: 745–758.

Hallett, M., Berardelli, A., Matheson, J., Rothwell, J., and Marsden, C.D. (1991). Physiological analysis of simple rapid movements in patients with cerebellar deficits. *J. Neurol. Neurosurg. Psychiatry.* 53: 124–133.

Hallett, M., Pascual-Leone, A., and Topka, H. (1996). Adaptation and skill learning: evidence for different neural substrates. In: J.R. Bloedel, T.J. Ebner, and S.P. Wise (eds.), *The Acquisition of Motor Behavior in Vertebrates.* Cambridge, MA: MIT Press, pp. 289–301.

Hallett, M., Shahani, B.T., and Young, R.R. (1975a). EMG analysis of stereotyped voluntary movements. *J. Neurol. Neurosurg. Psychiatry* 38: 1154–1162.

Hallett, M., Shahani, B.T., and Young, R.R. (1975b). EMG analysis of patients with cerebellar deficits. *J. Neurol. Neurosurg. Psychiatry* 38: 1163–1169.

Hamori, J., and Szentágothai, J. (1966). Identification under the electron microscope of climbing fibers and their synaptic contacts. *Exp. Brain Res.* 1: 65–81.

Hámori, J., and Takács, J. (1989). Two types of GABA-containing axon terminals in cerebellar glomeruli of cat: an immunogold-EM study. *Exp. Brain Res.* 74: 471–479.

Hámori, J., Takács, J., and Petrusz, P. (1996). Immunogold electron microscopic demonstration of glutamate and GABA in normal and deafferented cerebellar cortex: correlation between transmitter content and synaptic vesicle size. *J. Histochem. Cytochem.* 38: 1767–1777.

Hansel, C., and Linden, D.J. (2000). Long-term depression of the cerebellar climbing fiber–Purkinje neuron synapse. *Neuron* 26: 475–482.

Hanson, C.L., Chen, G., and Ebner, T.J. (2000). Role of climbing fibers in determining the spatial patterns of activation in the cerebellar cortex to peripheral stimulation: an optical imaging study. *Neuroscience.* 96: 317–331.

Harrington, D.L., and Haaland, K.Y. (1999). Neural underpinnings of temporal processing: a review of focal lesion, pharmacological, and functional imaging research. *Rev. Neurosci.* 10: 91–116.

Hartel, N.A. (1994). Induction of cerebellar long-term depression requires activation of glutamate metabotropic receptors. *Neuroreport* 5: 913–916.

Haruno, M., Wolpert, D.M., and Kawato, M. (1999). Multiple paired forward-inverse models for human motor learning and control. *Adv. Neural. Inf. Proc. Sys.* 11: 31–37.

Harvey, R.J., and Napper, R.M.A. (1988). Quantitative study of granular and Purkinje cells in the cerebellar cortex of the rat. *J. Comp. Neurol.* 274: 151–157.

Hashimoto, K., Watanabe, M., Kurihara, H., Offermanns, S., Jiang, H., Wu, Y., Jun, K., Shin, H.-S., Inoue, Y., Wu, D., Simon, M.I., and Kan, M. (2000). Climbing fiber synapse elimination during postnatal cerebellar development requires signal transduction involving $G\alpha q$ and phospholipase $C\beta 4$. *Progr. Brain Res.* 124: 31–48.

Hassul, M., and Daniels, P.D. (1977). Cerebellar dynamics: the mossy fiber input. *IEEE Trans. Biomed. Eng.* BME-24: 449–456.

Hawkes, R. (1997). An anatomical model of cerebellar modules. *Progr. Brain Res.* 114: 39–52.

Hawkes, R., and Eisenman, L.M. (1997). Stripes and zones: the origins of regionalization of the adult cerebellum. *Perspect. Dev. Neurobiol.* 5: 95–105.

Haykin, S. (1994). *Neural Networks: A Comprehensive Foundation* (2nd ed.). New York: Macmillan.

Haykin, S. (1995). Adaptive signal processing. In: M.A. Arbib (ed.), *The Handbook of Brain Theory and Neural Networks.* Cambridge, MA: MIT Press, pp. 82–85.

Haykin, S. (1996). *Adaptive Filter Theory* (3rd ed.). Upper Saddle River, NJ: Prentice Hall.

Hebb, D.O. (1949). *The Organization of Behaviour.* New York: John Wiley.

Heidary, H., and Tomasch, J. (1969). Neuron numbers and perikaryon areas in the human cerebellar nuclei. *Acta Anat.* 74: 290–296.

Helmuth, L.I., Ivry, R.B., and Shimizu, N. (1997). Preserved performance by cerebellar patients on tests of word generation, discrimination learning, and attention. *Learn. Mem.* 3: 456–474.

Hémart, N., Daniel, H., Jaillard, D., and Crépel, F. (1994). Properties of glutamate receptors are modified during long-term depression in rat cerebellar Purkinje cells. *Neurosci. Res.* 19: 213–221.

Hémart, N., Daniel, H., Jaillard, D., and Crépel, F. (1995). Receptors and second messengers involved in long-term depression in rat cerebellar slices in vitro: a reappraisal. *Eur. J. Neurosci.* 7: 45–53.

Herndon, R.H. (1963). The fine structure of the Purkinje cell. *J. Cell. Biol.* 18: 167–180.

Herrick, C.J. (1924a). *Neurological Foundations of Animal Behavior.* New York: Henry Holt.

Herrick, C.J. (1924b). Origin and evolution of the cerebellum. *Arch. Neurol. Psychiatry* 11: 621–652.

Hirano, T. (1990a). Depression and potentiation of the synaptic transmission between a granule cell and a Purkinje cell in rat cerebellar tissue. *Neurosci. Lett.* 119: 141–144.

Hirano, T. (1990b). Effects of postsynaptic depolarization in the induction of synaptic depression between a granule cell and a Purkinje cell in rat cerebellar culture. *Neurosci. Lett.* 119: 145–147.

Holdefer, R.N., Miller, L.E., Chen, L.L., and Houk, J.C. (2000). Functional connectivity between cerebellum and primary motor cortex in the awake monkey. *J. Neurophysiol.* 84: 585–590.

Holland, J.H. (1995). Can there be a unified theory of complex adaptive systems? In: H. Morowitz and J.L. Singer (eds.), *The Mind, The Brain, and Complex Adaptive Systems.* Reading, MA: Addison-Wesley, pp. 45–50.

Holmes, G. (1939). The cerebellum of man. *Brain* 62: 1–30.

Hopfield, J.J. (1982). Neural networks and physical systems with emergent collective computational abilities. *Proc. Natl. Acad. Sci. USA* 79: 2554–2558.

Hore, J., Wild, B., and Diener, H.-C. (1991). Cerebellar dysmetria at the elbow, wrist, and fingers. *J. Neurophysiol.* 65: 563–571.

Horn, K.M., van Kan, P.L.E., and Ruigrok, T.J.H. (1996). Inferior olive sensitivity is reduced by increased cerebellar output. *Soc. Neurosci. Abstr.* 22: 1092.

Horne, M.K., and Butler, E.G. (1995). The role of the cerebello-thalamo-cortical pathway in skilled movement. *Progr. Neurobiol.* 46: 199–213.

Houk, J.C. (1987). Model of the cerebellum as an array of adjustable pattern generators. In: M. Glickstein, C. Yeo, and J. Stein (eds.), *Cerebellum and Neuronal Plasticity.* New York: Plenum, pp. 249–260.

Houk, J.C., and Wise, S.P. (1995). Distributed modular architectures linking basal ganglia, cerebellum, and cerebral cortex: their role in planning and controlling action. *Cereb. Cortex* 5: 95–110.

Houk, J.C., Buckingham, J.T., and Barto, A.G. (1996). Models of the cerebellum and motor learning. *Behav. Brain Sci.* 19: 368–383.

Houk, J.C., Keifer, J., and Barto, A.G. (1993). Distributed motor commands in the limb premotor network. *Trends Neurosci.* 16: 27–33.

Houk, J.C., Singh, S.P., Fisher, C., and Barto, A.G. (1990). An adaptive sensorimotor network inspired by the anatomy and physiology of the cerebellum. In: W.T. Miller, R.S. Sutton, and P.J. Werbos (eds.), *Neural Networks for Control.* Cambridge, MA: MIT Press, pp. 301–348.

Imamizu, H., Miyauchi, S., Tamada, T., Sasaki, Y., Takino, R., Pütz, B., Yoshioka, T., and Kawato, M. (2000). Human cerebellar activity reflecting an acquired internal model of a new tool. *Nature* 403: 192–195.

Ioannou, P.A., and Sun, J. (1996). *Robust Adaptive Control.* Upper Saddle River, NJ: Prentice-Hall, p. 27.

Isermann, R., Lachmann, K.-H., and Matko, D. (1992). *Adaptive Control Systems.* New York: Prentice Hall.

Ito, M. (1970). Neurophysiological aspects of the cerebellar motor control system. *Int. J. Neurol. (Montevideo)* 7: 162–176.

Ito, M. (1972). Neural design of the cerebellar motor control system. *Brain Res.* 40: 81–84.

Ito, M. (1976a). Adaptive control of reflexes by the cerebellum. *Progr. Brain Res.* 44: 436–444.

Ito, M. (1976b). Cerebellar learning control of vestibulo-ocular mechanisms. In T. Desiraju (Ed.), *Mechanisms in Transmission of Signals for Conscious Behavior.* Amsterdam: Elsevier, pp. 1–22.

Ito, M. (1979). Is the cerebellum really a computer? *Trends Neurosci.* 2: 122–126.

Ito, M. (1982a). Cerebellar control of the vestibulo-ocular reflex – around the flocculus hypothesis. *Annu. Rev. Neurosci.* 5: 275–296.

Ito, M. (1982b). Questions in modeling the cerebellum. *J. Theoret. Biol.* 99: 81–86.

Ito, M. (1984). *The Cerebellum and Neural Control.* New York: Raven.

Ito, M. (1989). Long-term depression. *Annu. Rev. Neurosci.* 12: 85–102.

Ito, M. (1990). A new physiological concept on cerebellum. *Rev. Neurol. (Paris)* 146: 564–569.

Ito, M. (1993a). Cerebellar flocculus hypothesis (letter). *Nature* 363: 24–25.

Ito, M. (1993b). Neurophysiology of the nodulofloccular system. *Rev. Neurol. (Paris)* 149: 692–697.

Ito, M. (1993c). Movement and thought: identical control mechanisms by the cerebellum. *Trends Neurosci.* 16:448–450.

Ito, M. (1993d). Synaptic plasticity in the cerebellar cortex and its role in motor learning. *Can. J. Neurol. Sci.* 20 (suppl. 3): S70–S74.

Ito, M. (1996). Letter to the editor. *Trends Neurosci.* 19: 11–12.

Ito, M. (1998). Cerebellar learning in the vestibulo-ocular reflex. *Trends Cogn. Sci.* 2: 313–321.

Ito, M. (1999). The cerebellum, a gateway to modern neuroscience. *Brain Res. Bull.* 30: 33.

Ito, M. (2000). Neurobiology: internal model visualized. *Nature* 403: 153–154.

Ito, M., and Kano, M. (1982). Long-lasting depression of parallel fiber–Purkinje cell transmission induced by conjunctive stimulation of parallel fibers and climbing fibers in the cerebellar cortex. *Neurosci. Lett.* 33: 253–258.

Ito, M., Sakurai, M, and Tongroach, P. (1982). Climbing fibre induced depression of both mossy fibre responsiveness and glutamate sensitivity of cerebellar Purkinje cells. *J. Physiol. (Lond.)* 324: 113–134.

Ivry, R. (1993). Cerebellar involvement in the explicit representation of temporal information. *Ann. N. Y. Acad. Sci.* 682: 214–230.

Ivry, R.B. (1996). The representation of temporal information in perception and motor control. *Curr. Opin. Neurobiol.* 6: 851–857.

Ivry, R.B., and Diener, H.C. (1991). Impaired velocity perception in patients with lesions of the cerebellum. *J. Cogn. Neurosci.* 3: 355–366.

Ivry, R.B., and Fiez, J.A. (2000). Cerebellar contributions to cognition and imagery. In: M.S. Gazzaniga (ed.), *The New Cognitive Neurosciences.* Cambridge, MA: MIT Press, pp. 999–1011.

Ivry, R.B., and Keele, S.W. (1989). Timing functions of the cerebellum. *J. Cogn. Neurosci.* 1: 136–152.

Jeannerod, M., Arbib, M.A., Rizzolatti, G., and Sakata, H. (1995). Grasping objects: the cortical mechanisms of visuomotor transformation. *Trends Neurosci.* 18: 314–320.

Jenkins, I.H., Brooks, D.J., Nixon, P.D., Frackowiak, R.S.J., and Passingham, R.E. (1994). Motor sequence learning: a study with positron emission tomography. *J. Neurosci.* 14: 3775–3790.

Ji Z., Jin Q., and Vogel, M.W. (1997). Evidence of spinocerebellar mossy fiber segregation in the juvenile staggerer cerebellum. *J. Comp. Neurol.* 378: 354–362.

Jones, A., Paterlini, M., Wisden, W., and Merlo, D. (2000). Transgenic methods for directing gene expression to specific neuronal types: cerebellar granule cells. *Progr. Brain Res.* 124: 69–80.

Jordan, M.I., and Wolpert, D.M. (2000). Computational motor control. In M.S. Gazzaniga (ed.), *The New Cognitive Neurosciences.* Cambridge, MA: MIT Press, pp. 601–618.

Jueptner, M., and Weiller, C. (1998). A review of differences between basal ganglia and cerebellar control of movements as revealed by functional imaging studies. *Brain* 121:1437–1449.

Jueptner, M., Ottinger, S., Fellows, S.J., Adamschewski, J., Flerich, L., Müller, S.P., Diener, H.C., Thilmann, A.F., and Weiller, C. (1997). The relevance of sensory input for the cerebellar control of movements. *Neuroimage* 5: 41–48.

Jueptner, M.R., Rijntjes M., Weiller, C., Faiss, J.H., Timmann, D., Mueller, S.P., and Diener, H.C. (1995). Localization of a cerebellar timing process using PET. *Neurology* 45: 1540–1545.

Kaiserman-Abramof, I.R., and Palay, S.L. (1969). Fine structural studies of the cerebellar cortex in a mormyrid fish. In: R. Llinás (ed.), *Neurobiology of Cerebellar Evolution and Development*. Chicago: American Medical Association Educational and Research Foundation, pp. 171–205.

Kalil, K. (1979). Projections of the cerebellar and dorsal column nuclei upon the inferior olive of the rhesus monkey: an autoradiographic study. *J. Comp. Neurol.* 188: 43–62.

Kalman, R.E. (1960). A new approach to linear filtering and prediction problems. *J. Basic Eng. (ASME Trans. Ser. D)* 82: 35–45.

Kalman, R.E., and Bucy, R.S. (1961). New results in linear filtering and prediction theory. *J. Basic Eng. (ASME Trans. Ser. D)* 83: 95–108.

Kandel, E.R., Schwartz, J.H., and Jessell, T.M. (1991). *Principles of Neural Science* (3rd ed.). New York: Elsevier.

Kano, M. (1996). Long-lasting potentiation of GABAergic inhibitory synaptic transmission in cerebellar Purkinje cells: its properties and possible mechanisms. *Behav. Brain Sci.* 19: 354–361.

Kano, M., Hashimoto, K., Chen, C, Abeliovich, A., Aiba, A., Kurihara, H., Watanabe, M., Inoue, Y., and Tonegawa, S. (1995). Impaired synapse elimination during cerebellar development in PKC_{gamma} mutant mice. *Cell* 83: 1223–1231.

Kano, M., Hashimoto, K., Kurihara, H., Watanabe, M., Inoue, Y., Aiba, A., and Tonegawa, S. (1997). Persistent multiple climbing fiber innervation of cerebellar Purkinje cells in mice lacking mGluRl. *Neuron* 18: 71–79.

Kano, M., Rexhausen, U., Dreessen, J, and Konnerth, A. (1992). Synaptic excitation produces a long-lasting rebound potentiation of inhibitory synaptic signals in cerebellar cells. *Nature* 356: 601–604.

Kashiwabuchi, N., Ikeda, K., Araki, K., Hirano, T., Shibuki, K., Takayama, C., Inoue, Y., Kutsuwada, T., Yasgi, T., Kang, Y., Aizawa, S., and Mishina, M. (1995). Impairment of motor coordination, Purkinje cell synapse formation, and long-term-depression in GluRδ2 mutant mice. *Cell* 81: 245–252.

Katz, D.B., and Steinmetz, J.E. (1997). Single-unit evidence for eye-blink conditioning in cerebellar cortex is altered, but not eliminated, by interpositus nucleus lesions. *Learn. Mem.* 3: 88–104.

Kaufman, G.D., Mustarl, M.J., Miselis, R.R., and Perachio, A.A. (1996). Transneuronal pathways to the vestibulocerebellum. *J. Comp. Neurol.* 370: 501–523.

Kawano, K., and Shidara, M. (1993). The role of the ventral paraflocculus in ocular following in the monkey. In: N. Mano, I. Hamada, and M.R. DeLong (eds.), *Role of the Cerebellum and Basal Ganglia in Voluntary Movement*. Amsterdam: Elsevier, pp. 195–202.

Kawano, K., Shidara, M., Takemura, A., Inoue, Y., Gomi, H., and Kawato, M. (1996). Inverse-dynamics representation of eye movements by cerebellar Purkinje cell activity during short-latency ocular-following responses. *Ann. N. Y. Acad. Sci.* 781: 314–319.

Kawano, K., Takemura, A., Inoue, Y., Kitama, T, Kobayashi, Y., and Mustari, M.J. (1996). Visual inputs to cerebellar ventral paraflocculus during ocular following responses. *Progr. Brain Res.* 112: 415–422.

Kawato, M. (1990a). Computational schemes and neural network models for formation and control of multijoint arm trajectory. In W.T. Miller III, R.S. Sutton, and P.J. Werbos (eds.), *Neural Networks for Control*. Cambridge, MA: MIT Press, pp. 197–228.

Kawato, M. (1990b). Feedback-error-learning neural network for supervised motor learning. In R. Eckmiller (ed.), *Advanced Neural Computers*. Amsterdam: Elsevier, pp. 365–372.

Kawato, M. (1993). Optimization and learning in neural networks for formation and control of coordinated movement. In D.E. Meyer and S. Kornblum (eds.), *Attention and Performance XIV. Synergies in Experimental Psychology, Artificial Intelligence, and Cognitive Neuroscience*, Cambridge, MA: MIT Press, pp. 821–849.

Kawato, M. (1995). Cerebellum and motor control. In M.A. Arbib (ed.), *The Handbook of Brain Theory and Neural Networks*. Cambridge, MA: MIT Press, pp. 172–178.

Kawato, M. (1996a). Learning internal models of the motor apparatus. In J.R. Bloedel, T.J. Ebner, and S.P. Wise (eds.), *The Acquisition of Motor Behavior in Vertebrates*. Cambridge, MA: MIT Press, pp. 409–430.

Kawato, M. (1996b). The common inverse-dynamics motor command coordinates for complex and simple spikes. *Behav. Brain Sci.* 19: 462–464.

Kawato, M. (1997). Bidirectional theory approach to consciousness. In M. Ito, Y. Miyashita, and E.T. Rolls (eds.), *Cognition, Computation, and Consciousness*. Oxford, England: Oxford University Press, pp. 233–248.

Kawato, M. (1999). Internal models for motor control and trajectory planning. *Curr. Opin. Neurobiol.* 9: 718–727.

Kawato, M., and Gomi, H. (1992a). A computational model of four regions of the cerebellum based on feedback-error learning. *Biol. Cybern.* 68: 95–103.

Kawato, M., and Gomi, H. (1992b). The cerebellum and VOR/OKR learning models. *Trends Neurosci.* 15: 445–453.

Kawato, M., and Gomi, H. (1993). Feedback-error-learning model of cerebellar motor control. In: Mano, N., Hamada, I., and DeLong, M.R. (eds.), *Role of the Cerebellum and Basal Ganglia in Voluntary Movement*. Amsterdam: Elsevier, pp. 51–61.

Kawato, M., and Wolpert, D. (1998). Internal models for motor control. *Novartis Found. Symp.* 218: 291–307.

Kawato, M., Furukawa, K., and Suzuki, R. (1987). A hierarchical neural-network model for control and learning of voluntary movement. *Biol. Cybern.* 57: 169–185.

Keating, J.G., and Thach, W.T. (1995). Nonclock behavior of inferior olive neurons: interspike interval of Purkinje cell complex spike discharge in the awake behaving monkey is random. *J. Neurophysiol.* 75: 1329–1340.

Keating, J.G., and Thach, W.T. (1996). Non-clock-like discharge of cells in the deep cerebellar nuclei of the awake behaving monkey. *Soc. Neurosci. Abstr.* 22: 1092.

Keele, S.W., and Ivry, R. (1990). Does the cerebellum provide a common computation for diverse tasks? A timing hypothesis. *Ann. N. Y. Acad. Sci.* 608: 179–211.

Keifer, J., and Houk, J. (1994). Motor functions of the cerebellorubrospinal system. *Physiol. Rev.* 74: 509–542.

Kenyon, G.T. (1997). A model of long-term memory storage in the cerebellar cortex: a possible role for plasticity at parallel fiber synapses onto stellate/basket interneurons. *Proc. Natl. Acad. Sci. USA* 94: 14200–14205.

Kenyon, G.T., Medina, J.F., and Mauk, M.D. (1998a). A mathematical model of the cerebellar-olivary system I: self-regulating equilibrium of climbing fiber activity. *J. Comput. Neurosci.* 5: 17–33.

Kenyon, G.T., Medina, J.F., and Mauk, M.D. (1998b). A mathematical model of the cerebellar-olivary system II: adaptation through systematic disruption of climbing fiber equilibrium. *J. Comput. Neurosci.* 5: 71–90.

Kettner, R.E., Mahamud, S., Leung, H.-C., Sitkoff, N., Houk, J.C., Peterson, B.W., and Barto, A.G. (1997). Prediction of complex two-dimensional trajectories by a cerebellar model of smooth pursuit eye movement. *J. Neurophysiol.* 77: 2115–2130.

Kim, J.J., and Thompson, R.F. (1997). Cerebellar circuits and synaptic mechanisms involved in classical eyeblink conditioning. *Trends. Neurosci.* 20: 177–181.

Kim, S.-G., Ugurbil, K., and Strick, P.L. (1994). Activation of a cerebellar output nucleus during cognitive processing. *Science* 265: 949–951.

King, J.S. (1980). Synaptic organization of the inferior olivary complex. In J. Courville, C. de Montigny and Y. Lamarre (eds.), *The Inferior Olivary Nucleus: Anatomy and Physiology*. New York: Raven Press, pp. 1–32.

Kistler, W.M., and van Hemmen, J.L. (2000). Modeling synaptic plasticity in conjunction with the timing of pre- and postsynaptic action potentials. *Neural Comput.* 12: 385–405.

Kitazawa, S., Kimura, T., and Yin, P-B. (1998). Cerebellar complex spikes encode both destinations and error in arm movements. *Nature* 392: 494–497.

Kitzman, P.H., and Bishop, G.A. (1997). The physiological effects of serotonin on spontaneous and amino acid-induced activation of cerebellar nuclear cells: an in vivo study in the cat. *Progr. Brain Res.* 114: 209–223.

Kobayashi, Y., Kawano, K., Takemura, A., Inoue, Y., Kitama, T., Gomi, H., and Kawato, M. (1998). Temporal firing patterns of Purkinje cells in the cerebellar ventral paraflocculus during ocular following responses in monkeys II. Complex spikes. *J. Neurophysiol.* 80: 832–848.

Kolb, F.P., Irwin, K.B., Bloedel, J.R., and Bracha, V. (1997). Conditioned and unconditioned forelimb reflex systems in the cat: involvement of the intermediate cerebellum. *Exp. Brain Res.* 114: 255–270.

Kolston, J., Apps, R., and Trott, J.R. (1995). A combined retrograde tracer and GABA-immunocytochemical study of the projection from nucleus interpositus posterior to the posterior lobe c_2 zone of the cat cerebellum. *Eur. J. Neurosci.* 7: 926–933.

Konnerth, A., Dreessen, J., and Augustine, G.J. (1992). Brief dendritic calcium signals initiate long-lasting synaptic depression in cerebellar Purkinje cells. *Proc. Natl. Acad. Sci. USA* 89: 7051–7055.

Kornhuber, H.H. (1971). Motor functions of cerebellum and basal ganglia: the cerebellocortical saccadic (ballistic) clock, the cerebellonuclear hold regulator, and the basal ganglia ramp (voluntary speed smooth movement) generator. *Biol. Cybern.* 8: 157–162.

Kornhuber, H.H. (1974). Cerebral cortex, cerebellum, and basal ganglia: an introduction to their motor functions. In F.O. Schmitt and F.G. Worden (eds.), *The Neurosciences: Third Study Program*. Cambridge, MA: MIT Press, pp. 267–280.

Krupa, D.J., and Thompson, R.F. (1997). Reversible inactivation of the cerebellar interpositus nucleus completely prevents acquisition of the classically conditioned eye-blink response. *Learn. Mem.* 3: 545–556.

Kurihara, H., Hashimoto, K., Kano, M., Takayama, C., Sakimura, K., Mishina, M., Inoue, Y., and Watanabe, M. (1997). Impaired parallel fiber–Purkinje cell synapse stabilization during cerebellar development of mutant mice lacking the glutamate receptor ∂2 subunit. *J. Neurosci.* 17: 9613–9623.

Lalonde, R. (1994). Cerebellar contributions to instrumental learning. *Neurosci. Biobehav. Rev.* 18: 161–170.

Lalonde, R., and Botez-Marquard, T. (1997). The neurobiological basis of movement initiation. *Rev. Neurosci.* 8: 35–54.

Lalonde, R., and Hannequin, D. (1999). The neurobiological basis of time estimation and temporal order. *Rev. Neurosci.* 10: 151–173.

Landau, I.D., Lozano, R., and M'Saad, M. (1998). *Adaptive Control*. Berlin: Springer.

Lang, E.J., Sugihara, I., and Llinás, R. (1996). GABAergic modulation of complex spike activity by the cerebellar nucleoolivary pathway in rat. *J. Neurophysiol.* 76: 255–275.

Lansner, A., and Ekeberg, Ö. (1994). Neuronal network models of motor generation and control. *Curr. Opin. Neurobiol.* 4: 903–908.

Larsell, O. (1967). *The Comparative Anatomy and Histology of the Cerebellum* (2 vols.) Minneapolis: University of Minnesota Press.

Larsell, O., and Jansen, J. (1972). *The Comparative Anatomy and Histology of the Cerebellum: The Human Cerebellum, Cerebellar Connections, and Cerebellar Cortex*. Minneapolis: University of Minnesota Press.

Lasser-Ross, N., and Ross, W.N. (1992). Imaging voltage and synaptically activated sodium transients in cerebellar Purkinje cells. *Proc. Roy. Soc. Lond. B* 247: 35–39.

Lee, M., and Bower, J.M. (1990). A computer modeling approach to understanding the inferior olive and its relationship to the cerebellar cortex in rats. In: D.S. Touretsky (ed.), *Advances in Neural Information Processing Systems 2*. San Mateo, CA: Morgan Kaufmann Publishers, pp. 117–124.

Le Marec, N., and Lalonde, R. (2000). Treadmill performance of mice with cerebellar lesions 2: lurcher mutants. *Neurobiol. Learn. Mem.* 75: 195–206.

Legendre, A., and Courville, J. (1987). Origin and trajectory of the cerebello-olivary projection: an experimental study with radioactive and fluorescent tracers in the cat. *Neuroscience* 21: 877–891.

Leiner, H.C., and Leiner, A.L. (1997). How fibers subserve computing capabilities: similarities between brains and machines. *Int. Rev. Neurobiol.* 41: 535–553.

Leiner, H.C., Leiner, A.L. and Dow, R.S. (1986). Does the cerebellum contribute to mental skills? *Behav. Neurosci.* 100: 443–454.

Leiner, H.C., Leiner, A.L., and Dow, R.S. (1987). Cerebro-cerebellar learning loops in apes and humans. *Ital. J. Neurol. Sci.* 8: 425–436.

Leiner, H. C., Leiner, A.L., and Dow, R.S. (1991). The human cerebro-cerebellar system: its computing, cognitive, and language skills. *Behav. Brain Res.* 44: 113–128.

Leiner, H.C., Leiner, A.L., and Dow, R.S. (1993a). Cognitive and language functions of the human cerebrum. *Trends Neurosci.* 16: 444–447.

Leiner, H.C., Leiner, A.L., and Dow, R.S. (1993b). The role of the cerebellum in the human brain (reply). *Trends Neurosci.* 16: 453–454.

Lev-Ram, Jiang, T., Wood, J., Lawrence, D.S., and Tsien, R.Y. (1997). Synergies and coincidence requirements between NO, cGMP, and CA^{2+} in the induction of cerebellar long-term depression. *Neuron* 18: 1025–1038.

Lev-Ram, V., Nebyelul, Z., Ellisman, M.H., Huang, P.L., and Tsien, R.Y. (1997). Absence of cerebellar long-term depression in mice lacking neuronal nitric oxide synthase. *Learn. Mem.* 3: 169–177.

Linden, D.J. (1996a). A protein synthesis-dependent late phase of cerebellar long-term depression. *Neuron* 17: 483–490.

Linden, D.J. (1996b). Cerebellar long-term depression as investigated in a cell culture preparation. *Behav. Brain Sci.* 19: 339–346.

Linden, D.J. (1998). Synaptically evoked glutamate transport currents may be used to detect the expression of long-term potentiation in cerebellar culture. *J. Neurophysiol.* 79: 3151–3156.

Linden, D.J., and Connor, J.A. (1993). Cellular mechanisms of long-term depression in the cerebellum. *Curr. Opin. Neurobiol.* 3: 401–406.

Linden, D.J., and Connor, J.A. (1995). Long-term synaptic depression. *Annu. Rev. Neurosci.* 18: 319–357.

Linden, D.J., Dawson, T.M., and Dawson, V.L. (1995). An evaluation of the nitric oxide/cGMP/cGMP-dependent protein kinase cascade in the induction of cerebellar long-term depression in culture. *J. Neurosci.* 15: 5098–5105.

Linden, D.J., Smeyne, M., and Connor, J.A. (1993). Induction of cerebellar long-term depression in culture requires postsynaptic action of sodium ions. *Neuron* 11: 1093–1100.

Lisberger, S.G. (1994). Neural basis for motor learning in the vestibulo-ocular reflex of primates. III. Computational and behavioral analysis of the sites of learning. *J. Neurophysiol.* 72: 974–998.

Lisberger, S.G. (1996). Motor learning and memory in the vestibulo-ocular reflex: the dark side. *Ann. N. Y. Acad. Sci.* 781: 525–531.

Lisberger, S.G. (1995). A mechanism of learning found? *Curr. Biol.* 5: 221–224.

Lisberger, S.G., and Fuchs, A.F. (1978a). Role of primate flocculus during rapid behavioral modification of vestibuloocular reflex. I. Purkinje cell activity during visually guided horizontal smooth-pursuit eye movements and passive head rotation. *J. Neurophysiol.* 41: 733–763.

Lisberger, S.G., and Fuchs, A.F. (1978b). Role of primate flocculus during rapid behavioral modification of vestibuloocular reflex. II. Mossy fiber firing patterns during horizontal head rotation and eye movement. *J. Neurophysiol.* 41: 764–777.

Lisberger, S.G., and Seijnowski, T.J. (1992). Motor learning in a recurrent network model based on the vestibulo-ocular reflex. *Nature* 360: 159–161.

Lisberger, S.G., and Seijnowski, T.J. (1993). Cerebellar flocculus hypothesis (letter). *Nature* 363: 24–25.

Lisberger, S.G., Pavelko, T.A., and Broussard, D.M. (1994). Neural basis for motor learning in the vestibuloocular reflex of primates. I. Changes in the responses of brain stem neurons. *J. Neurophysiol.* 72: 928–953.

Lisberger, S.G., Pavelko, T.A., Bronte-Stewart, H.M., and Stone, L.S. (1994). Neural basis for motor learning in the vestibulo-ocular reflex of primates. II. Changes in the responses of horizontal gaze velocity Purkinje cells in the cerebellar flocculus and ventral paraflocculus. *J. Neurophysiol.* 72: 954–973.

Llinás, R. (1969). (ed.). *Neurobiology of Cerebellar Evolution and Development.* Chicago: American Medical Association Educational and Research Foundation.

Llinás, R. (1981a). Cerebellar modelling. *Nature* 291: 279–280.

Llinás, R. (1981b). Electrophysiology of the cerebellar networks. In V.B. Brooks (ed.), *Handbook of Physiology, Vol. II, Motor Control, Part 2.* Bethesda: American Physiological Society, pp. 831–876.

Llinás, R. (1982). Discussion of Tolbert, D.L. (1982). The cerebellar nucleocortical pathway. In S.L. Palay and V. Chan-Palay (eds.), *The Cerebellum, New Vistas.* Berlin: Springer-Verlag, pp. 296–319.

Llinás, R. (1995). Thorny issues in neurons. *Nature* 373: 107–108.

Llinás, R., and Hillman, D.E. (1969). Physiological and morphological organization of the cerebellar circuits in various vertebrates. In R. Llinás (ed.), *Neurobiology of Cerebellar Evolution and Development.* Chicago: American Medical Association Educational and Research Foundation, pp. 43–73.

Llinás, R., and Mühlethaler, M. (1988). Electrophysiology of guinea-pig cerebellar nuclear cells in the in vitro brain stem-cerebellar preparation. *J. Physiol. (Lond.)* 404: 241–258.

Llinás, R., and Sugimori, M. (1980a). Electrophysiological properties of in vitro Purkinje cell somata in mammalian cerebellar slices. *J. Physiol.* 305: 171–195.

Llinás, R., and Sugimori, M. (1980b). Electrophysiological properties of in vitro Purkinje cell dendrites in mammalian cerebellar slices. *J. Physiol.* 305: 197–213.

Llinás, R., and Sugimori, M. (1992). The electrophysiology of the cerebellar Purkinje cell revisited. In R. Llinás and C. Sotelo (eds.), *The Cerebellum Revisited.* New York: Springer, pp. 167–181.

Llinás, R., Baker, R., and Sotelo, C. (1974). Electrotonic coupling between neurons in cat inferior olive. *J. Neurophysiol.* 37: 560–571.

Llinás, R., Lang, E.J., and Welsh, J.P. (1997). The cerebellum, LTD, and memory: alternative views. *Learn. Mem.* 3: 445–455.

Lockery, S.R. (1992). Realistic neural network models using backpropagation: panacea or oxymoron? *Semin. Neurosci.* 4: 47–59.

Lorente de Nó, R. (1981). *The Primary Acoustic Nuclei*. New York: Raven Press, p. 24.

Luebke, A.E., and Robinson, D.A. (1992). Climbing fiber intervention blocks plasticity of the vestibulo-ocular reflex. *Ann. N. Y. Acad. Sci.* 656 (B. Cohen, D.L. Tomko, and F. Guedry [eds.]) *Sensing and Controlling Motion – Vestibular and Sensorimotor Function*, pp. 428–430.

Luebke, A.E., and Robinson, D.A. (1994). Gain changes of the cat's vestibulo-ocular reflex after flocculus deactivation. *Exp. Brain Res.* 98: 379–390.

Lukashin, A.V., Amirikian, B.B., Mozhaev, V.L., and Georgopoulos, A.P. (1995). Neural network modeling of motor cortical operations during mental rotation and memory scanning tasks. *Soc. Neurosci. Abstr.* 21: 2078.

Macchi, G., and Jones, E.G. (1997). Toward an agreement on terminology of nuclear and subnuclear divisions of the motor thalamus. *J. Neurosurg.* 86: 670–685.

Maekawa, K., and Simpson, J.I. (1973). Climbing fiber responses evoked in vestibulocerebellum of rabbit from visual system. *J. Neurophysiol.* 36: 649–666.

Maekawa, K., and Takeda, T. (1975). Mossy fiber responses evoked in the cerebellar flocculus of rabbits by stimulation of the optic pathway. *Brain Res.* 98: 590–595.

Makhoul, J. (1975). Linear prediction: a tutorial review. *Proc. IEEE* 63: 561–580.

Maler, L., and Mugnaini, E. (1993). Organization and function of feedback to the electrosensory lateral line lobe of gymnotiform fish, with emphasis on a searchlight mechanism. *J. Comp. Physiol. A.* 173: 667–670.

Maler, L., and Mugnaini, E. (1994). Correlating gamma-aminobutyric acidergic circuits and sensory function in the electrosensory lateral line lobe of a gymnotiform fish. *J. Comp. Neurol.* 345: 224–252.

Mann-Metzer, P., and Yarom, Y. (2000). Electrotonic coupling synchronized interneuron activity in the cerebellar cortex. *Progr. Brain Res.* 124: 107–114.

Mano, N., Kanazawa, I, and Yamamoto, K. (1986). Complex-spike activity of cerebellar P-cells related to wrist tracking movement in monkey. *J. Neurophysiol.* 56: 137–158.

Mano, N., Kanazawa, I., and Yamamoto, K. (1989). Voluntary movements and complex-spike discharges of cerebellar Purkinje cells. In P. Strata (ed.), *The Olivocerebellar System in Motor Control*. Berlin/Heidelberg: Springer-Verlag, pp. 265–280.

Markram, H., Lübke, J., Frotscher, M., and Sakmann, B. (1997). Regulation of synaptic efficacy by coincidence of postsynaptic APs and EPSPs. *Science* 275: 213–215.

Marr, D. (1969). A theory of cerebellar cortex. *J. Physiol. (Lond.)* 202: 437–470.

Marr, D. (1970). A theory for cerebral neocortex. *Proc. Roy. Soc. Lond. B.* 176: 161–234.

Marsden, C.D., Merton, P.A., Morton, H.B., Hallett, M., Adam, J., and Rushton, D.N. (1977). Disorders of movement in cerebellar disease in man. In: F.C. Rose (ed.), *Physiological Aspects of Clinical Neurology*. Oxford, England: Blackwell, pp. 179–199.

Martin, J.H., Cooper, S.C., Hacking, A., and Ghez, C. (2000). Differential effects of deep cerebellar nuclei inactivation on reaching and adaptive control. *J. Neurophysiol.* 83: 1886–1899.

Mason, C.R., Miller, L.E., Baker, J.F., and Houk, J.C. (1998). Organization of reaching and grasping movements in the primate cerebellar nuclei as revealed by focal muscimol inactivations. *J. Neurophysiol.* 79: 537–554.

Mauk, M.D. (1997). Roles of cerebellar cortex and nuclei in motor learning: contradictions or clues? *Neuron* 18: 343–346.

Mauk, M.D., and Donegan, N.H. (1997). A model of Pavlovian eyelid conditioning based on the synaptic organization of the cerebellum. *Learn. Mem.* 3: 130–158.

Mauk, M.D., Medina, J.F., Nores, W.L., and Ohyama, T. (2000). Cerebellar function: coordination, learning, or timing? *Curr. Biol.* 10: R522–R525.

Mauk, M.D., Steinmetz, J.E., and Thompson, R.F. (1986). Classical conditioning using stimulation of the inferior olive as the unconditional stimulus. *Proc. Natl. Acad. Sci. USA* 83: 5349–5353.

McCrea, R.A., Bishop, G.A., and Kitai, S.T. (1978). Morphological and electrophysiological characteristics of projection neurons in the nucleus interpositus of the cat cerebellum. *J. Comp. Neurol.* 181: 397–420.

McCulloch, W.S., and Pitts, W. (1943). A logical calculus of the ideas immanent in nervous activity. *Bull. Math. Biophys.* 5: 115–125.

McCurdy, M.L., Gibson, A.R., and Houk, J.C. (1992). *Neuroimage* 1: 23–41.

McCurdy, M.L., Houk, J.C., and Gibson, A.R. (1998). Organization of ascending pathways to the forelimb area of the dorsal accessory olive in the cat. *J. Comp. Neurol.* 392: 115–133.

McIntyre, J., and Bizzi, E. (1993). Servo hypotheses for the biological control of movement. *J. Mot. Behav.* 25: 193–202.

Medina, J.F., and Mauk, M.D. (1999). Simulations of cerebellar motor learning: computational analysis of plasticity at the mossy fiber to deep nucleus synapse. *J. Neurosci.* 19: 7140–7151.

Medina, J.F., Garcia, K.S., Nores, W.L., Taylor, N.M., and Mauk, M.D. (2000). Timing mechanisms in the cerebellum: testing predictions of a large-scale computer simulation. *J. Neurosci.* 20: 5516–5525.

Meek, J. (1992a). Comparative aspects of cerebellar organization: from mormyrids to mammals *Eur. J. Morphol.* 30: 37–51.

Meek, J. (1992b). Why run parallel fibers parallel? Teleostean Purkinje cells as possible coincidence detectors, in a timing device subserving spatial coding of temporal differences. *Neuroscience* 48: 249–283.

Meek, J., and Nieuwenhuys, R. (1991). Palisade pattern of mormyrid Purkinje cells: a correlated light and electron microscopic study. *J. Comp. Neurol.* 306: 156–192.

Melkonian, D.S., Mkrtchian, H.H., and Fanardjian, V.V. (1982). Simulation of learning processes in neuronal networks of the cerebellum. *Biol. Cybern.* 45: 79–88.

Miall, R.C. (1997). Sequences of sensory predictions. *Behav. Brain Sci.* 20: 258–259.

Miall, R.C. (1998). The cerebellum, predictive control and motor coordination. *Novartis Found. Symp.* 218: 272–290, (discussion) 284–290.

Miall, R.C., and Wolpert, D.M. (1995). The cerebellum as a predictive model of the motor system: a Smith predictor hypothesis. In W.R. Ferrell and U. Proske (eds.), *Neural Control of Movement*. New York: Plenum Press, pp. 215–223.

Miall, R.C., and Wolpert, D.M. (1996). Forward models for physiological motor control. *Neural Netw.* 9: 1265–1279.

Miall, R.C., Keating, J.G., Malkmus, M., and Thach, W.T. (1998). Simple spike activity predicts occurrence of complex spikes in cerebellar Purkinje cells. *Nature Neurosci.* 1: 13–15.

Miall, R.C., Malkmus, M., and Robertson, E.M. (1996). Sensory prediction as a role for the cerebellum. *Behav. Brain Sci.* 19: 466–467.

Miall, R.C., Weir, D.J., Wolpert, D.M., and Stein, J.F. (1993). Is the cerebellum a Smith predictor? *J. Mot. Behav.* 25: 203–216.

Middleton, F.A., and Strick, P.L. (1994). Anatomical evidence for cerebellar and basal ganglia involvement in higher cognitive function. *Science* 266: 458–461.

Middleton, F.A., and Strick, P.L. (1997). Dentate output channels: motor and cognitive components. *Progr. Brain Res.* 114: 553–556.

Middleton, F.A., and Strick, P.L. (1998). Cerebellar output: motor and cognitive channels. *Trends Cogn. Sci.* 2: 348–354.

Middleton, F.A., and Strick, P. (2000). Basal ganglia and cerebellar loops: motor and cognitive circuits. *Brain Res. Rev.* 31: 236–250.

Milaihoff, G.A., Kosinski, R.J., Azizi, S.A., Lee, H.S., and Border, B.G. (1992). The expanding role of the basilar pontine nuclei as a source of cerebellar afferents. In R. Llinás and C. Sotelo (eds.), *The Cerebellum Revisited*. New York: Springer, pp. 136–164.

Milak, M.S., Bracha, V., and Bloedel, J.R. (1995). Relationship of simultaneously recorded cerebellar nuclear neuron discharge to the acquisition of a complex, operantly conditioned forelimb movement in cats. *Exp. Brain Res.* 105: 325–330.

Milak, M.S., Shimansky, Y., Bracha, V., and Bloedel, J.R. (1997). Effects of inactivating individual cerebellar nuclei on the performance and retention of an operantly conditioned forelimb movement. *J. Neurophysiol.* 78: 939–959.

Miles, F.A., and Lisberger, S.G. (1981). Plasticity in the vestibulo-ocular reflex: a new hypothesis. *Annu. Rev. Neurosci.* 4: 273–299.

Miles, F.A., Fuller, J.H., Braitman, D.J., and Dow, B.M. (1980). Long-term adaptive changes in primate vestibuloocular reflex. III. Electrophysiological observations in flocculus of normal monkeys. *J. Neurophysiol.* 41: 1437–1476.

Miller, L.E., and Houk, J.C. (1995). Motor co-ordinates in primate red nucleus: preferential relation to muscle activation versus kinematic variables. *J. Physiol. (Lond.)* 488.2: 533–548.

Miller, W.T., III, Glanz, F.H., and Kraft, L.G., III. (1987). Application of a general learning algorithm to the control of robotic manipulators. *Int. J. Robotics Res.* 6(2): 84–98.

Montgomery, J.C., and Bodznick, D. (1994). An adaptive filter that cancels self-induced noise in the electrosensory and lateral line mechanosensory systems of fish. *Neurosci. Lett.* 174: 145–148.

Moore, J.K., and Osen, K.K. (1979). The cochlear nuclei in man. *Am. J. Anat.* 154: 393–418.

Moore, J.W., Desmond, J.E., and Berthier, N.E. (1989). Adaptively timed conditioned responses and the cerebellum: a neural network approach. *Biol. Cybern.* 62: 17–28.

Morgan, J.I., and Smeyne, R.J. (1997). Transgenic approaches to cerebellar development. *Perspect. Devel. Neurobiol.* 5: 33–41.

Mugnaini, E. (1983). The length of cerebellar parallel fibers in chicken and rhesus monkey. *J. Comp. Neurol.* 220: 7–15.

Mugnaini, E. (1985). GABA neurons in the superficial layers of the rat dorsal cochlear nucleus: light and electron microscopic immunocytochemistry. *J. Comp. Neurol.* 235: 61–81.

Mugnaini, E., and Maler, L. (1993). Comparison between the fish electrosensory lateral line lobe and the mammalian dorsal cochlear nucleus. *J. Comp. Physiol. A.* 173: 683–685.

Mugnaini, E., and Morgan, J.I. (1987). The neuropeptide cerebellin is a marker for two similar neuronal circuits in rat brain. *Proc. Natl. Acad. Sci. USA* 84: 8692–8696.

Mugnaini, E., Berrebi, A.S., Dahl, A.-L., and Morgan, J.I. (1987). The polypeptide PEP-19 is a marker for Purkinje neurons in cerebellar cortex and cartwheel neurons in the dorsal cochlear nucleus. *Arch. Ital. Biol.* 126: 41–67.

Mugnaini, E., Diño, M.R., and Jaarsma, D. (1997). The unipolar brush cells of the mammalian cerebellum and cochlear nucleus: cytology and microcircuitry. *Progr. Brain Res.* 114: 131–150.

Mugnaini, E., Osen, K.K., Dahl, A.-L., Friedrich, V.L., Jr., and Korte, G. (1980). Fine structure of granule cells and related interneurons (termed Golgi cells) in the cochlear nuclear complex of cat, rat and mouse. *J. Neurocytol.* 9: 537–570.

Mugnaini, E., Warr, W.B., and Osen, K.K. (1980). Distribution and light microscopic features of granule cells in the cochlear nuclei of cat, rat, and mouse. *J. Comp. Neurol.* 191: 581–606.

Nagao, S., Kitamura, T., Nakamura, N., Hiramatsu, T., and Yamada, J. (1997). Differences of the primate flocculus and ventral paraflocculus in the mossy and climbing fiber input organization. *J. Comp. Anat.* 382: 480–498.

Narendra, K.S. (1995). Adaptive control: neural network applications. In M.A. Arbib (ed.), *The Handbook of Brain Theory and Neural Networks.* Cambridge, MA: MIT Press, pp. 69–73.

Nelken, I., and Young, E.D. (1996). Why do cats need a dorsal cochlear nucleus? *J. Basic Clin. Physiol. Pharmacol.* 7: 199–220.

Nelson, B.J., and Mugnaini, E. (1989). Origins of GABAergic inputs to the inferior olive. In: P. Strata (ed.), *The Olivocerebellar System in Motor Control.* Berlin: Springer-Verlag, (Experimental Brain Research Series 17), pp. 86–107.

Nieuwenhuys, R. (1967). Comparative anatomy of the cerebellum. *Progr. Brain Res.* 25: 1–93.

Nieuwenhuys, R., and Nicholson, C. (1969a). A survey of the general morphology, the fiber connections and the possible functional significance of the gigantocerebellum of mormyrid fishes. In: R. Llinás (ed.), *Neurobiology of Cerebellar Evolution and Development.* Chicago: American Medical Association Educational and Research Foundation, pp. 107–134.

Nieuwenhuys, R., and Nicholson, C. (1969b). Aspects of the histology of the cerebellum of mormyrid fishes. In: R. Llinás (ed.), *Neurobiology of Cerebellar Evolution and Development.* Chicago: American Medical Association, pp. 135–169.

Nieuwenhuys, R., ten Donkelaar, H.J., and Nicholson, C. (1998). *The Central Nervous System of Vertebrates, Vol. 2.* Berlin: Springer.

Nieuwenhuys, R., Voogd, J., and van Huijzen, C. (1988). *The Human Central Nervous System: A Synopsis and Atlas* (3rd ed.). Heidelberg: Springer-Verlag.

Nixon, P.D., and Passingham, R.E. (1999). The cerebellum and cognition: cerebellar lesions do not impair spatial working memory or visual associative learning in monkeys. *Eur. J. Neurosci.* 11: 4070–4080.

Nunzi, M.-G., and Mugnaini, E. (2000). Unipolar brush cell axons form a large system of intrinsic mossy fibers in the postnatal vestibulocerebellum. *J. Comp. Neurol.* 422: 55–65.

Oberdick, J., Baader, S.L., and Schilling, K. (1998). From zebra stripes to postal zones: deciphering patterns of gene expression in the cerebellum. *Trends Neurosci.* 21: 383–390.

Olivier, J., Coenen, M.D., and Seijnowski, T.J. (1995). A model for how the cerebellum anticipates sensory inputs and modulates the vestibulo-ocular reflex (VOR). *Soc. Neurosci.* 21: 915.

Optican, L.M., and Robinson, D.A. (1980). Cerebellar-dependent adaptive control of the primate saccadic system. *J. Neurophysiol.* 44: 1058–1076.

Osborn, C.E., and Poppele, R.E. (1992). Parallel distributed network characteristics of the DSCT. *J. Neurophysiol.* 68: 1100–1112.

Oscarsson, O. (1969). The sagittal organization of the cerebellar anterior lobe as revealed by the projection patterns of the climbing fiber system. In: R. Llinás (ed.), *Neurobiology of Cerebellar Evolution and Development.* Chicago: American Medical Association Educational and Research Foundation, pp. 525–537.

Oscarsson, O. (1979). Functional units of the cerebellum – sagittal zones and microzones. *Trends Neurosci.* 2: 143–145.

Oscarsson, O. (1980). Functional organization of olivary projection to the cerebellar anterior lobe. In: J. Courville, C. de Montigny, and Y. Lamarre (eds.), *The Inferior Olivary Nucleus: Anatomy and Physiology.* New York: Raven Press, pp. 279–289.

Ozol, K.L., and Hawkes, R. (1997). Compartmentation of the granular layer of the cerebellum. *Histol. Histopathol.* 112: 171–184.

Palay, S.L., and Chan-Palay, V. (1974). *Cerebellar Cortex.* New York: Springer-Verlag.

Palkovits, M., Magyar, P., and Szentágothai, J. (1972). Quantitative histological analysis of the cerebellar cortex in the cat. IV. Mossy fiber–Purkinje cell numerical transfer. *Brain Res.* 45: 15–29.

Parent, A. (1996). *Carpenter's Human Neuroanatomy* (9th ed.). Baltimore: Williams & Wilkins.

Parkins, E.J. (1997). Cerebellum and cerebrum in adaptive control and cognition: a review. *Biol. Cybern.* 77: 79–87.

Parsons, L.M., Bower, J.M., Gao, J.-H., Xiong, J.-H., Li, J.-Q., and Fox, P.T. (1997). Lateral cerebellar hemispheres actively support sensory acquisition and discrimination rather than motor control. *Learn. Mem.* 4: 49–62.

Pastor, A.M., De la Cruz, R.R., and Baker, R. (1997). Characterization of Purkinje cells in the goldfish cerebellum during eye movement and adaptive modification of the vestibulo-ocular reflex. *Progr. Brain Res.* 114: 359–381.

Paulin, M. (1989). A Kalman filter theory of the cerebellum. In: M.A. Arbib and S.-I. Amari (eds.), *Dynamic Interactions in Neural Networks: Models and Data.* New York: Springer, pp. 239–259.

Paulin, M. (1996). Cerebellar theory out of control. *Behav. Brain Sci.* 19: 470–471.

Paulin, M. (1997). Neural representations of moving systems. In J.D. Schmahmann (ed.), *The Cerebellum and Cognition.* San Diego: Academic Press, pp. 515–533.

Paulin, M.G. (1993). The role of the cerebellum in motor control and perception. *Brain Behav. Evol.* 41: 39–50.

Paulin, M.G., Nelson, M.E., and Bower, J.M. (1989). Neural control of sensory acquisition: the vestibulo-ocular reflex. In D.S. Touretsky (ed.), *Advances in Neural Information Processing Systems I.* San Mateo, CA: Morgan Kaufmann Publishers, pp. 410–418.

Pellegrini, J.J., and Evinger, C. (1997). Role of cerebellum in adaptive modification of reflex blinks. *Learn. Mem.* 3: 77–87.

Pellionisz, A. (1970). Computer simulation of the pattern transfer of large cerebellar neuronal fields. *Acta Biochim. Biophys. Acad. Sci. Hung.* 5: 71–79.

Pellionisz, A. (1984). Coordination: a vector-matrix description of transformations of over-complete CNS coordinates and a tensorial solution using the Moore–Penrose generalized inverse. *J. Theoret. Biol.* 110: 353–375.

Pellionisz, A., and Graf, W. (1987). Tensor network model of the "three-neuron" vestibulo-ocular reflex-arc in cat. *J. Theoret. Neurobiol.* 5: 127–151.

Pellionisz, A. and Llinás, R. (1979). Brain modeling by tensor network theory and computer simulation. The cerebellum: distributed processor for predictive coordination. *Neuroscience* 4: 323–348.

Pellionisz, A., and Llinás, R. (1980). Tensorial approach to the geometry of brain function: cerebellar coordination via a metric tensor. *Neuroscience* 5: 1125–1136.

Pellionisz, A., and Llinás, R. (1982). Space-time representation in the brain. The cerebellum as a predictive space-time metric tensor. *Neuroscience* 7: 2949–2970.

Pellionisz, A., and Szentágothai, J. (1973). Dynamic single unit simulation of a realistic cere-bellar network model. *Brain Res.* 49: 83–99.

Pellionisz, A., and Szentágothai, J. (1974). Dynamic single unit simulation of a realistic cere-bellar network model. II. Purkinje cell activity within the basic circuit and modified by inhibitory systems. *Brain Res.* 68: 19–40.

Pellionisz, A., Peterson, B.W., and Tomko, D.L. (1990). Vestibular head-eye coordination: a geometrical sensorimotor neurocomputer paradigm. In R. Eckmiller, (ed.), *Advanced Neural Computers.* Amsterdam: Elsevier/North Holland, pp. 61–68.

Pennacchio, L.A., Boulev, D.M., Higgins, K.M., Scott, M.P., and Noebels, J.L. (1998). Progres-sive ataxia, myoclonic epilepsy and cerebellar apopotosis in cystatin B-deficient mice. *Nat. Genet.* 20: 251–258.

Peterson, B.W., and Houk, J.C. (1991). A model of cerebellar-brainstem interaction in the adaptive control of the vestibuloocular reflex. *Acta Otolaryngol. (Stockh).* Suppl. 481: 428–432.

Peterson, S.E., Fox, P.T., Posner, M.I., Mintun, M., and Raichle, M.E. (1989). Positron emission tomographic studies of the processing of single words. *J. Cogn. Neurosci.* 1: 133–170.

Pichitpornchai, C., Rawson, J.A., and Rees, S. (1994). Morphology of parallel fibers in the cerebellar cortex of the rat: an experimental light and electron microscopic study with biocytin. *J. Comp. Neurol.* 342: 206–220.

Pitts, W., and McCulloch, W.S. (1947). How we know universals: the perception of auditory and visual forms. *Bull. Math. Biophys.* 9: 127–147.

Poldrack, R.A., and Gabrieli, J. E. (1997). Functional anatomy of long-term memory. *J. Clin. Neurophysiol.* 14: 294–310.

Precht, W., and Llinás, R. (1969). Comparative aspects of the vestibular input to the cerebellum. In R. Llinás, (ed.), *Neurobiology of Cerebellar Evolution and Development*, Chicago: American Medical Association, pp. 677–702.

Qian, N. (1995). Generalization and analysis of the Lisberger-Seijnowski VOR model. *Neural Comput.* 7: 735–752.

Ramón y Cajal, S. (1995). *Histology of the Nervous System, 2 Vols.* (trans. from the 1909–1911 French edition by N. Swanson and L.W. Swanson). New York/Oxford: Oxford University Press.

Raphan, T., Dai, M.J., and Cohen, B. (1992). Spatial orientation of the vestibular system. *Ann. N. Y. Acad. Sci.* 656: 140–157.

Raymond, J.L., and Lisberger, S.G. (1997). Multiple subclasses of Purkinje cells in the primate floccular complex provide similar signals to guide learning in the vestibulo-ocular reflex. *Learn. Mem.* 3: 503–518.

Raymond, J.L., and Lisberger, S.G. (2000). Hypotheses about the neural trigger for plasticity in the circuit for the vestibulo-ocular reflex. *Progr. Brain Res.* 124: 235–246.

Raymond, J.L., Lisberger, S.G., and Mauk, M.D. (1996). The cerebellum: a neuronal learning machine? *Science* 272: 1126–1131.

Robinson, D.A. (1976). Adaptive gain control of vestibuloocular reflex by the cerebellum. *J. Neurophysiol.* 39: 954–969.

Robinson, D.A. (1981). Control of eye movements. In V.B. Brooks (ed.), *Handbook of Physiology, Vol, II, Motor Control, Part 2.* Bethesda: American Physiological Society, pp. 1275–1320.

Robinson, D.A. (1989). Integrating with neurons. *Annu. Rev. Neurosci.* 12: 33–45.

Robinson, D.A. (1992a). Implications of neural networks for how we think about brain function. *Behav. Brain Sci.* 15: 644–655.

Robinson, D.A. (1992b). How far into brain function can neural networks take us? *Behav. Brain Sci.* 15: 823–828.

Robinson, F.R., Straube, A., and Fuchs, A.F. (1997). Participation of caudal fastigial nucleus in smooth pursuit eye movements. II. Effects of mucimol inactivation. *J. Neurophysiol.* 78: 848–859.

Rolls, E.T., and Treves, A. (1998). *Neural Networks and Brain Function.* Oxford, England: Oxford University Press.

Rosenblatt, F. (1958). The Perceptron: a probabilistic model for information storage and organization in the brain. *Psychol. Rev.* 65: 386–408.

Rosenblatt, F. (1961). *Principles of Neurodynamical Perceptrons and the Theory of Brain Mechanisms.* Buffalo, NY: Cornell Aeronautical Laboratory (1962). Washington, DC: Spartan Books.

Ross, C.A. (1997). Intranuclear neuronal inclusions: a common pathogenic mechanism for glutamine-repeat neurodegenerative diseases? *Neuron* 19: 1147–1150.

Rossi, F., and Strata, P. (1995). Reciprocal trophic interactions in the adult climbing fibre–Purkinje cell system. *Progr. Neurobiol.* 47: 341–369.

Rothwell, J. (1994). *Control of Human Voluntary Movement* (2nd ed.). London: Chapman & Hall.

Rubia, F.J. (1992). A possible connection between the mossy and climbing fiber systems at precerebellar level. In: R. Llinás and C. Sotelo (eds.), *The Cerebellum Revisited.* New York: Springer, pp. 226–254.

Ruigrok, T.J.H. (1997). Cerebellar nuclei: the olivary connection. *Progr. Brain Res.* 114: 168–192.

Ruigrok, T.J.H., and Voogd, J. (1995). Cerebellar influence on olivary excitability in the cat. *Eur. J. Neurosci.* 7: 679–693.

Ruigrok, T.J.H., and Voogd, J. (2000). Organization of projections from the inferior olive to the cerebellar nuclei in the rat. *J. Comp. Neurol.* 426: 209–228.

Ruigrok, T.J.H., de Zeeuw, C.I., van der Burg, J., and Voogd, J. (1990). Intracellular labeling of neurons in the medial accessory olive of the cat: I. Physiology and light microscopy. *J. Comp. Neurol.* 300: 462–477.

Ruigrok, T.J.H., Osse, R.-J., and Voogd, J. (1992). Organization of inferior olivary projections to the flocculus and ventral paraflocculus of the rat cerebellum. *J. Comp. Neurol.* 316: 129–150.

Rumelhart, D.E. (1990). Series foreword. in: M.A. Gluck and D.E. Rumelhart (eds.), *Neuroscience and Connectionist Theory*. Hillsdale, NJ: Lawrence Erlbaum Associates, pp. ix–x.

Rumelhart D.E., Hinton, G.E., and Williams, R.J. (1986a). Learning internal representations by error propagation. In D.E. Rumelhart and J.L. McClelland (eds.), *Parallel Distributed Processing: Explorations in the Microstructure of Cognition, Vol. 1*. Cambridge, MA: MIT Press.

Rumelhart, D.E., Hinton, G.E., and Williams, R.J. (1986b). Learning representations by back-propagating errors. *Nature* 323: 225–228.

Russell, C.J., and Bell, C.C. (1978). Neuronal responses to electrosensory input in momyrid valvula cerebelli. *J. Neurophysiol.* 41: 1495–1510.

Rutherford, J.G., and Gwyn, D.G. (1980). A light and electron microscopic study of the inferior olivary nucleus of the squirrel monkey, *Saimiri sciureus*. *J. Comp. Neurol.* 189: 127–155.

Sadato, N., Ibañez, V., Deiber, M.-P., Campbell, G., Leonardo, M., and Hallett, M. (1996). Frequency-dependent changes of regional cerebral blood flow during finger movements. *J. Cereb. Blood Flow Metab.* 16: 23–33.

Saint-Cyr, J.A. (1983). The projection from the motor cortex to the inferior olive in the cat. *Neuroscience* 10: 667–684.

Sakurai, M. (1987). Synaptic modification of parallel fibre–Purkinje cell transmission in in-vitro guinea-pig cerebellar slices. *J. Physiol.* 394: 463–480.

Sakurai, M. (1989). Depression and potentiation of parallel fiber–Purkinje cell transmission in *in vitro* cerebellar slices. In P. Strata (ed.), *The Olivocerebellar System in Motor Control*. Berlin: Springer, pp. 221–230.

Salin, P.A., Malenka, R.C., and Nicoll, R.A. (1996). Cyclic AMP mediates a presynaptic form of LTP at cerebellar parallel fiber synapses. *Neuron* 16: 797–803.

Sanner, R.M., and Slotine, J.-J. E. (1993). Stable adaptive control of root manipulators using "neural" networks. *Neural Comput.* 7: 753–790.

Sasaki, K., Bower, J.M., and Llinás, R. (1989). Multiple Purkinje cell recording in rodent cerebellar cortex. *Eur. J. Neurosci.* 1: 572–586.

Scheibel, M.E., and Scheibel, A.B. (1955). The inferior olive: a Golgi study. *J. Comp. Neurol.* 102: 77–132.

Scheibel, M., Scheibel, A., Walberg, W., and Brodal, A. (1956). Areal distribution of axonal and dendritic patterns in inferior olive. *J. Comp. Neurol.* 106: 21–49.

Schild, R.F. (1980). Length of the parallel fibers in rat cerebellar cortex. *J. Physiol. (Lond.)* 303: 25P

Schilling, K. (2000). Lineage, development and morphogenesis of cerebellar interneurons. *Progr. Brain Res.* 124: 51–68.

Schlösser, R., Hutchinson, M., Joseffer, S., Rusinek, H., Saarimaki, A., Stevenson, J., Dewey, S.L., and Brodie, J.D. (1998). Functional magnetic resonance imaging of human brain activity in a verbal fluency task. *J. Neurol. Neurosurg. Psychiatry* 64: 492–498.

Schmahmann, J.D. (1991). An emerging concept. The cerebellar contribution to higher function. *Arch. Neurol.* 48: 1178–1187.

Schmahmann, J.D. (1992). In reply (letter to the editor). *Arch. Neurol.* 49: 1230.

Schmahmann, J.D. (1996). Dysmetria of thought: correlations and conundrums in the relationship between the cerebellum, learning, and cognitive processing. *Behav. Brain Sci.* 19: 472–473.

Schmahmann, J.D. (1997). (ed.). *The Cerebellum and Cognition (Int. Rev. Neurobiol.* 41). San Diego: Academic Press.

Schmahmann, J.D. (1998). Dysmetria of thought: clinical consequences of cerebellar dysfunction on cognition and affect. *Trends Cogn. Sci.* 2: 362–371.

Schmahmann, J.D., and Pandya, D.N. (1989). Anatomical investigation of projections to the basis pontis from posterior parietal association cortices in rhesus monkey. *J. Comp. Neurol.* 289: 53–73.

Schmahmann, J.D., and Pandya, D.N. (1991). Projections to the basis pontis from the superior temporal sulcus and superior temporal region in the rhesus monkey. *J. Comp. Neurol.* 308: 224–248.

Schmahmann, J.D., and Pandya, D.N. (1997a). Anatomic organization of the basilar pontine projections from prefrontal cortices in rhesus monkey. *J. Neurosci.* 17: 438–458.

Schmahmann, J., and Pandya, D.K. (1997b). The cerebrocerebellar system. In: J. Schmahmann (ed.), *The Cerebellum and Cognition.* San Diego: Academic Press (*Int. Rev. Neurobiol.* 41): 31–60.

Schmahmann, J.D., and Sherman, J.C. (1998). The cerebellar cognitive affective syndrome. *Brain* 121: 561–579.

Schmahmann, J.D., Doyon, J., Toga, A.W., Petrides, M., and Evans, A.C. (2000). *MRI Atlas of the Human Cerebellum.* San Diego: Academic Press.

Schnitzlein, B.N., and Faucette, J.R. (1969). General morphology of the fish cerebellum. In: R. Llinás (ed.), *Neurobiology of Cerebellar Evolution and Development,* Chicago: American Medical Association, pp. 77–106.

Schöner, G., and Kelso, J.A.S. (1988). Dynamic pattern generation in behavioral and neural systems. *Science* 239: 1513–1520.

Schreurs, B.G., and Alkon, D.L. (1993). Rabbit cerebellar slice analysis of long-term depression and its role in classical conditioning. *Brain Res.* 631: 235–240.

Schreurs, B.G., Oh, M.M., and Alkon, D.L. (1996). Pairing-specific long-term depression of Purkinje cell excitatory postsynaptic potentials results from a classical conditioning procedure in the rabbit cerebellar slice. *J. Neurophysiol.* 75: 1051–1060.

Schreurs, B.G., Tomsic, D., Gusev, P.A., and Alkon, D.L. (1997). Dendritic excitability microzones and occluded long-term depression after classical conditioning of the rabbit's nictitating membrane response. *J. Neurophysiol.* 77: 86–92.

Schweighofer, N., and Arbib, M.A. (1998). A model of cerebellar metaplasticity. *Learn. Mem.* 4: 421–428.

Schweighofer, N., Arbib, M.A., and Dominey, P.F. (1996a). A model of the cerebellum in adaptive control of saccadic gain. I. The model and its biological substrate. *Biol. Cybern.* 75: 19–28.

Schweighofer, N., Arbib, M.A., and Dominey, P.F. (1996b). A model of the cerebellum in adaptive control of saccadic gain. II. Simulation results. *Biol. Cybern.* 75: 29–36.

Schweighofer, N., Doya, K., and Kawato, M. (1999). Electrophysiological properties of inferior olive neurons: a compartmental model. *J. Neurophysiol.* 82: 804–817.

Schweighofer, N., Spoelstra, J., Arbib, M.A., and Kawato, M. (1998a). Role of the cerebellum in reaching movements in humans. I. Distributed inverse dynamics control. *Eur. J. Neurosci.* 10: 86–94.

Schweighofer, N., Spoelstra, J., Arbib, M.A., and Kawato, M. (1998b). Role of the cerebellum in reaching movements in humans. II. A neural model of the intermediate cerebellum. *Eur. J. Neurosci.* 10: 95–105.

Seeds, N.W., Williams, B.L., and Bickford, P.C. (1995). Tissue plasminogen activator induction in Purkinje neurons after cerebellar motor learning. *Science* 270: 1992–1994.

Seijnowski, T.J. (1977). Storing covariance with nonlinearly interacting neurons. *J. Math. Biol.* 4: 303–321.

Seitz, R.J., Canavan, A.G.M., Yagüez, L., Herzog, H., Tellmann, L., Knorr, U., Huang, Y.-X., and Hömberg, V. (1994). Successive roles of the cerebellum and premotor cortices in trajectorial learning. *Neuroreport* 5: 2541–2544.

Shambes, G.M., Gibson, J.M., and Welker, W. (1978). Fractured somatotopy in granule cell tactile areas of rat cerebellar hemispheres revealed by micromapping. *Brain Behav. Evol.* 15: 94–140.

Shibuki, C.A., and Okada, D. (1992). Cerebellar long-term potentiation under suppressed postsynaptic Ca^{2+} activity. *Neuroreport* 3: 231–234.

Shidara, M., Kawano, K., Gomi, H., and Kawato, M. (1993). Inverse-dynamics model eye movement control by Purkinje cells in the cerebellum. *Nature* 365: 50–52.

Shimansky, Y., Saling, M., Wunderlich, D.A., Bracha, V., Stelmach, G.F., and Bloedel, J.R. (1997). Impaired capacity of cerebellar patients to perceive and learn two-dimensional shapes based on kinesthetic cues. *Learn. Mem.* 4: 36–48.

Shinoda, Y., Futami, T., Sugiuchi, Y., Kakei, S., and Izawa, Y. (1993). Input–output organization of the cerebellar nuclei. In: N. Mano, I. Hamada, and M.R. DeLong (eds.), *Role of the Cerebellum and Basal Ganglia in Voluntary Movement.* Amsterdam: Elsevier, pp. 133–145.

Shinoda, Y., Izawa, Y., Sugiuchi, Y., and Futami, T. (1997). Functional significance of excitatory projections from the precerebellar nuclei to interpositus and dentate nucleus neurons for mediating motor, premotor and parietal cortical inputs. *Progr. Brain Res.* 114: 193–207.

Shinoda, Y., Sugihara, E., Wu, H.-S., and Sugiuchi, Y. (2000). The entire trajectory of single climbing and mossy fibers in the cerebellar nuclei and cortex. *Progr. Brain Res.* 124: 173–186.

Shmerling, D., Hegyi, I., Fischer, M., Blätter, T., Brandner, S., Götz, J., Rülicke, T., Flechsig, E., Cozzio, A., von Mering, C., Hangartner, C., Aguzzi, A., and Weissmann, C. (1998). Expression of amino-terminally truncated PrP [prion protein] in the mouse leading to ataxia and specific cerebellar lesions. *Cell* 93: 203–214.

Shynk, J.J. (1995). Adaptive filtering. In: M.A. Arbib (ed.), *The Handbook of Brain Theory and Neural Networks.* Cambridge, MA: MIT Press, pp. 74–78.

Silkis, I. (2000). Interrelated modification of excitatory and inhibitory synapses in three-layer olivary-cerebellar neural network. *Biosystems* 54: 141–149.

Silveri, M.C., Leggio, M.G., and Molinari, M. (1994). The cerebellum contributes to linguistic production: a case of agrammatic speech following a right cerebellar lesion. *Neurology* 44: 2047–2050.

Simpson, J.I., and Alley, K.E. (1974). Visual climbing fiber input to rabbit vestibulo-cerebellum: a source of direction-specific information. *Brain Res.* 82: 302–308.

Simpson, J.I., Graf, W., and Leonard, C.S. (1989). Three-dimensional representation of retinal image movement by climbing fiber activity. In P. Strata (ed.), *The Olivocerebellar System in Motor Control.* New York: Springer-Verlag, pp. 323–337.

Simpson, J.I., Van der Steen, J., and Tan, J. (1992). Eye movements and the zonal structure of the rabbit flocculus. In R. Llinás and C. Sotelo (eds.), *The Cerebellum Revisited.* New York: Springer Verlag, pp. 255–266.

Simpson, J.I., Wylie, D.R., and De Zeeuw, C.I. (1996). On climbing fiber signals and their consequence(s). *Behav. Brain Sci.* 19: 384–398.

Singer, J.L. (1995). Mental processes and brain architecture: confronting the complex adaptive systems of human thought (an overview). In: H. Morowitz and J.L. Singer (eds.), *The Mind, The Brain, and Complex Adaptive Systems.* Reading, MA: Addison-Wesley, pp. 1–9.

Sinkjær, T., Miller, L., Andersen, T., and Houk, J.C. (1995). Synaptic linkages between red nucleus cells and limb muscles during a multi-joint motor task. *Exp. Brain. Res.* 102: 546–550.

Siouris, G.M. (1993). *Aerospace Avionics Systems*. New York: Academic Press.

Slater, N.T., Rossi, D.J., and Kinney, G.A. (1997). Physiology of transmission at a giant glutamatergic synapse in cerebellum. *Progr. Brain Res.* 114: 150–163.

Smith, A.M. (1996). Does the cerebellum learn strategies for the optimal time-varying control of joint stiffness? *Behav. Brain Sci.* 19: 399–410.

Smolyaninov, V.V. (1971). Some special features of organization of the cerebellar cortex. In: I.M. Gelfand, V.S. Gurfinkel, S.V. Fomin, and M.L. Tsetlin (eds.), *Models of the Structural-Functional Organization of Certain Biological Systems* (translated from the Russian by C.R. Beard, translation reviewed by J.S. Barlow). Cambridge, MA: MIT Press, pp. 251–325.

Soechting, J.F., and Flanders, M. (1992). Moving in three-dimensional space: frames of reference, vectors, and coordinate systems. *Annu. Rev. Neurosci.* 15: 167–191.

Sotelo, C., and Chédotal, A. (1997). Development of the olivocerebellar projection. *Perspect. Devel. Neurobiol.* 5: 57–67.

Sotelo, C., Gotow, T., and Wassef, M. (1986). Localization of glutamic-acid-decarbolyxase-immunoreactive axon terminals in the inferior olive of the rat, with special emphasis on anatomical relations between GABAergic synapses and dendrodendritic gap junctions. *J. Comp. Neurol.* 252: 32–50.

Sotelo, C., Llinás, R., and Baker, R. (1974). Structural study of inferior olivary nucleus of the cat: morphological correlates of electrotonic coupling. *J. Neurophysiol.* 37: 541–559.

Stein, J.F. (1992). The representation of egocentric space in the posterior parietal cortex. *Behav. Brain Sci.* 15: 691–700.

Stein, J.F., and Glickstein, J.F. (1992). The role of the cerebellum in visual guidance of movement. *Physiol. Rev.* 72: 967–1017.

Stone, L.S., and Lisberger, S.G. (1989). Synergistic action of complex and simple spikes in the monkey flocculus in the control of smooth-pursuit eye movement. In P. Strata (ed.), *The Olivocerebellar System in Motor Control*. New York: Springer-Verlag, pp. 299–312.

Stone, L.S., and Lisberger, S.G. (1990). Visual responses of Purkinje cells in the cerebellar flocculus during smooth-pursuit eye movements in monkeys. I. Simple spikes. *J. Neurophysiol.* 63: 1241–1261.

Strata, P., and Rossi, F. (1998). Plasticity of the olivocerebellar pathway. *Trends Neurosci.* 21: 407–413.

Strata, P., Rossi, F., and Tempia, F. (1995). Inferior olive and the saccadic neural integrator. In W.R. Ferrell and U. Proskeu (eds.), *Neural Control of Movement*. New York: Plenum Press, pp. 241–249.

Strata, P., Tempia, F., Zagrebelsky, M., and Rossi, F. (1997). Reciprocal trophic interactions between climbing fibres and Purkinje cells in the rat cerebellum. *Progr. Brain Res.* 114: 263–282.

Sugawara, Y., Grant, K., Han, V., and Bell, C.C. (1999). Physiology of electrosensory lateral line lobe neurons in *Gnathonemus petersii*. *J. Exp. Biol.* 202: 1301–1309.

Sugihara, I., Lang, E.J., and Llinás, R. (1993). Uniform olivocerebellar conduction time underlies Purkinje cell complex spike synchronicity in the rat cerebellum. *J. Physiol.* 470: 243–271.

Sugihara, I., Lang, E.J., and Llinás, R. (1995). Serotonin modulation of inferior olivary oscillations and synchronicity: a multiple-electrode study in the rat cerebellum. *Eur. J. Neurosci.* 7: 521–534.

Sugihara, I., Wu, H.-S., and Shinoda, Y. (1999). Morphology of single olivocerebellar axons labeled with biotinylated dextran. *J. Comp. Neurol.* 414: 131–148.

Sutton, R.S., and Barto, A.G. (1981). Toward a modern theory of adaptive networks: expectation and prediction. *Psychol. Review* 88: 135–170.

Svensson, P., Ivarsson, M., and Hesslow, G. (1997). Effect of varying the intensity and train frequency of forelimb and cerebellar mossy fiber conditioned stimuli on the latency of conditioned eye-blink responses in decerebrate ferrets. *Learn. Mem.* 3: 105–115.

Svensson, P., Ivarsson, M., and Hesslow, G. (2000). Involvement of the cerebellum in a new temporal property of the conditioned eyeblink response. *Progr. Brain Res.* 124: 317–323.

Swenson, R.S., and Castro, A.J. (1983). The afferent connections of the inferior olivary complex in rats. An anterograde study using autoradiographic and axonal degeneration techniques. *Neuroscience* 8: 259–275.

Szentágothai, J. (1965). The use of degeneration methods in the investigation of short neuronal connexions. *Progr. Brain Res.* 14: 1–32.

Szentágothai, J. (1968). Structuro-functional considerations of the cerebellar network. *Proc. IEEE* 56: 960–968.

Takács, J., Gombos, G., Görcs, T., Becker, T., de Barry, J., and Hámori, J. (1997). Distribution of metabotropic glutamate receptor type 1a in Purkinje cell dendritic spines is independent of the presence of presynaptic parallel fibers. *J. Neurosci. Res.* 50: 433–442.

Tan, J., Epema, A.H., and Voogd, J. (1995). Zonal organization of the flocculovestibular nucleus projection in the rabbit: a combined axonal tracing and acetylcholinesterase histochemical study. *J. Comp. Neurol.* 356: 51–71.

Tan, J., Gerrits, N.M., Nanhoe, R., Simpson, J.I., and Voogd, J. (1995). Zonal organization of the climbing fiber projection to the flocculus and nodulus of the rabbit: a combined axonal tracing and acetylcholinesterase histochemical study. *J. Comp. Neurol.* 356: 23–50.

Tan, J., Simpson, J.I., and Voogd, J. (1995). Anatomical compartments in the white matter of the rabbit flocculus. *J. Comp. Neurol.* 356: 1–22.

Tauer, U., Volk, B., and Heimrich, B. (1996). Differentiation of Purkinje cells in cerebellar slice cultures: an immunochemical and Golgi EM study. *Neuropathol. Appl. Neurobiol.* 22: 361–369.

Teune, T.M., van der Burg, J., De Zeeuw, C.I., Voogd, J., and Ruigrok, T.J.H. (1998). Single Purkinje cell can innervate multiple classes of projection neurons in the cerebellar nuclei of the rat: a light microscopic and ultrastructural triple-tracer study in the rat. *J. Comp. Neurol.* 392: 164–178.

Teune, T.M., van der Burg, J., and Ruigrok, T.J.H. (1995). Cerebellar projections to the red nucleus and inferior olive originate from separate populations of neurons in the rat: a non-fluorescent double labeling study. *Brain Res.* 673: 313–319.

Thach, W.T. (1967). Somatosensory receptive fields of single units in cat cerebellar cortex. *J. Neurophysiol.* 30: 675–696.

Thach, W.T. (1972). Cerebellar output: properties, synthesis and uses. *Brain Res.* 40: 89–97.

Thach, W.T. (1980). Complex spikes, the inferior olive, and natural behavior. In: J. Courville, C. de Montigny, and Y. Lamarre (eds.), *The Inferior Olivary Nucleus: Anatomy and Physiology.* New York: Raven Press, pp. 349–360.

Thach, W.T. (1996a). A cerebellar role in acquisition of novel static and dynamic muscle activities in holding, pointing, throwing, and reaching. In: J.R. Bloedel, T.J. Ebner, and S.P. Wise (eds.), *The Acquisition of Motor Behavior in Vertebrates.* Cambridge, MA: MIT Press, pp. 223–234.

Thach, W.T. (1996b). On the specific role of the cerebellum in motor learning and cognition: clues from PET activation and lesion studies in man. *Behav. Brain Sci.* 19: 411–431.

Thach, W.T. (1996c). Q. Is the cerebellum an adaptive combiner of motor and mental/motor activities? A. Yes, maybe, certainly not, who can say? *Behav. Brain Sci.* 19: 501–503.

Thach, W.T. (1997). Context–response linkage. In: J. Schmahmann (ed.), *The Cerebellum and Cognition. (Int. Rev. Neurobiol.* 41: 599–611) San Diego: Academic Press.

Thach, W.T. (1998a). Combination, complementarity and automatic control: a role for the cerebellum in learning movement coordination. *Novartis Found. Symp.* 218: 219–232.

Thach, W.T. (1998b). A role for the cerebellum in learning movement coordination. *Neurobiol. Learn. Mem.* 70: 177–188.

Thach, W.T. (1998c). What is the role of the cerebellum in motor learning and cognition? *Trends Cogn. Sci.* 2: 331–337.

Thach, W.T., Goodkin, H.P., and Keating, J.G. (1992). The cerebellum and the adaptive coordination of movement. *Annu. Rev. Neurosci.* 15: 403–442.

Thach, W.T., Kane, S.A., Mink, J.W., and Goodkin H.P. (1992). Cerebellar output: multiple maps and modes of control in movement coordination. In: R. Llinás and C. Sotelo (eds.), *The Cerebellum Revisited.* New York: Springer, pp. 283–300.

Thach, W.T., Mink, J.W., Goodkin, H.P., and Keating, J.G. (1993). Combining versus gating motor programs: differential roles for cerebellum and basal ganglia? In N. Mano, I. Hamada, and M.R. DeLong (eds.), *Role of the Cerebellum and Basal Ganglia in Voluntary Movement.* Amsterdam: Elsevier, pp. 235–245.

Thach, W.T., Perry, J.G., Kane, S.A., and Goodkin, H.P. (1993). Cerebellar nuclei: rapid alternating movement, motor somatotopy, and a mechanism for the control of muscle synergy. *Rev. Neurol. (Paris)* 149: 607–628.

Their, P., Dicke, P.W., Haas, R., and Barash, S. (2000). Encoding of movement time by populations of cerebellar Purkinje cells. *Nature* 405: 72–76.

Thompson, R.F., Thompson, J.K., Kim, J.J., Krupa, D.J., and Shinkman, P.G. (1998). The nature of reinforcement in cerebellar learning. *Neurobiol. Learn. Mem.* 70: 150–176.

Timmann, D., Shimansky, Y., Larson, P.S., Wunderlich, D.A., Stelmach, G.E., and Bloedel, J.R. (1996). Visuomotor learning in cerebellar patients. *Behav. Brain Res.* 81: 99–113.

Tolbert, D.L., (1982). The cerebellar nucleocortical pathway. In S.L. Palay and V. Chan-Palay (eds.), *The Cerebellum – New Vistas.* Heidelberg: Springer, pp. 296–319.

Tolbert, D.L., and Bantli, H. (1979). An HRP and autoradiographic study of cerebellar corticonuclear-nucleocortical reciprocity in the monkey. *Exp. Brain Res.* 36: 563–571.

Tolbert, D.L., Bantli, H., and Bloedel, J.R. (1976). Anatomical and physiological evidence for a cerebellar nucleo-cortical projection in the cat. *Neuroscience* 1: 205–217.

Tolbert, D.L., Bantli, H., and Bloedel, J.R. (1977). The intracerebellar nucleocortical projection in a primate. *Exp. Brain Res.* 30: 425–434.

Tolbert, D.L., Bantli, H., and Bloedel, J.R. (1978). Organizational features of the cat and monkey cerebellar nucleocortical projection. *J. Comp. Neurol.* 182: 39–56.

Tolbert, D.L., Kultas-Ilinsky, K., and Ilinsky, I. (1980). EM-autoradiography of cerebellar nucleocortical terminals in the cat. *Anat. Embryol.* 161: 215–223.

Topka, H., Konczak, J., Schneider, K., Boose, A., and Dichgans, J. (1998). Multijoint arm movements in cerebellar ataxia: abnormal control of movement dynamics. *Exp. Brain Res.* 119: 493–503.

Topka, H., Konczak, J., and Dichgans, J. (1998). Coordination of multi-joint arm movements in cerebellar ataxia: analysis of hand and angular kinematics. *Exp. Brain Res.* 119: 483–492.

Trott, J.R., Apps, R., and Armstrong, D.M. (1990). Topographical organisation within the cerebellar nucleocortical projection to the paravermal cortex of lobule Vb/c in the cat. *Exp. Brain Res.* 80: 415–428.

Umetani, T. (1990). Topographic organization of the cerebellar nucleocortical projection in the albino rat: an autographic orthograde study. *Brain Res.* 507: 216–224.

Van der Neut, R. (1997). Targeted gene disruption: applications in neurobiology. *J. Neurosci. Methods* 71: 19–27.

van Kan, P.L.E., Gibson, A.R., and Houk, J.C. (1993). Movement-related inputs to intermediate cerebellum of the monkey. *J. Neurophysiol.* 69: 74–94.

Vemuri, V.R. (1992). *Artifical Neural Networks: Concepts and Control Applications.* Los Alamitos, CA: IEEE Computer Society Press.

Verhaagen, J., and Schrama, L.H. (1997). The application of gene transfer technology in neurobiology. *J. Neurosci. Methods* 71: vii.

Vetter, P., and Wolpert, D.M. (2000). Context estimation for sensorimotor control. *J. Neurophysiol.* 84: 1026–1034.

Victor, M., and Ropper, A.H. (2001). *Adams and Victor's Principles of Neurology* (7th ed.). New York: McGraw-Hill.

Viets, H.R., and Garrison, F.H. (1940). Purkinje's original description of the pear-shaped cells in the cerebellum. *Bull. Hist. Med.* 8: 1397–1398.

Vilis, T., and Hore, J. (1980). Central neural mechanisms contributing to cerebellar tremor produced by limb perturbations. *J. Neurophysiol.* 43: 279–291.

Vincent, P., and Marty, A. (1996). Fluctuations of inhibitory postsynaptic currents in Purkinje cells from rat cerebellar slices. *J. Physiol.* 494: 183–199.

von der Malsburg, C. (1997). The coherence definition of consciousness. In M. Ito, Y. Miyashita and E.T. Rolls (eds.), *Cognition, Computation, and Consciousness.* Oxford, England: Oxford University Press, pp. 193–204.

Voogd, J., and Bigaré, F. (1980). Topographical distribution of olivary and cortico nuclear fibers in the cerebellum: a review. In J. Courville, C. de Montigny and Y. Lamarre (eds.), *The Inferior Olivary Nucleus: Anatomy and Physiology.* New York: Raven Press, pp. 207–234.

Voogd, J., Gerrits, N.M., and Ruigrok, T.J. (1996). Organization of the vestibulocerebellum. *Ann. N. Y. Acad. Sci.* 781: 553–579.

Voogd, J., and Glickstein, M. (1998). The anatomy of the cerebellum. *Trends Neurosci.* 21: 370–375.

Voogd, J., and Ruigrok, T.J.H. (1997). Transverse and longitudinal patterns in the mammalian cerebellum. *Progr. Brain Res.* 114: 21–37.

Vos, B.P., Volny-Luraghi, A., Maex, R., and De Schutter, E. (2000). Precise spike timing of tactile-evoked cerebellar Golgi cell responses: a reflection of combined mossy fiber and parallel fiber activation? *Progr. Brain Res.* 124: 96–106.

Waespe, W., Cohen, B., and Raphan, T. (1985). Dynamic modification of the vestibulo-ocular reflex by the nodulus and uvula. *Science* 228: 199–202.

Wang, J., Zhou, T., Qiu, M., Du, A., Cai, K., Wang, Z., Zhou, C., Meng, M., Zhuo, Y., Fan, S., and Chen, L. (1999). Relationship between ventral stream for object vision and dorsal stream for spatial vision: an fMRI + ERP study. *Hum. Brain Mapp.* 8: 170–181.

Wang, J.-J., Shimansky, Y., Bracha, V., and Bloedel, J.R. (1998). Effects of cerebellar nuclear inactivation on the learning of a complex forelimb movement in cats. *J. Neurophysiol.* 79: 2447–2459.

Warr, W.B. (1982). Parallel ascending pathways from the cochlear nucleus: Neuroanatomical evidence of functional specialization. In W.D. Neff (ed.), *Contributions to Sensory Physiology, Vol. 7.* New York: Academic Press, pp. 1–38.

Webster, D.B. (1992). An overview of mammalian auditory pathways with an emphasis on humans. In D.B. Webster, A.N. Popper, and R. R. Fay (eds.), *The Mammalian Auditory Pathway: Neuroanatomy.* New York: Springer, pp. 1–22.

Weiss, C., Houk, J.C., and Gibson, A.R. (1990). Inhibition of sensory responses of cat inferior olive neurons produced by stimulation of red nucleus. *J. Neurophysiol.* 64: 1170–1185.

Welsh, J.P., and Harvey, J.A. (1989). Cerebellar lesions and the nictitating membrane reflex: performance deficits of the conditioned and unconditioned response. *J. Neurosci.* 9: 299–311.

Welsh, J.P., and Llinás, R. (1997). Some organizing principles for the control of movement based on olivocerebellar physiology. *Progr. Brain Res.* 114: 449–461.

Welsh, J.P., Lang, E.J., Sugihara, I., and Llinás, R. (1995). Dynamic organization of motor control within the olivocerebellar system. *Nature* 374: 453–457.

Werbos, P.J. (1975). *Beyond Regression: New Tools for Prediction and Analysis in the Behavioral Sciences.* Ph.D. Dissertation, Harvard University, Boston, MA.

Werbos, P.J. (1990). Backpropagation through time: what it does and how to do it. *Proc. IEEE* 78: 1550–1560.

White, S.A. (1975). An adaptive recursive digital filter. In S.-P. Chen (ed.), *Conference Record: Ninth Annual Asilomar Conference on Circuits, Systems, and Computers* (Nov. 3–5 1975), North Hollywood, CA: Western Periodicals Co. pp. 21–25.

Widrow, B. (1963). A statistical theory of adaptation. In: F.P. Caruthers and H. Levenstein (eds.), *Adaptive Control Systems*. New York: Macmillan, pp. 97–121.

Widrow, B., and Hoff, M.E., Jr. (1960). Adaptive switching circuits. *IRE WESCON Convention Record*, 96–104.

Widrow, B., and Lehr, M.A. (1990). Thirty years of adaptive neural networks: perceptron, madaline, and backpropagation. *Proc. IEEE* 78: 1415–1442.

Widrow, B., and Stearns, S.D. (1985). *Adaptive Signal Processing*. Englewood Cliffs, NJ: Prentice-Hall.

Widrow, B., and Stearns, S.D. (1985). Introduction to adaptive arrays and adaptive beamforming. In: *Adaptive Signal Processing*. Englewood Cliffs, NJ: Prentice-Hall, pp. 368–408.

Widrow, B., Glover, J.R., McCool, J.M., Kaunitz, J., Williams, C.S., Hearn, R.H., Zeidler, J.R., Dong, E., and Goodlin, R.C. (1975). Adaptive noise cancelling: principles and applications. *Proc. IEEE* 63: 1692–1716.

Widrow, B., Mantey, P.E., Griffiths, L.J., and Goode, B.B. (1967). Adaptive antenna systems. *Proc. IEEE* 55: 2143–2159.

Wiener, N. (1948). *Cybernetics or Control and Communication in the Animal and the Machine*. Cambridge, MA: MIT Press.

Wiener, N. (1950). *Extrapolation, Interpolation and Smoothing of Stationary Time Series*. Cambridge, MA: MIT Press/New York: John Wiley.

Wiener, N. (1961). *Cybernetics or Control and Communication in the Animal and the Machine* (2nd ed.) Cambridge, MA: MIT Press.

Wiener, S., and Berthoz, A. (1993). Forebrain structures mediating the vestibular contribution during navigation. In A. Berthoz (ed.), *Multisensory Control of Movement*. Oxford, England: Oxford University Press, pp. 427–456.

Williams, R.J., and Zipser, D. (1989). A learning algorithm for continually running fully recurrent neural networks. *Neural Comput.* 1: 270–280.

Wittmann, M. (1999). Time perception and temporal processing levels of the brain. *Chronobiol. Int.* 16: 17–32.

Wolpert, D.M., and Kawato, M. (1998). Multiple paired forward and inverse models for motor control. *Neural Netw.* 11: 1317–1329.

Wolpert, D.M., Goodbody, S.J., and Husain, M. (1998). Maintaining internal representations: the role of the human superior parietal lobe. *Nat. Neurosci.* 1: 529–533.

Wolpert, D.M., Miall, R.C., and Kawato, M. (1998). Internal models in the cerebellum. *Trends Cogn. Sci.* 2: 338–347.

Wolpert, M., and Kawato, M. (1998). Multiple paired forward and inverse models for motor control. *Neural Netw.* 11: 1317–1329.

Wouterlood, F.G., and Mugnaini, E. (1984). Cartwheel neurons of the dorsal cochlear nucleus: a Golgi-electron microscope study in rat. *J. Comp. Neurol.* 227: 136–157.

Wouterlood, F.G., Mugnaini, E., Osen, K.K., and Dahl, A.L. (1984). Stellate neurons in rat dorsal cochlear nucleus studies with combined Golgi impregnation and electron microscopy: synaptic connections and mutual coupling by gap junctions. *J. Neurocytol.* 13: 634–664.

Wullimann M.F., and Northcutt, R.G. (1990). Visual and electrosensory circuits of the diencephalon in mormyrids: an evolutionary perspective. *J. Comp. Neurol.* 297: 537–552.

Wylie, D.R., De Zeeuw, C.I., and Simpson, J.L. (1995). Temporal relations of the complex spike activity of Purkinje cell pairs in the vestibulocerebellum of rabbits. *J. Neurosci.* 15: 2875–2887.

Yamamoto, K., Kobayashi, Y., Takemura, A., Kawano, K., and Kawato, M. (1997). A mathematical model that reproduces vertical ocular following responses from visual stimuli by reproducing the simple spike firing frequency of Purkinje cells in the cerebellum. *Neurosci. Res.* 29: 161–169.

Yanagihara, D., and Kondo, I. (1996). Nitric oxide plays a key role in adaptive control of locomotion in cat. *Proc. Natl. Acad. Sci. USA* 93: 13292–13297.

Yeo, C.H., and Hardiman, M.J. (1992). Cerebellar cortex and eyeblink conditioning. *Exp. Brain Res.* 88: 623–638.

Yeo, C.H., and Hesslow, G. (1998). Cerebellum and conditioned reflexes. *Trends Cogn. Sci.* 2: 322–330.

Young, E.D., Nelken, I., and Conley, R.A. (1995). Somatosensory effects on neurons in the dorsal cochlear nucleus. *J. Neurophysiol.* 73: 743–765.

Young, E.D., Spirou, G.A., Rice, J.J., and Voigt, H.F. (1992). Neural organization and responses to complex stimuli in the dorsal cochlear nucleus. *Philos. Trans. R. Soc. Lond. B Biol. Sci.* 336: 407–413.

Yuen, G.L., Hockberger, J.C., and Houk, J.C. (1995). Bistability in cerebellar Purkinje cell dendrites modelled with high-threshold calcium and delayed-rectified potassium channels. *Biol. Cybern.* 73: 375–388.

Zagrebelsky, M., Rossi, F., Hawkes, R., and Strata, P. (1996). Topographically organized climbing fibre sprouting in the adult rat cerebellum. *Eur. J. Neurosci.* 8: 1051–1054.

Zipser, D., and Andersen, R.A. (1988). A back-propagation programmed network that simulates response properties of a subset of posterior parietal neurons. *Nature* 331: 679–684.

Index

(f = figure on the respective page)